Practical Psychiatry in the Long-Term Care Home

Practical Psychiatry in the Long-Term Care Home

A Handbook for Staff

Third Revised and Expanded Edition

Edited by
David K. Conn, Nathan Herrmann, Alanna Kaye, Dmytro Rewilak, Barbara Schogt

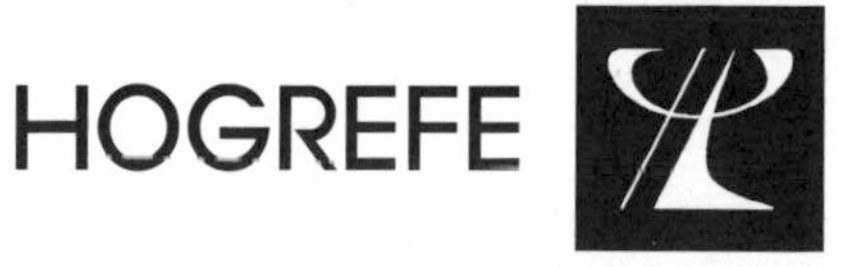

Library of Congress Cataloging-in-Publication Data

is available via the Library of Congress Marc Database under the LC Control Number 2007922290.

Library and Archives Canada Cataloguing in Publication

Practical psychiatry in the long-term care home: a handbook for staff / David K. Conn . . . [et al.], editors. – 3rd rev. & expanded ed.
Previously published under title: Practical psychiatry in the nursing home.
Includes bibliographical references and index.
ISBN 978-0-88937-341-9
1. Geriatric psychiatry. 2. Mentally ill older people—Institutional care. 3. Older people —Mental health services. 4. Psychotherapy for older people. 5. Nursing home care.
I. Conn, David K.
RC451.4.A5P73 2007 618.97'689 C2007-900943-3

PUBLISHING OFFICES
USA: Hogrefe & Huber Publishers, 875 Massachusetts Avenue, 7th Floor, Cambridge, MA 02139
Phone (866) 823-4726, Fax (617) 354-6875; E-mail info@hhpub.com
EUROPE: Hogrefe & Huber Publishers, Rohnsweg 25, 37085 Göttingen, Germany
Phone +49 551 49609-0, Fax +49 551 49609-88, E-mail hh@hhpub.com

SALES & DISTRIBUTION
USA: Hogrefe & Huber Publishers, Customer Services Department, 30 Amberwood Parkway, Ashland, OH 44805
Phone (800) 228-3749, Fax (419) 281-6883, E-mail custserv@hhpub.com
EUROPE: Hogrefe & Huber Publishers, Rohnsweg 25, 37085 Göttingen, Germany
Phone +49 551 49609-0, Fax +49 551 49609-88, E-mail hh@hhpub.com

OTHER OFFICES
CANADA: Hogrefe & Huber Publishers, 1543 Bayview Avenue, Toronto, Ontario M4G 3B5
SWITZERLAND: Hogrefe & Huber Publishers, Länggass-Strasse 76, CH-3000 Bern 9

Hogrefe & Huber Publishers. Incorporated and registered in the State of Washington, USA, and in Göttingen, Lower Saxony, Germany.

Printed and bound in the USA
ISBN: 978-0-88937-341-9

Foreword

Ira R. Katz

Why should there be a "Handbook for Staff" on practical psychiatry in the long term care facility? The answer is easy: It's because the overwhelming majority of nursing home residents have a diagnosable psychiatric disorder, most often a dementia such as Alzheimer's disease, or depression, usually as a complication of disabling medical conditions. Patients with chronic and severe mental illnesses that began for the first time earlier in life are present in nursing homes, but they are much less common.

Some have suggested that because of the high rates of psychiatric illness among their residents, nursing homes can, in fact, be viewed as psychiatric facilities. This might make sense in terms of the problems experienced by most of the residents. However, it is certainly not the case in terms of the design of nursing homes, the organization of the services provided, and the nature of staff training. It is in this context that this Handbook is an important book. It is designed to fill the gaps between what nursing home residents need, and the care that most facilities are designed to provide.

The Handbook can be viewed as a toolkit. It is a useful textbook on geriatric mental health that provides readable background information and practical guidance on the evaluation and management of the mental health problems that are common in nursing homes. It can also serve as an up to date text for courses on mental health in gerontology programs, and as a study guide that nurses, social workers, and administrators in nursing homes can use to educate themselves about these issues. In addition, the design of the Handbook makes it useful as a resource for educators and program directors. The key points listed at the start of each chapter can serve as outlines for in-service education, and the case examples spread throughout the book are valuable as discussion points for seminars or staff meetings. Finally, the family information sheets are important as tools for educating the residents' families about mental health treatment, and also as a means for facilitating communication between staff and families.

It is important for those working in nursing homes and other long-term care facilities to be knowledgeable about the psychiatric disorders of late life and to view their jobs in terms of their roles in what have been described as two separable but interacting mental health care systems within nursing homes. One is a professional or extrinsic system within which psychiatrists, psychologists, or other health or mental health care professionals evaluate, diagnose, and treat residents with specific psychiatric disorders. As described in the Handbook, this is the system that evaluates residents to look for medical causes for mental disorders and establishes psychiatric diagnoses. It provides psychotherapy or prescribes antidepressants for residents with depression, and designs behavioral treatment protocols and prescribes medications when they are needed for those with behavioral and psychological symptoms of dementia. For this system to work effectively, there must be close collaboration between the behavioral health professionals and the nursing home staff. To ensure that residents get the treatment they need, all staff members should be active in recognizing mental disorders and behavioral symptoms, and facilitating referrals for evaluation and treatment. Even after the referral, support and information from the staff is necessary to allow the mental health professional to establish diagnoses and plan treatments. If the clinical concern is the acute onset of confusion or a sudden worsening in cognitive status, a diagnosis of delirium requires staff input about the nature of the resident's deterioration and about the extent to which his or her behavior varies over the day. When the concern is about depression, staff input about the persistence of the resident's depressed mood and about symptoms such as mood reactivity, sleep, and appetite are necessary to complement the professional's own observations. When the concern is about psychological and behavioral symptoms of dementia, staff input about the nature of the behavioral symptoms, the presence or absence of hallucinations, delusions or depression, and behavioral observations about the frequency of specific behaviors, as well as their antecedents and consequences are needed to allow treatment planning. The staff's role also remains important after diagnosis and the initiation of treatment. Their role in the delivery of behavioral treatments is obvious. In addition, they are critical for educating patients and families about treatments, encouraging adherence, monitoring the outcome of treatment, and observing residents for early signs of drug side effects.

The second mental health care system is an intrinsic one. It is the sum total of the responses of nursing homes or care facilities in terms of policies, programs, and procedures for the delivery of care. Critical elements of this system for residents with dementia include activity programs that can help structure time for those who have lost their ability to initiate activities on their own. It also includes attention to each resident's cognitive deficits and residual abilities, staff communication and the way that basic nursing services are delivered. Everyone who has worked with patients suffering from dementia can recall interactions between residents and staff members that led to frustration or agitation. Perhaps the staff did not realize that the resident could not follow directions because they had an aphasia that prevented them from understanding verbal instructions, or possibly they had an apraxia that kept them from being able to translate thoughts into complex actions. All too often, residents become anxious because they can not understand what is being said or they can not perform what is being asked. In turn, the staff member repeats the request, perhaps accompanied by signs of frustration, and the resident's discomfort escalates, often with agitation or aggression. The best way to prevent such events is to be sure everyone who works in nursing homes can recognize the cognitive deficits that occur in dementia, and can adjust their interactions with residents accordingly. Other important skills include recognizing when residents are experiencing distress, and learning how to modify interactions to prevent escalation to agitation or aggression.

Another function of the intrinsic mental health system is to prevent demoralization, depression, and deterioration by helping residents experience a sense of control over their own lives. For cognitively intact residents who are dependent as a result of physical disabilities, it is a major challenge to deliver nursing care in a manner that helps to preserve a sense of autonomy and control. The key must be to honor the resident's preferences about daily routines and to provide as much choice as possible about care alternatives. When it is not possible to honor such preferences or provide choices, this should be explained, and residents should be given as much prior information as possible about the necessities of care. For residents with cognitive impairment, this challenge is even more difficult. Here, the task must be to provide as much choice as possible, but not so much as to overwhelm the resident's ability to make decisions. It might not, for example, be possible for a resident to answer the question, "What would you like to wear today?" and it might be more appropriate to ask, "Would you like to wear the blue sweater or the green one?" It is also important for staff members to know enough about who each resident is or was to be able to interact with them as unique individuals. Alzheimer's disease has been described as an illness in which cognitive deficits lead patients to lose their "sense of self." In this context, individualizing staff interactions with residents, referring to their biographical identities and helping them to maintain the preferences and patterns that were important to them, may help them to preserve this "sense of self," in spite of the progression of their dementia. For more intact residents, this may involve knowing and talking about their families, hobbies, or past work experiences. For more impaired residents, this may include behavioral approaches such as giving simplified arithmetic problems to a retired accountant, cloth for a tailor to sew, or laundry for a housekeeper to fold.

This Handbook provides the knowledge base to allow staff members of nursing homes and long-term care facilities to participate in both the professional and the intrinsic mental health systems. Which staff members should learn about mental health? Here, too, the answer is easy: Everyone. For nurses, administrators, and social workers, this knowledge is important; the Handbook should be required reading. For the nursing assistants or aides who have the most frequent direct contact with residents, it is even more critical. But the importance of knowledge about mental health is still broader. Everyone who has contact with residents, including those who work in food service, housekeeping, maintenance, and building security should be aware of the mental disorders of late life. They should know at least enough to help identify patients who may need medical evaluations or psychiatric referrals, by reporting acute changes in mental status or behavior which suggest the presence of depression or psychosis. In addition, as part of the intrinsic system, they should know enough to be able to recognize when their interactions with residents lead to agitation or suspiciousness, to understand that these are symptoms of mental disorders, and be aware of how to avoid further escalations. As a first step in disseminating knowledge about mental health throughout the long-term care facility, use of the Handbook as a toolkit should help to deliver the simplest possible messages to the largest possible group.

In using this Handbook as a resource, it is important to recognize that it is written to convey two basic messages. The first and most explicit is that psychiatric disorders are common in nursing homes and other long-term care facilities, and that their evaluation, diagnosis, and treatment can lead to a decrease in suffering and improvements in the quality of life for many residents. Although the focus of this Handbook is on the serious illnesses, the second message, mostly implicit, is highly optimistic. It *is* possible for nursing home residents to lead a good life, in spite of their illnesses and disabilities, if their mental health needs are met. This requires that the staff and mental health professionals work together effectively to ensure that psychiatric disorders such as delirium, depression, psychoses, and the behavioral and psychological symptoms of dementia are recognized and treated appropriately. It also requires that the day-to-day programming and the moment-to-moment care that characterize the intrinsic mental health system work, not just to manage behavioral disturbances, but to help residents maintain their autonomy and sense of self to the fullest possible extent.

Ira R. Katz, M.D., Ph.D.
Professor of Psychiatry, University of Pennsylvania; Director, Section of Geriatric Psychiatry, and Director, Mental Illness Research, Education and Clinical Center, Philadelphia VA Medical Center

Preface

The impetus for the original version of this book came from the positive response of staff who attended a seminar series entitled "Practical Psychiatry in Long-Term Care," presented by the Psychiatry Consultation-Liaison Team at Baycrest Centre for Geriatric Care in Toronto, Canada, in 1989. In view of the lack of available literature in this area, we decided to write a book based on the contents of this course with the addition of several new topics.

The first version of this book was published in 1992 with the title "Practical Psychiatry in the Nursing Home." In recognition of the widening range of institutions for the care of the elderly, the title of the second revised and expanded edition in 2001 was changed to "Practical Psychiatry in the Long-Term Care Facility." This third edition contains four new chapters focusing on alcohol use and misuse, sexuality and sexual behavior, group psychotherapy, and guidelines. Our intention has always been to produce a book that is practical, understandable, clinically relevant, "user friendly," and as jargon-free as possible. We hope that the book will continue to be useful for the staff of all long-term care facilities for the elderly, including nursing homes, homes for the aged, chronic care hospitals, and residential centres.

The prevalence of mental disorders in the residents of these facilities is very high and the staff, residents, and their families alike struggle with the problems associated with these disorders on a daily basis. We have aimed this book at all staff members and hope that it will be equally relevant to nurses, nursing aides, physicians, social workers, psychologists, occupational therapists, and all the other staff of these facilities. We are hopeful that the book will be used as a tool for both continuing education of staff and for the teaching of undergraduate students.

The book utilizes numerous clinical case examples, with an emphasis on practical management strategies. We have outlined questions that are frequently asked by staff and have attempted to respond to these questions. The chapters conclude with key points. We have avoided the use of excessive references and a list of suggested reading can be found at the end of each chapter. For several chapters we have added an information sheet, which can be photocopied and distributed to family members.

The case illustrations are composites of residents seen by the authors. They have been disguised to ensure anonymity. For the most part, we have preferred to use the term "resident" rather than "patient" in order to underline the fact that for these individuals the institution is their home, and like all of us, they are only "patients" when requiring medical care.

The authors include psychiatrists, nurses, a psychologist, and a social worker. We have tried to emphasize a biopsychosocial model throughout the book and a multidisciplinary approach to the management of these residents.

We are aware that the availability of mental health professionals in long-term care settings is variable, and often minimal. In the majority of institutions, front line staff have to "make do" without the help of consultants or staff trained to manage mental disorders. We are hopeful that the ideas and information contained in this book can be utilized by front line staff in their day-to-day management of residents with mental disorders. We have tried to emphasize that for any given problem there may be a variety of potential interventions. Often the best results occur following the introduction of several complementary management strategies. Because many of the problems in long-term care are by their very nature chronic, it is easy to slip into a pessimistic, or even nihilistic, frame of mind. This book tries to show that many of these problems can be managed successfully and that we *can* make a difference.

We have received a great deal of positive feedback regarding the usefulness of the first two editions. If you have any comments on how to improve future editions of this book, please contact David Conn at *dconn@baycrest.org* or at the Baycrest Centre for Geriatric Care, Department of Psychiatry, 3560 Bathurst Street, Toronto, Canada, M6A 2E1.

David Conn
Nathan Herrmann
Alanna Kaye
Dmytro Rewilak
Barbara Schogt

Acknowledgments

We are indebted to the long-term care residents with whom we have worked, and to their families. They have helped us to formulate our ideas and have given us valuable insights into the world of the institution.

We would like to thank our colleagues at Baycrest, Sunnybrook, and other facilities, who have helped us to understand the often difficult work of the frontline staff.

We greatly appreciate the contribution of Shelly Clancy, Malerie Feldman, Paula Ferreira, Marci Fromstein, Ruby Nishioka, Dilshad Ratansi, Betty Rychlewski, and Anna Virdo for their work in preparing this and /or previous manuscripts.

Finally, we would like to acknowledge the support and enthusiasm of Robert Dimbleby, Dr. Christine Hogrefe, and the staff of Hogrefe & Huber Publishers with regard to this project.

Contributors

David K. Conn, M.B., B.Ch., F.R.C.P.C.
Psychiatrist-in-Chief, Department of Psychiatry, Baycrest Geriatric Health Care System; Associate Professor, Department of Psychiatry, University of Toronto, and Cochair, Canadian Coalition for Seniors' Mental Health

Maggie Gibson, Ph.D, C.Psych.
Psychologist, Veterans Care Program, St. Joseph's Health Care London, Ontario; Associate Scientist, Lawson Health Research Institute; Adjunct Clinical Professor, Department of Psychology, University of Western Ontario

Etta Ginsberg-McEwan, M.S.W.
Formerly Director, Department of Social Work, Baycrest Geriatric Health Care System

Nathan Herrmann, M.D., F.R.C.P.C.
Director of Geriatric Psychiatry, Sunnybrook Health Sciences Centre; Professor, Department of Psychiatry, University of Toronto

Ira R. Katz, M.D., Ph.D.
Professor of Psychiatry, University of Pennsylvania; Director, Section of Geriatric Psychiatry, and Director, Mental Illness Research, Education and Clinical Center, Philadelphia VA Medical Center

Alanna Kaye, R.N., B.ScN., M.HSc. (candidate)
Formerly Nurse Clinician, Department of Psychiatry, Baycrest Geriatric Health Care System

Susan Lieff, M.D., F.R.C.P.C.
Staff Psychiatrist, Baycrest Geriatric Health Care System; Director, Education Scholars Program, Centre for Faculty Development, Faculty of Medicine and Associate Professor, Department of Psychiatry, University of Toronto

Robert Madan, M.D., F.R.C.P.C.
Staff Psychiatrist and Coordinator of Postgraduate Education, Department of Psychiatry, Baycrest Geriatric Health Care System; Coordinator of Postgraduate Education, Division of Geriatric Psychiatry and Assistant Professor, Department of Psychiatry, University of Toronto

David Myran, M.D., F.R.C.P.C.
Coordinator, Geriatric Psychiatry Community Service, Baycrest Geriatric Health Care System, and Assistant Professor, Department of Psychiatry, University of Toronto

Dmytro Rewilak, Ph.D.
Staff Psychologist, Baycrest Geriatric Health Care System

Anne Robinson, R.N.
Formerly Nurse Clinician, Department of Psychiatry, Baycrest Geriatric Health Care System

Joel Sadavoy, M.D., F.R.C.P.C.
Cecilia and Raymonde Sacklyn Chair in Applied General Psychiatry, and Head of Geriatric Psychiatry Program, Mount Sinai Hospital; Professor, Department of Psychiatry, University of Toronto

Barbara Schogt, M.D., F.R.C.P.C.
Formerly Staff Psychiatrist, Baycrest Geriatric Health Care System and Lecturer, Department of Psychiatry, University of Toronto

Ken Schwartz, M.D., F.R.C.P.C.
Co-Coordinator, Psychiatric Day Hospital, Baycrest Geriatric Health Care System, and Assistant Professor, Department of Psychiatry, University of Toronto

Michel Silberfeld, M.D., F.R.C.P.C.
Formerly Coordinator, Competency Clinic, Department of Psychiatry, Baycrest Geriatric Health Care System, and Assistant Professor, Department of Psychiatry, University of Toronto

Ivan Silver, M.D., F.R.C.P.C.
Staff Psychiatrist, Sunnybrook Health Sciences Centre; Vice Dean of Continuing Education, and Professor, Department of Psychiatry, University of Toronto

Marcia Sokolowski, M.A. Ph.D. (candidate)
Clinical ethicist, Baycrest Geriatric Health Care System

Table of Contents

1 Mental Health Issues in Long-Term Care Facilities

David K. Conn

Key Points

- The prevalence of mental disorders in residents of long-term care facilities is at least 80%.
- Common problems include depression and behaviors associated with dementia, such as verbal and physical aggression, wandering, and physical resistance to care.
- Very few residents ever receive care from mental health professionals.
- The biopsychosocial model of care is helpful both in the understanding of the problems and in the planning of individualized care.
- Staff vigilance and the use of screening instruments can facilitate the early recognition and prevention of psychiatric/emotional disorders.

History

The characteristics of long-term care facilities for the elderly have changed dramatically over the past 100 years. Until the 20th century most facilities for the aged were primitive, badly run, and offered only custodial care.

Institutions for the disabled and infirm date all the way back to the third or fourth century AD [1]. Such facilities developed initially in the Middle East, and over many centuries the concept subsequently spread to Western Europe. By medieval times it was common that the aged and sick were cared for by a variety of religious orders in monasteries, often in remote locations.

In England and Wales, as monasteries disappeared in the 1500s, responsibility for the poor was gradually taken on by the local parishes. Under the Poor Relief Act in 1601, poor houses were established for those who were blind, disabled, mentally or physically ill, as well as the destitute. These poor houses were also referred to as work houses because they were a source for cheap labor. By the nineteenth century between one-third and one-half of the occupants in a typical work house were elderly or "impotent" persons.

With the development of our modern concept of a hospital in the nineteenth century, the primary emphasis was placed on the treatment of the acutely sick, rather than the chronically ill, and completely separate institutions were established for "the insane." In other institutions, the elderly, the poor, the chronically sick, and the disabled were crowded together in appalling conditions, often with vagrants and the destitute. By the beginning of the twentieth century, there was clearly a growing need for convalescent and chronic care beds. It was only at this point that the modern concept of the nursing home was firmly established, modeled on the general principles of the sanatorium. The early nursing homes were occasionally attached to general hospitals, but more frequently they were built as completely separate institutions, usually some distance from the closest city.

Trends

With the growth of the elderly population in modern industrial countries, the number of people receiving care in nursing homes has been rising dramatically. In the United States, for example, the number of beds in such facilities has more than tripled during the past 25 years, and now totals over 1.7 million. This growth in the number of nursing home beds (1963–1995) is shown in **Figure 1**. The average length of stay in a nursing home is 2.5 years and approximately 25% of the population will be admitted to a nursing home at some point during their lives.

The continuing growth of the elderly population in the U.S. is shown in **Figures 2 and**

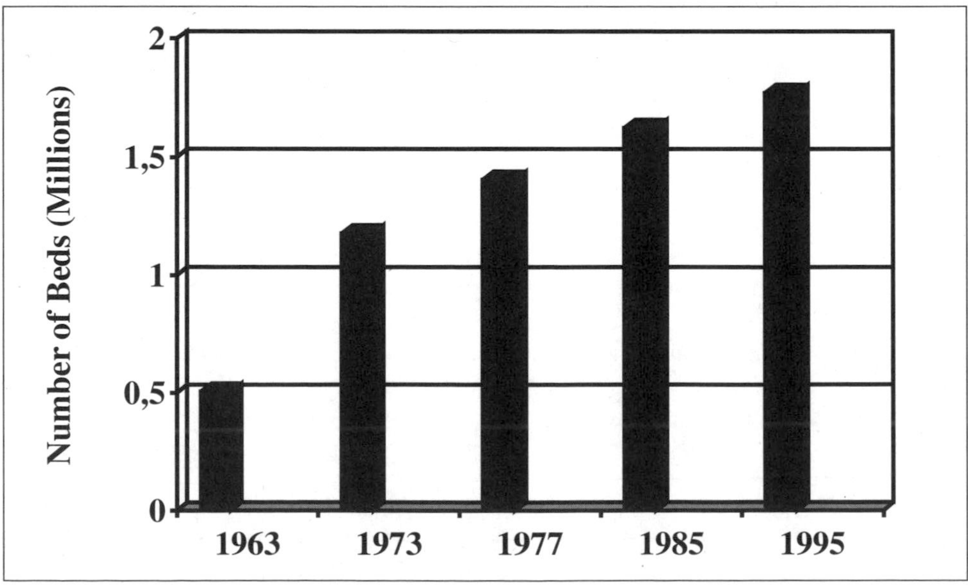

Figure 1 Number of Nursing Home Beds, United States, 1963–1995. [Refs. 3, 29, 30]

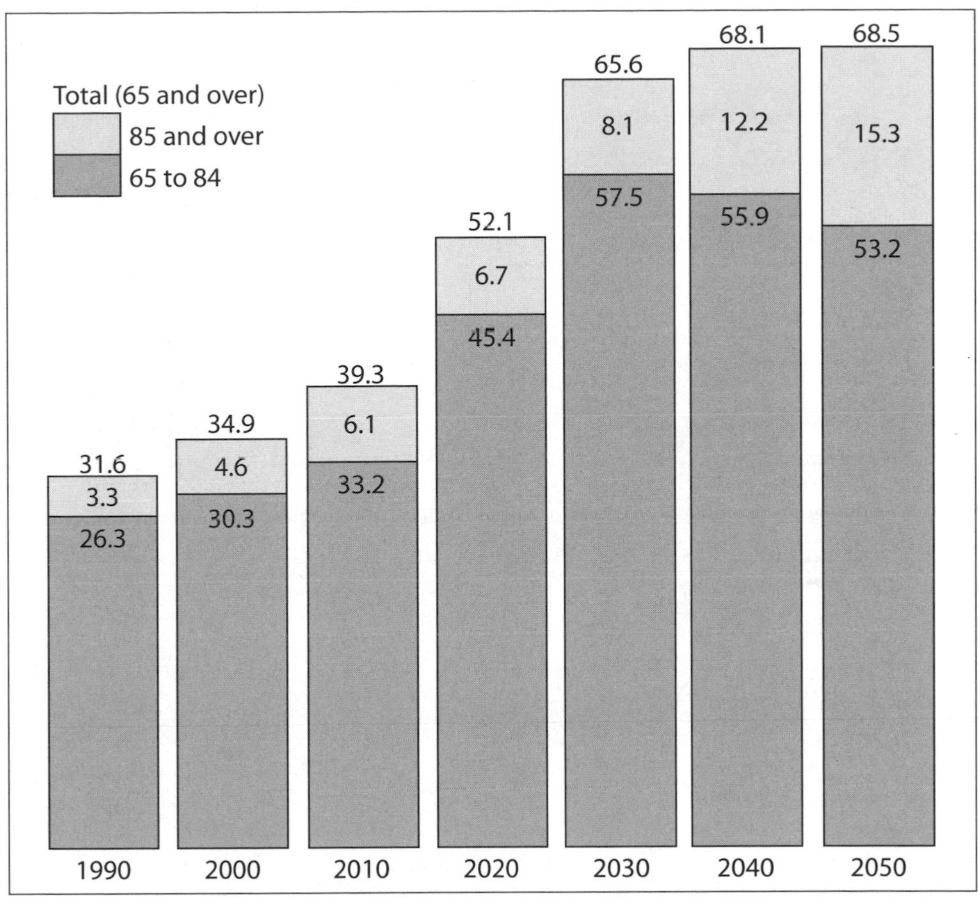

Figure 2 Projections of Elderly Population, by Age, 1990–2050 (Middle Series Projections, in Millions). [Ref. 31]

3. It is projected that the population 65 years and over will grow at a sustained 1.2% per year until 2010. After 2010, however, the rate of growth will increase in a more striking manner as the Baby Boom generation enters old age.

The phenomenal projected growth of the population 85 years and over is shown in **Figure 3**. It is of course this age group that is most likely to require long-term care. The continuing increase in life-expectancy at age 65 is demonstrated in **Figure 4**. Accordingly the projected growth in requirements for nursing home and other long-term care beds is illustrated in **Figure 5**.

There are many important trends in this field which are particularly influenced by these changing demographics. Seven of these trends, which will have a critical impact on the future of long-term care include:

- A growth in the physical size of facilities
- A greater focus on the need to optimize the environment (physical space and activities)

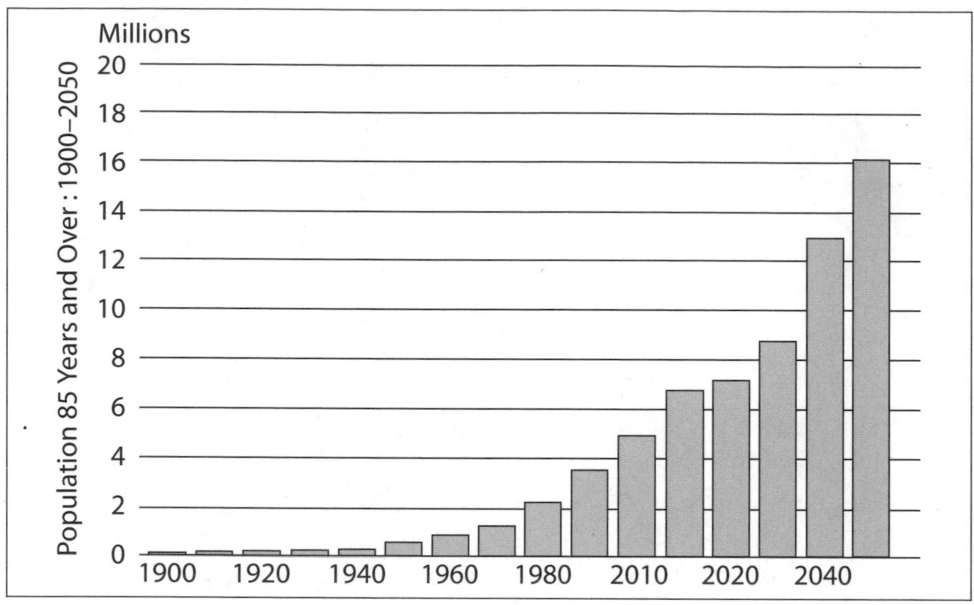

Figure 3 Population 85 Years and over, 1990–2050. [Ref. 32]

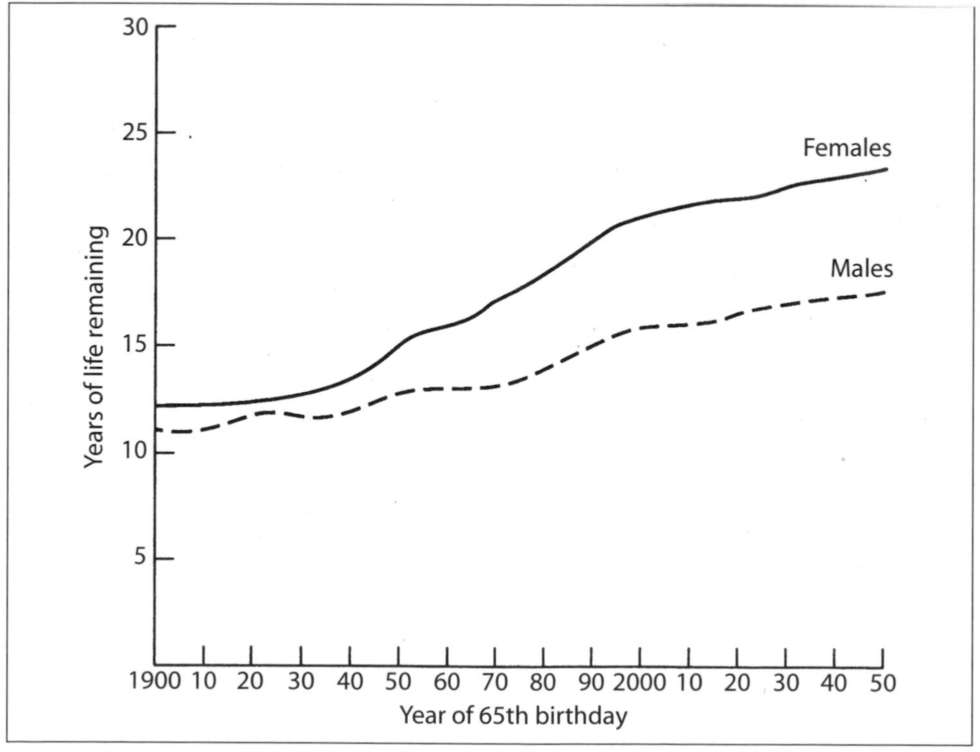

Figure 4 Life Expectancy at Age 65. [Ref. 32]

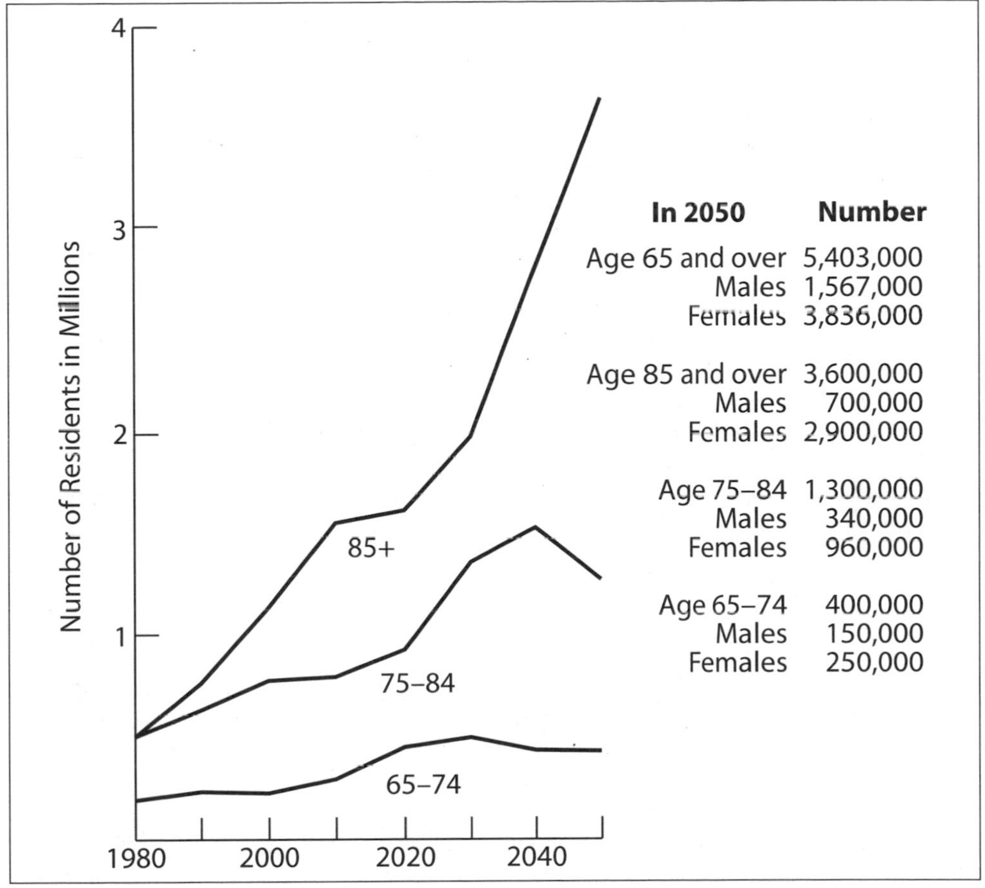

Figure 5 Projected Number of Nursing Home Residents in the United States by Age, 1980–2050. [Ref. 33]

- An increase in the availability of high levels of care
- A significantly greater percentage of residents with dementia and severe cognitive impairment
- More residents with psychiatric and behavioral disorders
- Greater involvement of university programs in nursing homes, with the development of the so-called "teaching nursing home"
- Increased legislation (e.g., OBRA 1987 in the U.S.) to ensure higher standards of care and the development of best practice guidelines

The Residents

There is considerable evidence that most elderly residents of nursing homes do in fact need a great deal of care and assistance. For example in the 1995 U.S. National Nursing Home

Survey 96.9% of residents required assistance with at least one activity of daily living [2]. 96% required assistance in bathing, 86% in dressing, 58% in toileting, and 45% in eating. It is clear that one's ability or inability to perform the activities of normal daily living contributes substantially to the final decision regarding admission to a nursing home.

As of 1995 there were approximately 16,700 nursing homes operating in the United States, consisting of a total of 1.77 million beds [3]. These institutions are categorized federally as Skilled Nursing Facilities (SNFs) and Intermediate Care Facilities (ICFs). It is estimated that currently, 1 in 10 persons aged 75 and older, and 1 in 5 aged 85 and older are living in nursing homes. Expenditures for nursing home care in 1997 in the U.S. were estimated at 82.8 billion dollars, out of a total of 1.1 trillion dollars in personal health care. In this context, about 38% of this expenditure was private spending and the rest was public.

To deal with these powerful demographic and economic forces, various governments are trying new approaches. For example, in Canada the province of Ontario has attempted to reform long-term care based on certain key guiding principles, one of which states that:

> "an increasing proportion of the elderly and people with physical disabilities who require health and social services will receive them in their own homes, to avoid both inappropriate use of acute care beds and unnecessary growth in the number of extended and chronic care beds."

But in spite of this well-founded goal of attempting to maintain the elderly in the community for as long as possible by increasing the availability of community care and supports, the unstoppable demographic realities we now face, as well as the cumulative ravages of illness and old age, will lead to an increased requirement for long-term care beds.

In dealing with these strategic planning issues, it is often suggested that children frequently abandon or ignore their elderly parents, but this is just a myth. In fact families remain the primary source of care for the vast majority of frail parents, and this burden is especially carried by daughters, who are themselves also often trying to care for young children. However, as the demand for care increases, most often as a result of progressive mental impairment, it frequently becomes an impossible burden for the family, and institutional care becomes a necessity.

Prevalence of Psychiatric/Behavioral Disturbances

Studies suggest that while 80% or more of elderly nursing home residents suffer from some form of mental disorder, only a very small percentage ever receive any care from mental health professionals. During the 1960s hundreds of thousands of psychiatric patients were discharged from state mental hospitals, especially in the U.S. This happened partly because of pressure from groups who felt that such individuals should live in the community, and partly because advances in drug therapy allowed even severely ill patients to function at reasonable levels. But many of these former patients, especially those who were elderly, were not able to care for themselves, and as a result ended up being transferred to nursing homes, which were expected to continue the appropriate care and management of these patients, even though such homes were not staffed or funded to provide mental health care.

The U.S. National Center for Health Statistics reported in 1977 that approximately 20% of all nursing home residents had a mental disorder (psychiatric illness or dementia) as their primary source of disability, and that nearly 70%, which was more than 900,000 residents, had a chronic mental disorder which contributed to social dependency, functional impairment, and need for nursing home care [4]. Two thirds of all residents were found to have behavioral problems, most commonly agitation or apathy. In one important study, Rovner and his colleagues found that 76% of their sample of nursing home residents showed at least one problem behavior, while 40% displayed five or more such difficulties [5]. Another study, performed in New York City [6], found that the three most common behavior problems in nursing homes for the aged, were verbal abuse, physical resistance to care, and physical aggressiveness.

Similarly, a survey in Ontario, Canada [7] found that the most common behavior problems were agitation, wandering, and depression, whereas the problem of greatest concern for staff was physical aggression. Yet in spite of these statistics, surveys suggest that few patients with a diagnosable mental disorder receive care from mental health professionals.

In addition to the distinct lack of psychiatric care for nursing home residents, several investigations suggest that psychotropic drugs are overused in this population: 50% to 80% of residents commonly receive psychotropic agents [8, 9]. A study of physicians' prescribing practices surveyed the records of 173 nursing homes and revealed that 43% of almost 6,000 residents had prescriptions for an antipsychotic medication [10]. Incredibly, the average dose per resident turned out to be directly related to the size of the nursing home, and the size of the prescribing physicians' caseload. It is clear that more research is needed in order to determine the appropriate use of these medications.

Common Psychiatric and Emotional Problems

It appears that the majority of residents with psychiatric problems in the nursing home setting suffer from some form of underlying primary brain disease. The most common of these disorders is dementia, and the most common cause of dementia is Alzheimer's disease, followed by vascular dementia. Dr. Alzheimer himself, in his initial description of dementia, emphasized the development of behavioral disturbances. His descriptions included paranoid delusions, hallucinations, unfounded jealousy, hiding of objects, and screaming. Dementing disorders are often associated with disruptive behavior, including physical and verbal aggression, anger, paranoid ideation, wandering, insomnia, and incontinence. A study of 126 patients with dementia [11] found that 83% of them exhibited one or more such behavior problems. Rovner et al. reported the prevalence of specific psychiatric disorders in 454 consecutive nursing home admissions (see **Table 1**) [12]. 67.4% had a dementia and 10% had an affective disorder. 40% of patients with dementia had additional psychiatric syndromes.

Depression is another common mental problem in the nursing home setting. Depressive symptoms occur in approximately 15% of the elderly in the general community, although the prevalence rate for major clinical depression is probably 2% to 4%. In contrast, studies

Table 1 Prevalence of Dementia and Other Psychiatric Disorders in New Admissions to Nursing Homes (*N* = 454)

Diagnosis	*n*	%
Dementias complicated by depression, delusions, or delirium		
Primary degenerative dementia of the Alzheimer's type		
with delusions/hallucinations	43	9.5
with depression	7	1.5
with delirium	15	3.3
Multiinfarct dementia		
with delusions/hallucinations	14	3.1
with depression	8	1.7
with delirium	14	3.1
Dementia plus depression	14	3.1
Other dementias		
with delusions/hallucinations	4	0.9
with delirium	4	0.9
Subtotal	(123)	(27.1)
Dementia only		
Primary degenerative dementia of Alzheimer's type	122	26.9
Multiinfarct dementia	59	13.0
Other dementias	2	0.4
Subtotal	(183)	(40.3)
Other psychiatric disorders		
Affective disorders	47	10.4
Schizophrenia/other	11	2.4
Subtotal	(58)	(12.8)
No psychiatric disorder	90	19.8
TOTAL	454	100.0

From B.W. Rovner et al. (1990). The prevalence and management of dementia and other psychiatric disorders in nursing homes. International Psychogeriatrics, 2:13–24. Reprinted with permission of Cambridge University Press.

suggest that between 15% and 25% of nursing home residents have symptoms of major depression, and another 25% have depressive symptoms of lesser severity [13, 14]. The recognition and diagnosis of depression is particularly important because it is a treatable condition; unfortunately, on occasion untreated depression can lead to extreme morbidity and ultimately to death.

Diagnostic Classifications

The diagnoses used in this book are based on the American Psychiatric Association's diagnostic system, entitled DSM-IV-TR [15]. It is a multi-axial system with Axis I containing the major psychiatric diagnosis, Axis II containing personality traits and disorders, Axis III the medical illnesses, Axis IV the level of psychosocial stress, and Axis V the level of functioning of the individual. **Table 2** lists common DSM-IV-TR diagnoses seen in long-term care residents.

Table 2 Common Psychiatric Diagnoses in Residents of Long-Term Care Facilities

- Dementia
- Delirium
- Mood disorder due to a general medical condition
- Psychotic disorder due to a general medical condition
- Personality change due to a general medical condition
- Major depression
- Dysthymic disorder
- Adjustment disorder
- Personality disorder

Models of Care

The "biopsychosocial" model, in contrast to the biomedical approach, is the model of choice in both geriatrics and psychiatry. In formulating a clinical situation, it is often helpful to categorize etiological factors into biological (physical), psychological, and social categories, as illustrated in **Figure 6**. The category "social" includes both cultural and environmental factors. This model then allows for the design of treatment interventions aimed at a variety of factors.

In some institutions models which favor one or another professional orientation, such as a "social work model" or a "nursing model," are preferred. It is the conclusion of the authors of this book that a biopsychosocial approach, which attempts to understand a resident's problems from a variety of different perspectives, makes the most sense. Inherent in any model of nursing home care is an acceptance of reasonable goals, and an emphasis on "care not cure." Lawton tries to define "the good life" for nursing home residents, and outlines the components of such an experience, which include behavioral competence, psychological well-being, and quality of life and of the objective environment [16]. These are translated into goals of health, happiness, satisfaction with daily life, and a comfortable environment.

Case Illustration

Mrs. A., an 89-year-old widow, had been admitted to the nursing home two months previously. She was born in England, emigrated to Canada shortly before the First World War, and had worked as a secretary prior to her marriage to a tailor. They had a "solid," happy marriage, and two children. Mr. A. had died one year earlier of a stroke. Mrs. A. was having difficulty functioning in her own apartment, and was neglecting herself to the point that finally her daughter arranged for an application and placement at the home. Mrs. A. had not adjusted well to the new environment, and had been weepy, distressed, and agitated at times. She appeared unmotivated and disinterested in activities and programs. She was sleeping poorly, not eating, and stated clearly that she wanted to die. Her daughter was away in Florida, and her son lived out of town. Mrs. A. had a past history of hypothyroidism and of postpartum depression. Her own mother was described as having had "bad nerves," and her son had required treatment for depression. Mrs. A. had a history of losses early in life, including the death of her mother when she was 8 years old. She was cared for by an aunt until her father remarried, and she subsequently had a poor relationship with her stepmother. Mrs. A. described frequent episodes of mild depression for many years but never sought professional help. It was worthy of note that the unit itself was under some stress due to illness among the staff, including the head nurse. There was also some disruption on the floor because of renovations that were underway.

Comment

In order to understand the possible reasons for Mrs. A.'s depression and grief it is helpful to use the framework described in Figure 6. This approach can be helpful both in understanding the situation and in developing a management plan. In the case of Mrs. A., predisposing factors for depression include a biological vulnerability based on a positive family history of mood disorder, and a previous history of hypothyroidism. She is also psychologically predisposed because of her early life losses, especially the death of her mother, and deprivation. Major precipitants include her recent admission to the institution and the death of her husband one year earlier, producing an "anniversary reaction." Recent problems on the unit may also have led to less available support from staff. Factors which could perpetuate the depression include her poor adjustment to the home, her apparent inability to develop new relationships, and her long-standing history of depression. Management steps based on our approach would include medical investigations, such as thyroid function, antidepressant medication, supportive psychotherapy, and attempts to encourage her to participate in recreation programs. With the introduction of appropriate treatment, the return of her daughter from vacation, and the restabilization of the unit, her prognosis would probably be good.

	Biological	Psychological	Social
Predisposing			
Precipitating			
Perpetuating			

Figure 6 The Biopsychosocial Model: A Grid for Formulation

What Are the Components of Good Care?

Attempts to understand and support the biological, psychological, and social needs of the resident provide a solid foundation for good care. Edelson and Lyons emphasize the need to individualize care and promote a sense of mastery in the residents in order that they can feel a sense of trust in and some control over their environment [17]. They stress in particular the importance of understanding the meaning in the impaired resident's behavior. They also point out that an understanding of "the system" is critical and that an institution is like a living organism. One must battle against nihilism, cynicism, and resistance to change which is often present in geriatric institutions. Borson and colleagues note that long-term care "emphasizes maintenance of functional capacity, delaying the progress of disease when possible, and the creation of a safe, supportive environment that promotes maximal autonomy and life satisfaction. The over-arching philosophy of good long-term care is the preservation of dignity and purpose in the face of dependency and decline" [18].

Potential Problems in the Care of Nursing Home Residents

There has been growing public criticism regarding care in nursing homes. A series of books with titles such as "Warehouses of Death" have presented searing indictments of nursing home care [19]. There have been accounts of mistreatment and abuse of the elderly, poor medical/nursing care, and even greed, particularly in the private sector. In spite of this, considering the funds available, the staff of the majority of nursing homes do an admirable job under trying conditions. However, there are still problems to be solved, and these problems include:

- Poor staff/resident ratios
- Lack of qualified professional staff
- Low morale among staff
- Poorly designed and aging facilities
- Lack of commitment from society and government to direct appropriate funds to this population

Legislation and Regulations in the United States

Concerns about poor care, misuse of physical restraints and psychotropic medications, as well as inappropriate placement of some residents led to Federal legislation in the United States, termed the Omnibus Budget Reconciliation Act of 1987 (OBRA 87). The Health Care Financing Administration (HCFA) issue regulations [20] and individual states are responsible for enforcing these laws. This is achieved by the use of surveys based on operational criteria.

The regulations require Preadmission Screening and Annual Resident Review (PASARR). If an applicant is found to suffer from a serious mental disorder, then a determination of treatment needs and appropriate level of care must be made. The requirement for comprehensive assessment led to guidelines for the administration of the Minimum Data Set (MDS), or equivalent instrument. One potential weakness of the MDS is a tendency for the instrument to misrepresent the degree of mood or behavior disturbance present [21]. The results of the MDS may trigger the use of Resident Assessment Protocols (RAPs) that define common disorders, disabilities or functional impairments and outline procedures for appropriate evaluation and management. RAPs, which are particularly relevant to mental disorders, include cognitive loss/dementia, delirium, psychosocial well-being, mood state, behavior problems, psychotropic drug use, and physical restraints. The regulations also restrict the use of physical restraints and provides strict guidelines for the use of psychotropic medications, particularly antipsychotics (see Chapter 12)

Creation of Best Practice Guidelines and Consensus Statements

In several countries guidelines which focus on mental health problems in long-term care homes have been created, generally by multidisciplinary groups [22, 23, 24]. Canadian guidelines, which were released in 2006 are described in Chapter 16.

Special Problems in the Nursing Home Setting

Behavior Problems

One of the major challenges for staff is the management of disruptive behaviors, especially those resulting from dementia and other organic mental syndromes. Although control of these problems can be difficult to obtain, very specific pharmacological, psychological, behavioral, and environmental modifications can often be quite helpful. Several chapters in this book will address these approaches.

Relocation

There has been a considerable interest in the issue of the impact of relocation, i.e., simply changing one's place of residence, and conflicting literature has developed with regard to the potential dangers of moving an elderly person into an institution. Some research has suggested that relocation per se is dangerous. Other studies suggest that relocation is only a serious problem when individuals are moved without their knowledge and participation. There is evidence to suggest that orientation of the person to the nursing home ahead of time will decrease the stress of relocation.

Roommate Incompatibility

Most of the adults admitted to an institution are accustomed to their privacy. The prospect of sharing living quarters with a complete stranger would be unappealing to most of us. In spite of this, most nursing homes do not have the luxury of predominantly private rooms. Private rooms are often sought after like gold dust. One of the difficult tasks for administrators can be the distribution of private rooms, and staff often spend a considerable amount of time trying to decide on the best combination of roommates.

Death and Dying

For white Americans, the nursing home is now the second most common place in which to die. Staff often become emotionally attached to residents over a number of years and it can be difficult when death finally arrives. Birkett [25] notes that there are a variety of different categories of residents who die in nursing homes including:

- Patients who are severely demented and whose consciousness is impaired
- Patients who are physically ill but whose need for specific medical measures cannot be established
- Patients who are critically ill but for whom hospital care would have a negative effect or whose lives would not be prolonged by medical measures
- Patients whose lives might be saved by medical measures at a higher level of care but

this care is withheld because of concurrent illness, the patient's advanced age, or poor quality of life, or as a result of the patient's expressed wishes

Decision-making with regard to the degree of medical interventions to be undertaken can be problematic. When the resident is no longer competent, family members or other substitute decision-makers are asked to make decisions. It is important to know the family ahead of time and to have been able to establish a route of communication to the family spokesperson. Sometime families have difficulties reaching a consensus and meetings are necessary to clarify the wishes of the family members.

Detecting Behavioral Problems that May Require Intervention

With increased education of staff in the nursing home setting the early recognition and even prevention of some psychiatric/emotional problems may be possible. There is no doubt that for illnesses such as depression early intervention may be critical. A variety of screening instruments such as the Geriatric Depression Scale [26] and the Folstein Mini-Mental State Exam [27] may be of particular help, and can be easily administered by most staff members following a short period of training. This is discussed in some detail in Chapter 2. Most importantly, staff should rely on their own experience, judgment, and vigilance to determine when intervention is necessary. This book attempts to guide the staff member at the bedside with some basic information regarding the assessment and management of these problems.

Future Directions in Nursing Home Care

Future directions will include the development of newly designed facilities that offer a more appropriate physical environment for the elderly impaired resident. New technologies, such as interactive videoconferencing, will allow for increased consultation and education to long-term care homes [28]. There is a developing movement toward the involvement of academic institutions in nursing homes, and the term "teaching nursing home" has become popular. This will offer exciting new opportunities for us to develop a greater understanding of the kinds of problems experienced by residents and their families in the nursing home setting. These developments will hopefully generate improvements in clinical care and education and lead to the establishment of expanded research programs for this rapidly growing population. The authors of this book particularly hope that extra funding will be available to increase the availability of mental health professionals in the long-term care setting.

References

1. Forbes, W.F., Jackson, J.A., Kraus, A.S. (1987). Institutionalization of the elderly in Canada. Toronto: Butterworth.
2. U.S. National Center for Health Statistics. (1997). The national nursing home survey: 1995. Advance data No. 289. Hyattsville, Maryland.
3. U.S. National Center for Health Statistics. (1997). The national nursing home survey: 1995. Advance data No. 280. Hyattsville, Maryland.
4. U.S. National Center for Health Statistics. (1979). The national nursing home survey: 1977. Summary for the United States. Vital and Health Statistics, Serial 13, Number 43. Washington, DC: U.S. Government Printing Office.
5. Rovner, B.W., Kafonek, S., Filipp, L., Lucas, M.J., Folstein, M.F. (1986). Prevalence of mental illness in a community nursing home. American Journal of Psychiatry, 143:1446–1449.
6. Zimmer, J.A., Watson, N., Treat, A. (1984). Behavioral problems among patients in skilled nursing facilities. American Journal of Public Health, 74:1118–1121.
7. Conn, D.K., Lee, V., Steingart, A., Silberfeld, M. (1992). Psychiatric Services: A survey of nursing homes and homes for the aged in Ontario. Canadian Journal of Psychiatry, 37:525–530.
8. Glasscote, R.M., Beigel, A., Butterfield, A., Clark, E., Cox, B.A., Elpers, J.R., et al. (1976). Old folks at homes: A field study of nursing and board and care homes. Washington, DC: Joint Information Service of the American Psychiatric Association and the National Association for Mental Health.
9. Prien, R.F. (1980). Problems and practices in geriatric psychopharmacology. Psychosomatics, 21:213–223.
10. Ray, W.A., Federspiel, C.F., Schaffner, W. (1980). A study of antipsychotic drug use in nursing homes: Epidemiological evidence suggesting misuse. American Journal of Public Health, 70: 485–491.
11. Swearer, J.M., Drachman, D.A., O'Donnell, B.F., Mitchell, A.L. (1988). Troublesome and disruptive behaviors in dementia: Relationships to diagnosis and disease severity. Journal of the American Geriatrics Society, 36:784–790.
12. Rovner, B.W., German, P.S., Broadhead, J., Morriss, R.K., Brant, L.J., Blaustein, J., Folstein, M.F. (1990). The prevalence and management of dementia and other psychiatric disorders in nursing homes. International Psychogeriatrics, 2:13–24.
13. Katz, I.R., Lesher, E., Kleban, M., Jethanandani, V., Parmelee, P. (1989). Clinical features of depression in the nursing home. International Psychogeriatrics, 1:5–15.
14. Ames, D. (1991). Epidemiological studies of depression among the elderly in residential and nursing homes. International Journal of Geriatrics Psychiatry, 6:347–354.
15. American Psychiatric Association. (2000). Diagnostic and statistical manual of mental disorders (4th Ed. – Text Revision). Washington, DC: American Psychiatric Association.
16. Lawton, M.P. (1983). Environment and other determinants of well-being in older people. Robert W. Kleemeier Memorial Lecture. Gerontologist, 23:349–357.
17. Edelson, J.S., Lyons, W. (1985). Institutional care of the mentally impaired elderly. New York: Van Nostrand Reinhold Company.
18. Borson, S., Liptzin, B., Nininger, J., Rabins, P. (1987). Psychiatry and the nursing home. American Journal of Psychiatry, 144:1412–1418.
19. Baum, D.J. (1987). Warehouses of death: The nursing home industry. Don Mills, ON: Burns and MacEachern.
20. Health Care Financing Administration. (1991). Medicare and Medicaid: Requirements for Long-Term Care Facilities, Final Regulations. Federal Register 56:48865–48921, September 26.
21. Lawton, M.P., Casten R., Parmelee P.A., Van Haitsma K., Corn J., Kleban M.H. (1998). Psycho-

metric characteristics of the minimum data set II: Validity. Journal of the American Geriatrics Society, 46:736–744.

22. Canadian Coalition for Seniors' Mental Health (CCSMH). (2006). National Guidelines for Seniors' Mental Health: The Assessment and Treatment of Mental Health Issues in Long Term Care Homes. Toronto: CCSMH. Available at www.ccsmh.ca.
23. American Geriatrics Society, American Association for Geriatric Psychiatry (AGS/AAGP). (2003). Consensus statement on improving the quality of mental health care in U.S. nursing homes; management of depression and behavioral symptoms associated with dementia. Journal of the American Geriatrics Society, 51(9):1287–1298.
24. Department of Health, New South Wales. (2006). Aged Care: Working with People with Challenging Behaviours in Residential Aged Care Facilities. North Sydney: NSW Health.
25. Birkett, D.P. (1988). The life-threatened patient in the long-term care facility. In Klagsbrun, S.C., Goldberg, I.K., Rawnsley, M.M., Kutscher, A.H., Marcus, E.R., Siegel, A. (Eds.), Psychiatric aspects of terminal illness. Philadelphia: The Charles Press.
26. Yesavage, J.A., Brink, T.L., Rose, T.L., Lum, D., Huang, V., Adey, M., Leirer, V.O. (1983). Development and validation of a geriatric depression screening scale: A preliminary report. Journal of Psychiatric Research, 17:37–49.
27. Folstein, M.F., Folstein, S.E., McHugh, P.R. (1975). "Mini-Mental State:" A practical method for grading the cognitive state of patients for the clinician. Journal of Psychiatric Research, 12:189–198.
28. Shulman, B., Conn, D.K., Elford, R. (2006). Geriatric telepsychiatry and telemedicine: A literature review. Canadian Journal of Geriatrics, 9:139–146.
29. Strahan, G. (1985). Nursing home characteristics: preliminary data from the 1985 National Nursing Home Survey. Advance data 131. Hyattsville, MD: National Center for Health Statistics.
30. Bryant, E., Taube, C. (1966). Utilization of institutions for the aged and chronically ill. United States: April–June 1963. Hyattsville, MD: National Center for Health Statistics.
31. U.S. Department of Commerce: Bureau of the Census. (1989). Population profile of the United States. Series P-23. No. 159. Washington, DC: U.S. Government Printing Office.
32. U.S. Department of Commerce: Bureau of the Census. (1983). America in Transition: An aging society. Series P-23. No. 128. Washington, DC: U.S. Government Printing Office.
33. Brody, J.A., Foley, D.J. (1985). Epidemiologic considerations. In E.L. Schneider (Ed.), The teaching nursing home. New York: Raven Press.

Suggested Readings

1. Streim, J.E., Katz, I.R. (2005). Psychiatric aspects of nursing home care. In J. Sadavoy, L.F. Jarvik, G.T. Grossberg, B.S. Meyers (Eds.), Comprehensive Textbook of Geriatric Psychiatry, Third Ed. New York: W.W. Norton & Company.
   A useful overview of psychiatric issues in long-term care.
2. Reichman, W.E., Katz, P.R. (1996). Psychiatric Care in the Nursing Home. New York: Oxford University Press.
   An excellent multiauthored textbook reviewing major disorders and treatment approaches. A new edition will be released shortly.

2 The Mental Status Examination

Barbara Schogt and Dmytro Rewilak

Key Points

- The purpose of the Mental Status Examination (MSE) is to observe and describe mental functioning.
- Most mental status data can be gathered unobtrusively during the course of routine interactions with the resident.
- Clinical judgment is used in determining how detailed the MSE should be. The decision is based on the purpose for which the information is being gathered, and what the resident can tolerate.
- When doing an MSE it is useful to refer back to a mental checklist of the major areas that need to be covered (see **Tables 1 and 2**).

The Mental Status Examination (MSE) provides an organized approach to observing and describing important aspects of an individual's mental functioning. It is based on observations that are made at a particular point in time regarding the individual's appearance, behavior, feeling, and thinking.

Skilled professionals make numerous observations about the residents with whom they work. Whether contact with a resident is a casual greeting in the hall or a more formal work-related interaction, the opportunity to make observations is always present. Based on their training, experience, and prior knowledge of the resident, staff interpret these observations to assess changes in the resident, to guide further information gathering, and to make management decisions. Mental status data are most helpful when they are placed within the context of other available clinical information, including the individual's socio-cultural background, medical history, and current physical and laboratory status. A comprehensive understanding of the resident both guides interviewers and observers as they perform the MSE and provides a background against which to interpret observations.

It is important to adopt an organized approach to making and recording these naturally occurring observations for the following reasons:

The MSE guides and sharpens observational skills. By following a mental checklist of areas that need to be assessed, the observer becomes more attentive and is less likely to omit important areas in gathering information. There is also less likelihood of confusing the process of observing and recording data with the process of interpreting and analyzing these data. For example, to observe that, "Mrs. P. seems a bit off today," is to give a general impression that something may be wrong with her. Much more information is made available, however, if the observer identifies what it was about Mrs. P. that made him or her say that she seemed "off." The observer may have noticed a change in Mrs. P.'s appearance, such as a deterioration in her usually meticulous grooming, or a change in her behavior such as increased irritability. Mrs. P. may have expressed uncharacteristically gloomy feelings or shown evidence of rambling speech and disorganized thinking. Each of these observations suggests different possibilities, resulting in different courses of action to investigate further why Mrs. P. is "a bit off."

The MSE facilitates communication of information. The use of a standard approach to assessing residents and recording observations has several practical consequences:

- It is easier for members of the staff to understand and build on the observations made by others
- It is easier to identify changes in a resident's condition over time
- The observations provide a basis for making comparisons between residents or groups of residents
- An accurate record is established that, apart from its clinical value, may be useful for research and/or administrative purposes

This chapter describes the components of the MSE (see **Table 1**). Concepts relating to mental functioning are defined and case examples are used to illustrate important points. Our goal is to provide the professional working within a long-term care setting with the information necessary to perform and record an accurate and clinically useful MSE. The chapter also includes a brief discussion of standardized assessment instruments and their role in a clinical setting. Two case examples of complete MSEs are presented at the end of the chapter.

Table 1 Components of the MSE

- Behavioral observations
- Mood and affect
- Thought
- Perception
- Cognition

General Considerations

Before proceeding with a detailed description of each component of the MSE, a few general questions should be addressed.

When and How Should Information Be Gathered?

As noted above, every contact with a resident provides an opportunity for information gathering. Much of the mental status data can be gathered unobtrusively, in an nonthreatening manner. Sometimes, however, questions have to be posed that are more difficult to weave into the course of a routine interaction. Posing such questions can be associated with considerable discomfort for caregivers, and residents may perceive the inquiries as jarring, intrusive, and threatening to their self-esteem. Prior contact and especially the presence of a good rapport with the resident can facilitate the gathering of this information. Even when assessing someone for the first time, however, the examiner can introduce potentially threatening material without disturbing the flow of the interaction. Examples will be given later in the chapter.

The organization shown in **Table 1** is the one used when recording a MSE and is useful to keep in mind as a mental checklist when assessing residents, but the information may be gathered in any order. This flexibility helps reduce the anxiety sometimes associated with the MSE, both for staff and residents.

How Comprehensive Should the MSE Be?

The MSE ranges from a cursory 5-minute survey of cognitive functioning to a detailed evaluation that is administered by a psychologist and requires several hours. The amount of detail required depends on the purpose for which the information is to be used. For example, assessing a resident's cognitive potential for rehabilitation following a stroke is a much more complex task than establishing that an individual has become disoriented following an increase in medication.

The comprehensiveness of the MSE also depends on what the resident can tolerate. A formal MSE, especially the evaluation of cognitive (intellectual) functions, requires that the resident be able to participate in an interview situation. In the case of a highly agitated individual, questions may have to be kept to a minimum or avoided altogether, as the information necessary to manage the situation can be gathered on the basis of observation alone.

How Should Information Be Recorded in the Chart?

The chart is used by staff as a source of information and a vehicle for communication. It is also a legal document. Mental status information is most informative when it is recorded in the form of descriptions, using quotations in the resident's own words, rather than as interpretations by the observer. For example, coworkers learn more from an entry in the chart that states., "Mrs. T. was afraid that her coffee had been tampered with, but she ate her sandwich and took her medication" than from the entry, "Mrs. T. is paranoid." Judgmental, pejorative, and critical comments are inappropriate and have no place on the chart, but sensitive information must be recorded, especially if not having a record of the information places others at risk. To write that, "Mr. G. behaved in his usual rude and offensive manner," is both inappropriate and uninformative. However, recording that, "Mr. G. grabbed me by the arm, tried to kiss me as I bent over to give him his medication, and used sexually explicit language," provides important clinical information to other caregivers.

Components of the MSE

Behavioral Observations

The MSE is usually introduced with a general description of the resident. This includes observations about the individual's appearance, verbal and nonverbal behavior, and attitude.

Appearance

When observing and describing appearance, attention to detail and the liberal use of adjectives allows the observer to paint a picture of an individual that brings that individual to life in the minds of others. Visual cues play a major part in the initial impression we form of others. The person's general appearance (e.g., height, weight, complexion, state of health) and details of self-care (e.g., grooming, make-up, clothing) are involved in creating this impression. Especially in long-term care settings, where changes in residents are so gradual as to be almost imperceptible, a glance back in the chart to a description recorded several years earlier provides useful clinical information.

Behavior

An accurate description of nonverbal behavior is particularly relevant in working with the elderly. The overall level of activity ranges from agitation, restlessness and pacing to a slowing, where movements are hesitant, delayed or almost absent. Gait, a crucial variable in determining the level of independence, also deserves comment and may be described, for example, as unsteady, stiff, or shuffling. Abnormal postures and movements, such as various tremors and facial movements, are frequently seen in this population.

Speech

Difficulties in communication that may affect other sections of the MSE are noted here. These can include language barriers in nonnative speakers, hearing impairment, and speech that is unintelligible because it is too soft, hoarse, or poorly articulated.

Attitude

Included in the general description is an impression of the way in which the resident relates to the observer. The resident's attitude may be friendly, suspicious, demanding, hostile, overly familiar, inattentive, or withdrawn. It must be kept in mind that many variables affect the resident's attitude, including characteristics of the caregiver, and the circumstances of the interaction. All caregivers, for example, have their bad days when they may be too tired, busy, or preoccupied to respond to those around them in their usual manner. Residents will pick up these fluctuations in staff and their own responses will be affected accordingly.

Some residents seem to create an atmosphere of chaos around them. Staff members working with a resident like this may find themselves developing strong views that contradict those of coworkers and result in major conflicts centered around the resident. Intense feelings of anger and helplessness are evoked in caregivers. This problem is discussed in detail in Chapter 8, "The Resident with Personality Disorder." For the purpose of the MSE, it is important for observers to learn to monitor their subjective responses to residents and use these reactions as a valuable source of data.

Mood and Affect

An individual's dominant feeling state over a period of hours, days, or even weeks is called mood. Affects are the various emotions displayed by the individual in the course of an interaction. Miss J. may have an overall mood of depression but display anxiety, fear, and irritability as well as sadness during a particular interview. These affects may be conveyed through tone of voice, gesture, facial expression, physiological reactions to emotion, such as crying or flushing, and content of speech.

Affects can be classified not just according to type, but also according to quality. Emotions may be experienced intensely or be shallow and less deeply felt. Lability of affect refers to rapidly fluctuating emotional states. Subjective feelings can be elicited by asking questions such as, "How would you describe your feelings?" It is also important, however, to watch for nonverbal emotional behaviors such as facial expression and postures that may be at odds with what the individual is saying about his or her feelings. When Mr. M. whispers with tears in his eyes that everything is fine or Mrs. E. mutters through clenched teeth that she is not at all angry, their words clearly are not the whole story.

The question of suicidal ideation must be addressed whenever the interviewer has even the slightest concern in this area. Not just depressed individuals, but also those who are frightened, anxious, or apparently resigned to their fate may be suicidal. Many clues, other than those available through the mental status, can alert staff to the risk of self-harm or suicide. These are discussed in Chapter 6, "The Suicidal Resident."

Asking people whether they are suicidal can be uncomfortable. Society has traditionally regarded the taking of one's own life as taboo and in contravention of religious and natural laws. Suicide is associated with fear and shame. Moreover, some caregivers believe that by enquiring into suicidal ideation they can drive residents to commit suicide because they are giving the residents ideas they never had in the first place. This belief is not borne out through clinical experience. The majority of individuals who have suicidal thoughts welcome the opportunity to share their frightening, isolating feelings with others. People who are not suicidal will say so and are rarely resentful or threatened by having been asked. When inquiring into suicidal ideation, the topic may be approached gradually, beginning with such questions as, "Have you ever felt your life was not worth living?," moving to, "Have you ever felt so low that you wanted to end your life?," and finally posing more direct questions, "Do you have any thoughts of killing yourself?" If suicidal thoughts are present, the resident should then be asked whether the thoughts are accompanied by a wish or intent to die, whether any suicide plans have been made, and if so, whether the means are available to put the plan into action.

Encountered less frequently than suicidal ideation are thoughts of harming others. If there is any suspicion that such thoughts or plans may exist, however, the question must be explored in the same way as that of suicidal ideation.

An inquiry into the somatic functions that are often disturbed in mood disorders is sometimes included in this section of the MSE. These include changes in sleep, appetite, weight, and libido (sex drive). Clearly, in an ill, elderly population, any findings in this area will be confounded by the many disorders other than depression that can interfere with these functions. This point is dealt with in Chapter 5, "Mood and Anxiety Disorders."

Thought

In assessing the individual's thinking, attention is focused on two main areas. These are the individual's thought process (how the individual thinks) and thought content (what the individual thinks).

Thought Process

Access to what others are thinking comes primarily through their speech. Abnormalities in thought process are reflected in disturbances in the rate, quantity, and form of speech. Excessively rapid or slowed speech, lack of spontaneous speech, and speech limited to one word answers are examples of disturbed thought process. Circumstantial speech refers to a pattern of responding to questions in an overinclusive manner. A tangential response is one in which the original questions is never answered and the individual, through a series of associations, ends up talking about an unrelated topic. Thinking may be disorganized to an even greater degree, resulting in a complete loss of logical connections between ideas. Individuals may jump from topic to topic without following any apparent pattern or connect words through rhyming. In its most extreme form, disorganized thinking results in speech that consists of a series of apparently random words. Because abnormal thought process can result in speech that sounds bizarre, it can be extraordinarily difficult for the listener to quote, even minutes after hearing it. It is useful to jot down an example immediately so that the quote can be recalled for later charting. Disorders in thought process occur in illnesses such as schizophrenia and mania. They must be distinguished from the disturbed communication resulting from brain lesions such as strokes and tumors.

Thought Content

The content of thought can be disturbed in a variety of ways. Individuals can become preoccupied with a particular idea or subject. Obsessions (repetitive unwanted thoughts) and phobias (irrational fears), although recognized by their sufferers as being illogical, exert considerable control over mental life and behavior. Miss L., for example, experiences a compulsion (an uncontrollable impulse) to wash her hands, because she cannot rid herself of the obsessional idea that, as soon as she touches something, she is contaminated. Even though she knows it makes no sense, Miss L. scrubs her hands to the point where they bleed and she experiences great anxiety whenever she cannot get to a sink. Mrs. R., who has had a lifelong fear of heights and elevators, has had to settle for a less favorable room on the ground floor so that she can walk to the dining room and participate in activities without having to confront her fear.

Delusions

Another example of disturbed thought content are false beliefs that the individual does not recognize as irrational. These are called delusions. The ideas are so fixed, that the person cannot be talked out of them even when presented with logical evidence that refutes the ideas. Delusions may be disorganized and fleeting or highly structured and held for many years. There may be a single delusional belief such as the idea that a spouse is having affairs. In other cases an elaborate system of beliefs is created to encompass the individual's entire world, with new information constantly being incorporated into the delusional belief system. For example, Mrs. O. says, "There is a conspiracy to take control of this building. The telephones are bugged, they are listening through the vents, and now they have bribed the cleaning staff. I know that, because for the last three days they have started cleaning at the other end of the hall and they never used to do that."

The presence of a delusion is indicative of psychosis (loss of touch with reality). Other manifestations of psychosis include the disorders of thought form described above and perceptual disturbances (see below). Psychotic symptoms can occur in many different disorders, including delirium, dementia, schizophrenia, and mood disorders.

Asking residents whether they have delusions can feel awkward. The interviewer may feel threatened by exploring a realm of ideas that in layman's terms would be called "crazy." Many psychotic individuals reveal their delusional beliefs spontaneously or behave in a manner that clearly suggests that they are out touch with reality. In other cases, however, the delusions begin to emerge only after careful questioning by the interviewer. Examples of questions eliciting information about delusions include, "Do you have any ideas that might seem unusual to others?," "Have you ever thought people might be trying to harm you in some way?," and "Have you ever thought that you were special and in some way different from other people?"

Some psychotic people are uncomfortable discussing their delusions. In these cases, the interviewer may still suspect that an individual has delusions although the delusions have not been identified.

When deciding whether a belief meets the criteria for a delusion, the observer must remember that certain religious and cultural ideas held by large groups of people are considered irrational in other societies. For example when Mrs. G. accuses Mrs. O. of having caused her fall by placing "the evil eye" on her, Mrs. G.'s background must be considered before concluding that she is suffering from a persecutory delusion.

Perception

Perception is the complex process of obtaining information about the world. It begins with sensations, but involves many other variables as well. For example, a child sees that he has cut himself but is not aware of any pain until he sees blood and hears his parent's concerned response. Information received by the child through his visual, tactile, and auditory senses is interpreted at a higher level to form the perception of a cut that hurts. The perceptual process may be distorted in a number of different ways.

Illusions

These are formed when a real stimulus is misinterpreted. For example, Mr. F., who is hard of hearing, has the repeated experience of hearing his name mentioned, as he walks by groups of people engaged in conversation. Miss G., who is suffering from toxic levels of medication, misinterprets the image of the duvet flung over the chair as a man sitting in her room. Sensory deficits as well as higher level cognitive difficulties increase the risk of developing illusions.

Hallucinations

These are perceptions that occur in the absence of any appropriate external stimulus. They may involve any sensory modality. Mrs. C. may hear voices accusing her of being an unworthy person, Mr. R. sees little people running through his room, and Mrs. D. smells a horrible odor emanating from the vents.

Illusions and hallucinations vary not just in their content and in the sensory modality involved, but also in how they are understood by their sufferers. At times, individuals recognize that their perceptions are distorted but are frightened nevertheless. At other times, individuals develop delusional interpretations of the abnormal perceptions. Mrs. D., for example, may interpret the horrible odor as evidence of a plot to poison her or drive her out of the institution.

Information regarding abnormal perceptual experience is elicited with questions like, "Have you ever had an unusual experience such as hearing voices when nobody was there, or seeing something that nobody else could see?" When abnormal perceptions occur is important since hallucinations can occur in the absence of any neurological or psychiatric disturbance. It is nor unusual for people to experience abnormal perceptions as they are falling asleep or waking up. Hallucinations occurring at other times usually suggest the presence of a mental disorder.

Cognition

Cognition refers to the mental processes involved in the acquisition, processing, and utilization of knowledge or information. The assessment of cognitive functions is an important component of the MSE. These functions are listed in **Table 2**.

Table 2 Cognitive Functions

- Attention and concentration
- Language
- Memory
- Abstraction
- Constructional ability

General Comments

As noted earlier in the chapter, the comprehensiveness of the cognitive assessment depends on the purpose for which the information is being gathered and the resident's ability to tolerate the assessment. Being confronted with evidence of cognitive impairment can be painful both for the impaired resident and for staff who have worked closely with the resident on a daily basis, sometimes for many years. Because of this, there may be a tendency to gloss over or even omit this part of the MSE in order to protect everyone involved. When residents respond to the cognitive assessment with outrage that someone would dare to ask them "silly questions" or try to dodge questions by joking or by distracting the interviewer. This often indicates problems in the area of cognition that need to be pursued if at all possible.

Care should be taken in every case to prepare residents for this part of the assessment. If this is not done residents become understandably upset when someone begins asking them, apparently out of the blue, if they know where they are and whether they can do some arithmetic. The following example illustrates one way of introducing the cognitive assessment in a nonthreatening manner:

Interviewer: *Mrs. A., you mentioned earlier that you have noticed some difficulty in remembering names.*
Mrs. A.: *That's right. It's so annoying. They come back to me eventually but at the time I feel so silly.*
Interviewer: *Have you noticed any other problems with your memory or thinking?*
Mrs. A.: *Well, not really . . . but I do worry about it sometimes.*

Interviewer: *Maybe we can look into this problem a bit further. I'd like to ask you a few questions now to check your memory and your thinking . . ..*

Occasionally, even when a careful approach has been taken, an impaired resident will become anxious and distressed when faced with a task he or she cannot do. This kind of response is referred to as a catastrophic reaction, and requires that the resident be reassured and the cognitive assessment be postponed to a more appropriate time.

A number of factors affect performance on the cognitive assessment. Some of these include intelligence, level of education, cultural considerations, sensory deficits, fatigue, pain, anxiety, poor motivation, an altered level of consciousness, and a noisy or otherwise distracting environment. These factors should be considered both in the administration of the cognitive assessment and in the interpretation of its results.

Impairment in one area of cognition affects the efficiency of other cognitive processes. This interdependency of cognitive abilities needs to be borne in mind when administering and interpreting test data. If, for example, an individual cannot attend to what is being said because of pain, or is unable to comprehend spoken language as a result of a stroke, it will be difficult to assess that person's memory accurately, since memory tests require a capacity for sustained attention and intact language capabilities.

Attention and Concentration

Attention is the foundation of cognition. It usually is tested early in the course of the assessment since impairments in this area will result in problems throughout the cognitive assessment. These problems may be attributed mistakenly to other impairments if the attentional deficit has not been identified.

Attention can be disturbed as a result of a decreased level of consciousness. A note is made, therefore, whether the individual is alert or drowsy.

Excessive distractibility is another form of attentional disturbance, reflecting limitations in the individual's span of attention. This aspect of attention is tested through digit recall. The interviewer recites a series of random numbers at a rate of one digit per second and asks the resident to repeat the series back to him. The length of the series is increased each time the resident gives a correct response. Different numbers are used on every trial. The task can be made more demanding by asking the resident to repeat the series backwards. Now, the individual not only has to keep the series of digits in mind, but he also has to mentally juggle the digits around. Normal individuals are able to repeat five digits forwards and four backwards.

A measure of concentration is the subtraction of serial sevens. The individual is asked to subtract 7 from 100, then keep subtracting 7 from each succeeding answer.

Language

Language functions are also tested early in the cognitive assessment. Aphasic disturbances, disorders of language comprehension and/or expression, are distinguished from dysarthrias, problems with the mechanical articulation of speech (e.g., slurring).

Throughout the assessment, the interviewer makes note of the individual's spontaneous speech. Problems in spontaneous speech include word-finding difficulties, circumlocutions, word substitutions, and impaired fluency.

Testing of repetition involves asking the individual to repeat single words, phrases, and sentences of increasing complexity. Individuals with language difficulties may omit words and alter word sequences. Individuals with dysarthria slur and stumble over words.

Screening for possible comprehension deficits requires the resident to respond to a series of "Yes–No" questions (e.g., "Does a bird fly?") and commands of increasing complexity such as, "Point to the door," and, "Close your eyes and open your mouth." To test for higher order deficits, the resident can be given a construction such as, "If the lion and the tiger have a fight and the tiger kills the lion," then asked the question, "Who is killed?"

Difficulties in naming are identified by asking residents to name objects that are pointed out to them. Failure to recall high frequency words such as chair and pencil indicates a greater degree of impairment than difficulty with low frequency words such as shoelace and key-chain.

Aspects of oral and written language are tested by asking residents to read aloud, explain the content of what they have read, copy sentences, and write spontaneously.

Memory

Memory may be classified into three types: immediate, recent, and remote. Immediate memory, referred to as short-term memory by psychologists, is the process of holding events, objects, or ideas in immediate awareness without necessarily committing them to memory. A good example of immediate memory is the operation of locating a phone number in the directory, keeping it in mind and dialling it without subsequently retaining it. Clinically, it can be examined through recall of digits which has already been described in the section on attention.

Recent memory is the ability to learn new information. Orientation to place and time requires registration and retention of new information on an ongoing basis and depends on the intactness of recent memory. Residents are asked to give their exact location, the day of the week, date, month, and year. While incorrect responses may suggest an impaired ability to learn new information, they could reflect the resident's restricted contact with the outside world. A simple test of recent memory involves presenting the individual with three or four unrelated words or objects until he has learned them and asking him to recall them after a five and 20 minute delay. If the individual has difficulty recalling the items spontaneously, providing him with cues (e.g., "The third one was a vegetable.") might assist his recall. If he benefits from cueing, this might suggest problems retrieving rather than storing new information.

Remote memory involves the recall of information that has been known for a long time. It can be tested by questions about birthdays, names of family members, famous political figures and actors, and important historical events. General knowledge questions are sometimes asked, but it is important to bear in mind that the resident's background and education will influence responses.

Abstraction

The ability to think at an abstract level is a good indicator of overall intellectual functioning. Residents are asked to give similarities between two items (e.g., an apple and an orange, or a statue and a poem), or to interpret proverbs. Like general knowledge, interpretation of similarities and proverbs is influenced by the individual's educational and cultural background.

Constructional Ability

Copying a two- or three-dimensional figure, such as two intersecting pentagons or a cube, requires the ability to perceive the visual stimulus, plan the drawing, and then execute it. Residents who have problems with this task may show other manifestations of impaired visuospatial functioning, such as difficulty finding their way around the institution.

Clock drawing is a frequently used measure of constructional ability. The resident is asked to draw a clock, place all the numbers in their correct position, and set the hands for 10 minutes after 11. Should the resident have difficulty spontaneously drawing the clock, he is presented with a predrawn circle and then asked to put in the numbers and set the time. Clock-drawing is sensitive in picking up a number of abnormalities (e.g., constructional deficits, spatial neglect, planning difficulties) that are differentially related to different neurological conditions.

It may assist in picking up frontal lobe dysfunction which is often not detected on basic screening tests like the Mini-Mental State Examination (MMSE).

Praxis

Praxis is the ability to perform voluntary purposeful movements. The inability to do so, in the absence of any sensory, motor, or comprehension deficits, is called an apraxia. The resident may be able to perform an activity automatically (e.g., blowing out a match), but begins to experience difficulty when he tries to place the movement under conscious control. In the typical examination for disorders of praxis, the resident is asked to make symbolic movements (e.g., blow a kiss), use actual objects, and pantomime the use of objects without the real object (e.g., using a comb) both to imitation and to command.

Insight and Judgment

Insight involves the capacity to understand a situation, and judgment is used in planning a response. One way of assessing these abilities is by asking residents how they understand relevant aspects of their situation (e.g., their institutionalization or an illness) and how they plan to respond, based on that understanding.

Standardized Assessment Instruments in the MSE

Many questionnaires, scales, and tests have been developed to assess different areas of mental status functioning. As long as these are not used as the sole basis for making diagnostic and management decisions, they can enrich the clinical assessment by providing additional and corroborating information. A number of cautionary statements need to be made, however, regarding their use in clinical settings.

Assessment instruments are best used as an adjunct to, and not a replacement for, the clinical assessment. When used, care should be taken that the instrument was developed for clinical as opposed to research or epidemiological purposes, that it is reliable, and that standards are available for the population to which it is being applied. The application in the elderly of depression instruments, such as the Hamilton Depressing Rating Scale [1] and the Beck Depression Scale [2], has been criticized; some of the symptoms used as evidence of depression in a younger population, such as loss of appetite and sleep disturbance, are common in the elderly for reasons other than depression. The Geriatric Depression Scale [3] is a scale that has been developed specifically for the rating of depression in the elderly. It focuses on the cognitive and affective features of depression and consists of 30 yes/no items. Higher scores are associated with more severe levels of depression. The scale is listed in Appendix 1 to this chapter.

The Mini-Mental State Examination (MMSE) [4] is a widely used and practical tool that screens for cognitive impairment. It consists of items that assess orientation, attention/concentration, language, constructional ability, and immediate and delayed recall, and takes 5 to 10 minutes to administer. Recently, population-based norms for the MMSE by age and educational level have been reported for both an American [5] and Canadian [6] sample of individuals.

The Montreal Cognitive Assessment (MoCA) [7] is another cognitive screening tool that was designed to assist first-line professionals to detect the presence of mild cognitive impairment (MCI), a clinical state that lies between normal aging and dementia and shows an accelerated progression to dementia. The initial criteria for MCI focused on the presence of a memory impairment in the context of essentially intact nonmemory cognitive functions, such as language and visuospatial skills, and largely intact everyday functional competencies. The criteria were modified in time to allow for clinical subtypes, based on either the presence (amnestic MCI) or absence (nonamnestic MCI) of memory impairment as the most prominent deficit, and variable outcomes depending on the underlying etiology [8]. With the advent of treatments for dementia, early detection is crucial for early intervention, and the MoCA attempts to address the fact that most individuals meeting clinical criteria for MCI score in the range of normal elderly individuals.

While the MoCA screens for impairment in most of the cognitive domains that are included in the MMSE (i.e., orientation, attention, language, memory, visuospatial ability), albeit in a different or expanded way in some instances, it contains additional items assessing executive function and abstraction. It takes 10 minutes to administer. Its greatest value lies in the availability of normative data with suggested cut-offs for normal controls, individuals with MCI, and individuals with Alzheimer's disease. The MoCA test protocol together with test instructions, normative data, and references may be downloaded (www.mocatest.org) and used without permission for clinical and educational noncommercial purposes.

A more detailed and diagnostically informative characterization of an individual's cognitive functioning is achieved through neuropsychological testing (see Chapter 13 under Cognitive Assessment for a brief discussion of the value of neuropsychological assessment).

The use of both the MMSE and neuropsychological tests in the evaluation of patients with suspected dementia reflects the fact that dementia (see Chapter 3) is characterized mainly by the presence of multiple cognitive deficits. There is increasing recognition, however, that the behavioral (e.g., aggressive behaviors, wandering) and psychological (e.g., delusions, hallucinations) signs and symptoms of dementia are a function of neurobiological abnormalities just as the cognitive deficits are. Not only that, the greatest opportunity for intervention and alleviation of patient suffering and caregiver burden appears to be within the domain of these behavioral and psychological signs and symptoms of dementia. Recognition of this has led to the development of many different scales and measures that are proving to be clinically useful in the monitoring of these symptoms and their progression. The most useful appear to be those that target specific categories of behavior, such as the Cohen-Mansfield Agitation Inventory [9] and the Neuropsychiatric Inventory [12], which are included in Appendices 2 and 3 to this chapter.

Case Illustration

Mr. G. was lying on his bed. His sparse gray hair was uncombed, he was not wearing his dentures, and his stained pajama top was half undone. He looked pale and sweaty. He was short of breath and rolled his head from side to side moaning. When first addressed, he appeared startled and suspicious, his eyes darting from one interviewer to the other. After the purpose of the meeting was explained, he became calmer but continued to startle easily and was constantly distracted by noises in the hall.

He appeared anxious and fearful. He was not feeling suicidal. Mr. G.'s thinking was rambling and difficult to follow. He seemed to be preoccupied with the idea that bad people were coming to take him away and kill him, although it was not clear who these people were or where they would take him. He did not express any other delusional ideas. When he heard the medication cart rolling down the hall, he said "It's them! They're coming! I know it!," but he was reassured when told that it was only the medication cart. These was no evidence that he was suffering from hallucinations.

Mr. G. was disoriented to time, thinking it was shortly after breakfast when it was eleven o'clock at night. He identified the year as 1947 and could not tell the examiner where he was. He was unable to perform serial sevens, but was able to list the days of the week backwards until Friday at which point he was distracted by a car honking outside. Given his impaired concentration and agitated state, further cognitive testing was not attempted.

Comment

On the basis of the MSE and data from his history, physical exam, and laboratory status, Mr. G. was diagnosed as having a delirium (see Chapter 4, Delirium) resulting from pneumonia. The mental status data would predict that he will become very frightened and possibly put up a struggle when the ambulance attendants arrive to transfer him to hospital, but that he may respond positively to reassurance and a calm explanation to what is happening.

Case Illustration

At the time of the examination, Miss J. was sitting in her room, staring down at her hands. She was neatly dressed in a tweed skirt and silk blouse. Her slight, brittle-looking frame was dwarfed by the armchair in which she sat. She had little interest in her surroundings and avoided eye contact during the meeting, responding to questions with brief answers, speaking so softly that at times she was barely audible.

Miss J. appeared deeply depressed. She became tearful when talking about her past life, especially her mother. She expressed feelings of hopelessness, worthlessness, and guilt. She wished her life were over and admitted to having thoughts about killing herself, but did not think she had the courage to act on the thoughts. Her appetite was poor, she had lost weight and was no longer sleeping well at night. There was no evidence of a thought or perceptual disorder.

Miss J. participated reluctantly in the cognitive assessment, sighing frequently and complaining that she was too tired. She was oriented except to the exact date. She refused to continue subtracting serial sevens after two correct subtractions and recalled two out of three objects after five minutes. She copied two intersecting pentagons without difficulty, and wrote the sentence, "I am sad." Miss J. felt she was beyond help, but did agree to participate in the treatment plan that was discussed with her.

Comment

The above is a description of a depressed individual (see Chapter 5). The treatment plan was based not only on the MSE, but also on information regarding previous episodes of depression, and the absence of abnormal findings on a recent physical examination.

References

1. Hamilton, M. (1967). Development of a rating scale for primary depressive illness. British Journal of Social and Clinical Psychiatry, 6:278–296.
2. Beck, A.T., Ward, C.H., Mendelson, M., Mock, J., Erbaugh, J. (1961). An inventory for measuring depression. Archives of General Psychiatry, 4:561–571.
3. Yesavage, K., Brink, T.L., Rose, T.L., Lum, O., Huang, V., Adey, M., Leirer, O. (1983). Development and validation of a geriatric depression screening scale: A preliminary report. Journal of Psychiatric Research, 17:37–49.
4. Folstein, M.F., Folstein, S.W., McHugh, P.R. (1975). "Mini-mental state." A practical method of grading the cognitive states of patients for the clinician. Journal of Psychiatric Research, 12:189–198.
5. Crum, R.M., Anthony, J.C., Bassett, S.S., Folstein, M.F. (1993). Population-based norms for the Mini-Mental State Examination by age and educational level. Journal of the American Medical Association, 269:2386–2391.
6. Tombaugh, T.N., McDowell, I., Krisjansson, B., Hubley, A.M. (1996). Mini-Mental State Examination (MMSE) and the modified MMSE (3MS): A psychometric comparison and normative data. Psychological Assessment, 8:48–59.
7. Nasreddine, Z.S., Phillips, N.A., Bédirian, V., Charbonneau, S., Whitehead, V., Collin, I., Cummings, J.L., & Chertkow, H. (2005). The Montreal Cognitive Assessment, MoCA: A brief screening tool for mild cognitive impairment. Journal of the American Geriatrics Society, 53, 695–699.

8. Petersen, R.C. (2005). Mild cognitive impairment: Where are we? Alzheimer's disease and associated disorders, 19:166–169.
9. Cohen-Mansfield, J., Marx, M.S., Rosenthal, A.S. (1989). A description of agitation in a nursing home. Journal of Gerontology, 44:M77–M84.
10. Cohen-Mansfield, J. (1986). Agitated behaviors in the elderly II. Preliminary results in the cognitively deteriorated. Journal of the American Geriatrics Society, 34:722–727.
11. Cohen-Mansfield, J. (1991). Instruction manual for the Cohen-Mansfield Agitation Inventory (CMAI). Rockville, MD: The Research Institute of the Hebrew Home of Greater Washington.
12. Cummings, J.L., Mega, M., Gray, K., Rosenberg-Thompson, S., Carusi, D.A., Gornbein, J. (1994). The Neuropsychiatric Inventory: Comprehensive assessment of psychopathology in dementia. Neurology, 44:2308–2314.

Suggested Readings

1. Leon, R.L., Bowden, C.L., Faber, R.A. (1998). The Psychiatric Interview, History and Mental Status Examination. In M.J. Kaplan, B.J. Saddock (Eds.), Comprehensive Textbook of Psychiatry (5th Ed., Vol. 1, pp. 449–461). Baltimore: Williams and Wilkins.
   Provides an excellent overview of how to conduct a thorough mental status examination.
2. Strub, R.L., Black, F.W. (1977). The Mental Status Examination in neurology. Philadelphia: F.A. Davis.
   Offers more comprehensive and detailed information on the assessment of cognitive abilities.
3. Finkel, S.I. (Ed.). (1996). Behavioral and psychological signs and symptoms of dementia: Implications for research and treatment. International Psychogeriatrics, 8 (Supplement 3).

Appendix 1: Geriatric Depression Scale[1]

Instructions

These questions are about your everyday mood, attitudes and feelings. I would like to know how you have been feeling over the past week, including today. As I read them to you, please answer "Yes" or "No."

1. Are you basically satisfied with your life?	yes/**no**
2. Have your dropped many of your activities and interests?	**yes**/no
3. Do you feel that your life is empty?	**yes**/no
4. Do you often get bored?	**yes**/no
5. Are you hopeful about the future?	yes/**no**
6. Are you bothered by thoughts you can't get out of your head	**yes**/no
7. Are you in good spirits most of the time?	yes/**no**
8. Are you afraid that something bad is going to happen to you?	**yes**/no
9. Do you feel happy most of the time?	yes/**no**
10. Do you often feel helpless?	**yes**/no
11. Do you often get restless and fidgety?	**yes**/no
12. Do you prefer to stay at home, rather than going out and doing new things?	**yes**/no
13. Do you frequently worry about the future?	**yes**/no
14. Do you feel you have more problems with memory than most?	**yes**/no
15. Do you think it is wonderful to be alive now?	yes/**no**
16. Do you often feel downhearted and blue?	**yes**/no
17. Do you feel pretty worthless the way you are now?	**yes**/no
18. Do you worry a lot about the past?	**yes**/no
19. Do you find life very exciting?	yes/**no**
20. Is it hard for you to get started on new projects?	**yes**/no
21. Do you feel full of energy?	yes/**no**
22. Do you feel that your situation is hopeless?	**yes**/no
23. Do you think that most people are better off than you are?	**yes**/no
24. Do you frequently get upset over little things?	**yes**/no
25. Do you frequently feel like crying?	**yes**/no
26. Do you have trouble concentrating?	**yes**/no
27. Do you enjoy getting up in the morning?	yes/**no**
28. Do you prefer to avoid social gatherings?	**yes**/no
29. Is it easy for you to make decisions?	yes/**no**
30. Is your mind as clear as it used to be?	yes/**no**

N.B. Responses associated with depression are in **bold**.

Suggested Ratings: Normal	0–10
Mild depression:	11–20
Moderate to severe depression:	21–30

1 Reprinted from Journal of Psychiatric Research, 17:37–49, Yesavage, K. et al., Development and validation of a geriatric depression screening scale: A preliminary report, 1983, with permission from Elsevier.

Appendix 2: Cohen-Mansfield Agitation Inventory (CMAI) – Long Form[1]

1. Pace, aimless wandering
2. Inappropriate dress or disrobing
3. Spitting (include at meals)
4. Cursing or verbal aggression
5. Constant unwarranted request for attention or help
6. Repetitive sentences or questions
7. Hitting (including self)
8. Kicking
9. Grabbing onto people
10. Pushing
11. Throwing things
12. Strange noises (weird laughter or crying)
13. Screaming
14. Biting
15. Scratching
16. Trying to get into a different place (e.g., out of the room, building)
17. Intentional falling
18. Complaining
19. Negativism
20. Eating/drinking inappropriate substances
21. Hurt self or others (cigarette, hot water, etc.)
22. Handling things inappropriately
23. Hiding things
24. Hoarding things
25. Tearing things or destroying property
26. Performing repetitious mannerisms
27. Making verbal sexual advances
28. Making physical sexual advances
29. General restlessness

Rating:

As manifest during last fortnight

1 = Never	2 = < 1 × week
3 = 1–2 × per week	4 = Several times a week
5 = Once or twice per day	6 = Several times per day
7 = Several times an hour	

1 [Refs. 9, 10, 11]. Note: For instructions concerning administration and scoring, consult the CMAI Manual, © by Jiska Cohen-Mansfield, all rights reserved. Reprinted with permission of the author.

Appendix 3: Neuropsychiatric Inventory (NPI)[1]

The NPI consists of 12 behavioral areas:

Delusions	Apathy
Hallucinations	Disinhibition
Agitation	Irritability
Depression	Aberrant motor behavior
Anxiety	Night-time behaviors
Euphoria	Appetite and eating disorders

Frequency is rated as:
1 – Occasionally – less than once per week
2 – Often – about once per week
3 – Frequency – several times a week but less than every day
4 – Very frequently – daily or essentially continuously present

Severity is rated as:
1 – Mild – produce little distress in the patient
2 – Moderate – more disturbing to the patient but can be redirected by the caregiver
3 – Severe – very disturbing to the patient and difficult to redirect

Distress is scored as:
0 – No distress
1 – Minimal
2 – Mild
3 – Moderate
4 – Moderately severe
5 – Very severe or extreme

For each domain there are 4 scores. Frequency, severity, total (frequency × severity), and caregiver distress. The total possible score is 144 (i.e., A maximum of 4 in the frequency rating × 3 in the severity rating × 12 remaining domains). This relates to changes, usually over the 4 weeks prior to completion.

1 Source: Cummings J.L., Mega M., Gray K., Rosenberg-Thompson S., Carusi D.A., Gornbein J. (1994). The Neuropsychiatric Inventory: Comprehensive assessment of psychopathology in dementia. Neurology, 44: 2308–2314. [Ref. 12]. © Jeffrey L. Cummings (1994). Reprinted with the permission of the author. Permission to use this inventory must be obtained from Jeffrey L. Cummings, Reed Neurological Research Center, UCLA School of Medicine, 710 Westwood Plaza, Los Angeles, CA 90095-1769, USA.

3 Alzheimer's Disease and Other Dementias

Nathan Herrmann and Robert Madan

Key Points

- Dementia is the most common mental disorder affecting residents in long-term care.
- Residents with dementia will demonstrate cognitive impairment that significantly impairs their daily functioning and their relationships with other people.
- Residents with dementia show behavioral disturbances such as apathy, agitation, depression, delusions, hallucinations, wandering, and aggression, that can significantly affect their care and their quality of life.
- Alzheimer disease is the most common cause of dementia, but there are other causes, some of which are potentially treatable.
- The general principles of management of residents with dementia include:
  – setting realistic goals and expectations,
  – providing consistent care within a highly structured environment, and
  – constructing care plans that utilize a resident's remaining strengths and abilities.
- The management of specific behavioral disturbances must be comprehensive. Treatment considerations include environmental manipulations, behavioral or psychological interventions, and drug therapy.
- Residents with dementia have an increased susceptibility to side-effects from psychoactive drugs; drug therapy must be closely monitored and reevaluated at regular intervals.

Overview

Residents with dementia demonstrate cognitive impairment that is persistent, progressive, and affects the way in which they function. *Cognitive impairment* refers to a loss of previous mental abilities and can include problems with orientation, concentration, memory, language, calculation, insight, and judgment. *Impairment of functioning* refers to a change in social or occupational functioning, or a reduced ability to perform the activities of daily living including grooming, dressing, feeding, and toileting. Although dementias are best known for the disturbance of memory, staff in long-term care are often more concerned about the accompanying behavioral problems such as agitation, wandering, shouting, and suspiciousness.

Between 5–10% of people over age 65 and 20–30% of people over 80 years of age will suffer from dementia. These figures, which demonstrate how the risk of developing the illness increases with advancing age, are likely underestimates. Studies have shown the prevalence rates in nursing homes to be in excess of 50%, making dementia the most common mental disorder affecting this population.

Diagnosis

The diagnosis of dementia is made clinically on the basis of the history, neuropsychological assessment, investigations, and physical examination. Many diagnostic classification systems exist, the most commonly used in North America being the Diagnostic and Statistical Manual of the American Psychiatric Association (DSM-IV-TR). The DSM-IV-TR diagnostic criteria for dementia are listed in **Table 1**.

The presence of impaired memory is essential for a diagnosis of dementia as defined by the DSM. Short-term memory impairment refers to an inability to learn new information and can be tested by asking the person to recall three objects after five minutes. Long-term

Table 1 Diagnostic Criteria for Dementia

A. 1. Memory impairment, AND
   2. At least one of the following:
      a) Disorder of language (aphasia)
      b) Inability to carry out motor activities (apraxia)
      c) Inability to recognize objects (agnosia)
      d) Impairment of abstract thinking, judgment, planning (executive functioning)

B. The disturbance in A1 and 2 significantly interferes with work or usual social activities or relationships with others.

C. Course is marked by gradual onset and continuing decline.

Adapted from DSM-IV-TR, American Psychiatric Association, 2000.

memory impairment is indicated if the person is unable to recall personal information or items of general knowledge that were known previously. While memory impairment occurs early in most dementias, some dementias, such as frontotemporal dementias, may present initially with impulsive and socially inappropriate behaviors, with memory impairment occurring later in the illness. The resident must also show other evidence of cognitive impairment such as impaired judgment, inability to think abstractly, speech and language difficulties, and the inability to recognize or correctly use common objects. The resident's personality may change (e.g., a previously quiet and withdrawn person may become outgoing and rude) or become accentuated (e.g., the somewhat suspicious resident may develop fixed and false beliefs of being persecuted, or, in other words, may develop "persecutory delusions"). The diagnosis of dementia requires that these features significantly interfere with the resident's social activities, relationships with other people, or daily functioning.

Several short, simple, easily administered tests are available to screen for cognitive impairment. The Mini-Mental State Examination (MMSE) is a reliable, valid, and widely used measure of cognitive impairment that can be performed in 10 minutes by any staff member (see Chapter 2). The cut-off score for dementia has traditionally been 24 out of a maximum of 30 points on the MMSE. Performance on this test is influenced by age and education. A standardized version of the MMSE has been designed in order to ensure reliability in administration and scoring [1]. The clock drawing test is sensitive to cognitive impairment and is widely used for assessment of cognitive function. Although screening exams like these help to identify cognitive impairment, the diagnosis of dementia should not be based on test scores alone, but also on the resident's history and functional status.

Alzheimer's Disease

Approximately 50% of people with dementia have Alzheimer's disease. This progressive illness usually begins in mid to late life, and becomes increasingly common with aging. Some people die within one year of diagnosis, but most survive for up to five to ten years. The disease progresses through a number of stages. Initially these residents may have trouble with short-term memory, forgetting appointments or misplacing belongings. They may experience difficulty with speech, frequently searching for the correct word, or have problems naming objects. In the early stages the residents may be aware of their difficulties, and begin to restrict their activities or become depressed. As the illness progresses, the memory problems become much more severe, while speech becomes more vague and less grammatically correct. Residents often lose track of time and become disoriented. Their ability to read, write, and calculate is impaired at this stage. They may lose the ability to use common objects or perform common tasks (referred to as "apraxia"). This often leads to further dependence on staff. Insight is usually lost at this stage, and residents may complain of their belongings being stolen, or of seeing intruders in their rooms. In the final stages of Alzheimer's disease residents become almost totally dependent. They may be incontinent, bedridden, and totally unable to feed themselves. Speech, if present, is fragmented, garbled, and incomprehensible. Death usually results from the physical deterioration and infections such as pneumonia or a urinary tract infection that occur at this stage.

The diagnosis of Alzheimer's disease is made on the basis of the criteria outlined previously, and only after other causes of dementia have been ruled out. There are no laboratory tests or x-rays that specifically identify this illness as a cause of dementia, and a definitive diagnosis can only be made at autopsy. Microscopic examination of the brain reveals several characteristic changes including neuronal loss, senile plaques, and neurofibrillary tangles. The brain is shrunken or "atrophied." Brain atrophy can be seen on CT scans or MRI while the person is alive, but it is not specific for Alzheimer's disease, and may also occur in normal elderly.

The cause of Alzheimer's disease is not known. A small percentage of individuals with Alzheimer's disease will have a familial form of the illness, with a significant number of family members suffering from the disease in every generation. Research has indicated that these individuals will have abnormalities of specific genes on chromosomes such as 21, 1, and 14. Studies have documented that genetics may also play a significant role in the much more common, nonfamilial types of Alzheimer's disease with genetic variations acting as risk factors for developing the illness (e.g., variations to the APOE gene on chromosome 19). At the present time there is no agreement about etiology, and it may be that Alzheimer's disease has a number of causes.

Table 2 Causes of Dementia

Causes of Dementia
Alzheimer disease
Dementia with Lewy bodies
Mixed dementia (Alzheimer's and cerebrovascular disease)
Vascular dementia
Alcoholic and other toxic dementias
Frontotemporal dementia (including Pick's disease)
Normal pressure hydrocephalus
Dementias secondary to metabolic disturbances:
– Thyroid disease
– Vitamin B_{12} deficiency
Dementia with other neurologic illness:
– Parkinson's disease
– Huntington's disease
– Wilson disease
– Multiple sclerosis
Infectious dementias:
– Syphilis
– Creutzfeldt-Jakob disease
Dementia from head trauma
Dementia from brain tumors
Dementia syndrome of depression

Other Dementias

Although Alzheimer's disease represents at least 50% of dementias, other causes need to be considered (**Table 2**). Dementia caused by cerebral circulation problems and/or repeated small strokes is referred to as vascular dementia. Pure vascular dementia without Alzheimer's disease is extremely rare. What is much more common is a combination of Alzheimer's disease and cerebrovascular disease (mixed dementia). Dementia with Lewy bodies has become recognized as a fairly frequent cause of dementia. It is marked by progressive cognitive decline with some combination of either fluctuations, Parkinsonism, or visual hallucinations. Many neurological illnesses such as Parkinson's disease, Huntington's chorea, and multiple sclerosis are also associated with dementia.

Some dementias are potentially at least partially reversible, including dementia secondary to vitamin B12 deficiency, and thyroid disease. The consistent use of certain types of medications is the most common cause of reversible dementia. For example, medications that reduce the neurotransmitter acetylcholine in the brain can cause cognitive impairment in the elderly. A classic example is the class of medication called tricyclic antidepressants. However, many other common nonpsychiatric medications can reduce acetylcholine in the brain to varying degrees. These can even include common over-the-counter cough and cold preparations that utilize older sedating antihistamines like diphenhydramine and dimenhydrinate. Psychiatric disorders, most notably depression, can present with cognitive impairment and other manifestations of dementia. The dementia syndrome of depression, previously referred to as "pseudodementia," is at least potentially partially reversible with adequate treatment for the depression. There is some evidence, though, that elderly patients with the dementia of depression, even if initially reversible, may go on to develop Alzheimer's disease at high rates. Onset of a first episode of depression in late life is recognized as a possible prodrome to Alzheimer's disease.

Behavioral Disturbances in Dementia

Behavioral disturbances in persons with dementia are common and are often the reason why families have decided on institutionalization. They are difficult for staff to deal with and frequently lead to psychiatric consultation. **Table 3** provides a list of some of the typical behavioral disturbances associated with dementia. It is crucial for caregivers to understand that these behaviors are due to the underlying dementia, and not to blame the patient.

Table 3 Behavioral Disturbances in Dementia

Agitation	Catastrophic reactions
Restlessness	Incontinence
Wandering	Phobias/fears
Mood disorder	Shouting/screaming
Delusions	Sleep disturbances
Misidentification syndromes	Sundowning
Hallucinations	Disinhibition
Rage and violence	Sexual behaviors
Compulsive/repetitive/bizarre behaviors	

Mood Disturbances

Depression in people with documented dementia has been identified as a common treatable form of excess morbidity. The diagnosis is based on mood, changes in sleep and appetite, and changes in activity and energy. Because many of these signs and symptoms can occur in demented patients without depression, staff should be vigilant for recent changes in any of these areas that could signify the coexistence of these two disorders. It is important to recognize that sadness, while a feature of depression, is not in itself diagnostic of a depressive disorder. The presence of at least some of the other symptoms of depression is necessary for the diagnosis. Criteria for the diagnosis of depression in Alzheimer's disease have been proposed for research purposes [2]. The criteria are broader than DSM-IV-TR, recognizing that depression in someone with dementia is not the same illness as depression in a young cognitively intact adult.

Displays of inappropriate affect are occasionally associated with dementia. Residents may show excessive tearfulness, laughter, or crying that is abruptly turned on and off, or affect that is incongruous with their underlying mood. These behaviors, referred to as "emotional incontinence," "pathological laughter/crying," or "pseudobulbar affect," are sometimes associated with depression, but can also occur as a direct result of injury to the brain (e.g., stroke). Residents with this type of inappropriate affect may not have any of the other signs and symptoms of a depressive illness.

Apathy States

Changes in the activity levels of demented residents are common and are often functionally limiting. Residents may become withdrawn, slowed-down, and want to spend the day lying in bed or sitting in a chair. These individuals are suffering from a lack of motivation (or "apathy"), and while the dementia may contribute significantly to this condition, so too can things like institutionalization, lack of reward or role, or lack of interesting and stimulating activities. Apathy can occur with depression, but may occur in the absence of depressive symptoms entirely.

Agitation and Aggression

At the other extreme are the agitated residents who wander and require constant redirection and attention from staff.

Agitation can present in many ways ranging from direct expressions of anxiety, to repetitive shouting or screaming. Displays of physical aggression are of particular concern. Agitation can be triggered when residents experience frustrations and stresses which overwhelm them. Episodes of acute agitation are referred to as "catastrophic reactions," and occasionally lead to aggression. Seemingly minor events, such as being unable to string beads in an activity group or being bathed, may provoke aggressive, agitated reactions in residents who are unable to verbalize their frustrations. Physical aggression toward nursing staff and caregivers often occurs in the context of personal care such as dressing, toileting, or bathing.

Psychosis

Delusions and hallucinations frequently coexist and may occur in more than 25% of residents at some stage of the dementia. The delusions of dementia tend to be fleeting, poorly structured, and often involve themes of belongings being stolen, or of being the victims of persecution. The delusions, which are secondary to disruption of brain function, are sometimes viewed as psychological defenses. The resident who cannot find his glasses may feel "better" believing they have been stolen, rather than admitting his memory is failing. When a resident believes she is the victim of persecution, the implication may be that she is an important person who inspires jealousy. Occasionally the delusions are more elaborate and involve the institution, staff members, or other residents. These false beliefs are probably best conceptualized as psychotic, rather than defensive phenomenon, as they are associated with changes in brain functioning and often respond to treatment with antipsychotic medication.

Hallucinations are most commonly visual or auditory and may involve seeing people or animals, or hearing voices or noises. The hallucinations may or may not be frightening or disturbing to the resident.

Sexual Disturbances

While many residents with dementia lose interest in sex, some do not. The disinhibition and lack of social judgment that accompanies dementia may lead to masturbation and disrobing in public, or even solicitation of sex from staff or other residents.

Management

General Management Principles

There are several general principles which can facilitate the management of residents with dementia:

Expectations and Goals

The primary goal in dealing with cognitively impaired individuals is to help them function at the highest level physically, emotionally, and intellectually, for as long as possible. This goal implies that staff must acknowledge the cognitive impairment and behavioral disturbances so that expectations are neither too high nor too low. The staff need to recognize that disturbed behavior is a direct expression of the underlying brain disease; this prevents behavior from being interpreted as "manipulative" or "attention-seeking," and the resident from being labeled as a "bad" person. The resident's premorbid personality and functioning also need to be considered in order to establish reasonable and realistic expectations.

Case Illustration

Mr. A. was a 72-year-old resident with a history of a stroke which affected the right side of his body and caused problems with his speech. He was reasonably self-sufficient in his daily activities, and even organized a weekly trip by taxi to a local pub. Mr. A. constantly argued with the nursing staff and his physician, demanding more of the medications which had been prescribed for him. On several occasions he left the home to get prescriptions for these medications from unknowing physicians in the community. Staff confronted him several times to explain the danger of taking too much medication, but the behavior persisted. Frustrated, the team and nursing home administration threatened him with discharge if he could not abide by the home's rules. He was referred for a psychiatric consultation that revealed significant cognitive impairment. His level of comprehension was poor, and his behavior was ritualistic and repetitive. He repeatedly stated that his doctors had told him the medications were essential for his health, which led him to erroneously conclude that "if some was good, more was better." With a better understanding of Mr. A.'s impairment the staff redesigned a management plan which took his cognitive deficits into account and was successful in resolving the conflicts.

Communication

Because dementia can significantly affect the ability of residents to comprehend language and express themselves, a consideration of communication is essential. Staff should speak slowly, in short clear sentences, and be concrete, avoiding ambiguous messages. Questions should be structured in a way that limits choices and allows the resident to respond with "yes/no" answers. Nonverbal communication can be useful and may include gesturing, emotional inflection in the voice, and the use of touch. The resident should be allowed ample time to respond. A resident's inability to communicate is a source of frustration that can result in agitation and anxiety. Supportive comments, such as "This must be very frustrating for you . . ." often reduce agitation by validating the resident's distress.

Consistency and Structure

Residents with dementia have difficulty tolerating change and adapting to new situations. For the cognitively impaired elderly, the long-term care institution can provide consistent care within the context of a structured environment and a daily schedule. This combination is often sufficient for controlling agitation and other disorders of behavior.

Focus on Strengths and Abilities

In order to maximize functional capacity and independence, care plans should be tailored to the residents' remaining strengths and abilities, rather than focusing only on their disability. Tasks of daily living can be broken down into steps that allow residents to perform the components they are still able to do. For example, while some residents may be unable

Case Illustration

Mr. B. was an 86-year-old widower with Alzheimer disease who was admitted to hospital with pneumonia. He was agitated, often striking out at staff when they attempted to care for him. Although his pneumonia cleared quickly, his family decided to place him in a nursing home. While awaiting placement, he was moved several times within the hospital. On each occasion he became acutely agitated and would often require physical restraints and sedatives. Following transfer to the nursing home, he was a major management problem because of his verbal abuse, shouting, and aggressive behavior. A psychiatric consultation was requested which identified change of environment as the precipitant of his episodes of acute agitation. This predictable pattern was discussed with the staff who agreed to view the ensuing couple of weeks as a period of adjustment for Mr. B. He was placed on a structured daily schedule, which involved care by a consistent primary nurse, and careful monitoring of his activities to avoid over-stimulation. An antipsychotic was prescribed as needed for episodes of severe agitation. Over the next month his behavior settled and he adapted well to the daily routine without the need for continued medication.

to choose suitable clothing, they may be able to dress themselves. Other residents may not be able to use a knife to cut food, but may be able to use a spoon and a fork. Residents who have lost the ability to speak coherently may still be able to sing well. Detailed knowledge of the resident's premorbid personality, skills, and interests enhances the effectiveness of this approach.

Case Illustration

Miss C., a 72-year-old woman with a three-year history of dementia, was agitated, wandered most of the day, and slept poorly at night. Knowledge that she had been a professional tennis player and instructor for many years, helped the team to devise a schedule which included allowing her to hit a tennis ball against a wall in a secluded courtyard for a period of time each day. This activity helped to reduce her daytime agitation and improve her sleep at night.

Teamwork

Clinicians working in isolation are at risk of focusing too narrowly on their own perspectives or approaches, and do not benefit from the observations and expertise of their colleagues. A team meeting can allow sharing of ideas and builds a sense of working together, which is very helpful in managing the stresses that can occur when working with behaviorally challenging residents (and their families).

Case Illustration

Mrs. I., a 76-year-old woman with severe dementia, would spend much of her day disrobing and yelling out. Her daughter was greatly distressed, and tended to blame the nursing staff. The psychiatrist felt pressured to "do something." A routine medical work-up did not provide any obvious metabolic cause for her behavior, and treatment with risperidone, at increasing doses, was begun with some benefit. At a subsequent team meeting the staff observed that the resident seemed to be itchy, and repeat metabolic testing done by the family physician raised the possibility of a liver-related skin condition. Treatment with a medication to control the itchiness led to the ability to decrease the risperidone. The staff and the daughter were much less distressed.

Comment

This case illustrates the need for team support, problem-solving, and the wide-range of expertise that only a team can provide. Focusing only on "usual" medications, such as risperidone, would have missed this treatable medical cause of Mrs. I.'s agitation.

Other Treatment Considerations

The management of residents with dementia requires a consideration of their cognitive impairment, functional disability, and behavioral disturbances. At the present time a diagnosis of dementia implies that cognitive impairment is progressive and permanent. Sudden changes in cognitive function, or in mood and behavior, warrant a thorough medical assessment as even relatively minor illnesses such as respiratory or urinary tract infections may cause these changes and significantly impair a resident's functioning.

More gradual deterioration in cognition and functioning usually reflects the underlying progression of dementia. Treatments are available to improve cognition, function, and behavior and possibly delay disease progression. These drugs include the cholinesterase inhibitors (donepezil, rivastigmine, galantamine), and memantine (NMDA antagonist) (see Chapter 11). The cholinesterase inhibitors have mainly been studied in subjects with mild to moderate dementia, often in community settings. There are fewer studies for this class of medication in severe dementia and in the nursing home, however there are data which suggest they can be effective in this population. Memantine has been studied in subjects with moderate to severe dementia and appears to provide similar modest benefits for cognition, function, and behavior.

Management of Behavioral Disturbances

The management of behavioral disturbances always requires a multi-modal approach that includes environmental manipulations, behavioral or psychological interventions, and use of medications (**Table 4**).

Table 4 Management of Behavioral Disturbances

1. Assessment
   - document behavior including frequency, severity, antecedents, and consequences
   - review recent changes in environment
   - review recent medication changes
   - medical assessment (physical examination and laboratory investigations)
   - assess safety of resident, coresidents, and staff
2. Optimize medical conditions and Improve sensory impairment
3. Nonpharmacological Interventions:
   - environmental interventions (Snoezelen, music, light, sound, activity, room change, etc.)
   - behavioral interventions (see Chapter 13)
4. Pharmacotherapy:
   - choose appropriate medication
   - measure effectiveness
   - monitor for side-effects
   - taper and withdraw if possible

Generally speaking, it is most reasonable to do a comprehensive multidisciplinary assessment of the problem, and then implement a nonpharmacologic strategy prior to starting a medication. Behavioral management techniques and caregiver education are essential components to treatment. Should nonpharmacologic treatments fail to ameliorate the symptoms sufficiently, or if there is clear urgency and/or risk to the patient or others, pharmacologic treatment will be necessary. One must consider the use of psychoactive medications quite carefully in this population. Treatment guidelines and reviews have listed the atypical antipsychotics risperidone and olanzapine as first line medications for aggression and psychosis in dementia [3–6]. However, it is clear that these medications are not risk free. Recent research has highlighted the concern of a threefold increased risk of stroke in subjects being treated for dementia and behavioral symptoms with risperidone or olanzapine (see Chapter 11). Reviews of pooled data reveal a 1.5–1.7 fold increased risk of death with the use of atypical antipsychotics in the demented elderly. The risks need to be balanced against the possible benefits. The elderly, and particularly those with underlying brain disease, have an increased sensitivity to the effects of these medications, and side-effects may accrue over time. Staff should constantly monitor their usefulness and be vigilant for adverse side-effects. Continuous reappraisal and regular attempts to withdraw these medications are indicated at least every three to six months.

Family, staff, and physicians alike are often reluctant to discontinue a medication which they feel has helped with a resident's problematic behavior. However, the dementias are progressive illnesses, and behaviors which may occur at one stage of the illness may not last forever. Behavioral problems may be transient, as some are due to temporary condi-

Case Illustration: Dementia, Agitation, and Aggression

Mr. D., an 80-year-old resident, had a 5-year history of progressive memory loss, disorientation, and speech difficulties. He could no longer recognize his wife, and referred to the staff as if they were his long-time business associates. Mr. D. was agitated and often struck out at nursing staff. He would walk into other residents' rooms and frighten them with his loud aggressive speech.

Comment

What kind of information would be useful in designing a care plan for this gentleman?
Mr. D.'s wife indicated that prior to the onset of the dementia, he was an action-oriented person who was always busy. He controlled a leather-goods company and was a workaholic. He had a large circle of male friends and tended to have a low opinion of women. His only pastime was listening to classical music. Based on this information, an appropriate care plan was devised. Whenever possible, male nurses and attendants were used. Exercise and walking were encouraged. In activity group, Mr. D. was given leather and tools for a simple crafts activity, meant to be reminiscent of his previous work. His wife brought in a tape recorder with a collection of his favorite symphonies. He was also encouraged to wear a small portable cassette tape-player with headphones during the day, as the sounds of classical music seemed effective in reducing his agitation.

Can the violent outbursts be controlled?
The staff was asked to observe all episodes of violence and record the precipitants, the nature of the act, and the consequences for the resident. It became apparent that the violence was limited to occasions when he was showered or bathed. Using a male attendant during these interactions helped reduce the agitation. At other times, when female nurses bathed him, the knowledge that this was a particularly difficult time for Mr. D. helped staff to anticipate the agitation and avoid injury.

Can anything else be done to control agitation?
There are residents with dementia whose agitation and aggressive outbursts remain a significant problem despite all interventions. In Mr. D's case the behavioral strategies were supplemented by treatment with an antipsychotic. Because his agitation was worse during the day, a relatively nonsedating antipsychotic, risperidone, was chosen and started in low doses. After several weeks of treatment, the agitation improved and the antipsychotic was withdrawn six months later.

tions such as medical illness or environmental change. Careful research has shown that beliefs about medications may influence opinion about their value. For example, placebo response rates in studies of antipsychotic medications used to control agitation in dementia are usually in the range of 40% or higher. It is quite unlikely that a placebo is causing the behavioral change, but more likely it is the staff's hopes for the medication to work, or a spontaneous change in the residents' behavior, that is responsible for this high placebo response rate. Despite beliefs about the value of medications, trials of discontinuation are absolutely necessary; clearly careful monitoring for relapse of behavioral problems is essential.

Case Illustration: Dementia and Wandering

Mrs. E., an 84-year-old widow with vascular dementia, had been a resident in the nursing home for over two years. From the time of admission she tended to wander around the floor in an aimless manner, often entering other residents' rooms and lying down on their beds.

Comment

What kind of care does the wandering resident require?
The primary consideration for a resident who wanders is to ensure their safety. Ideally, a resident like Mrs. E., who is a known wanderer, should be on a floor which can be locked or monitored with an alarm system, and is designed to allow for wandering in a nonrestrictive and obstruction-free manner. Where this type of structure is unavailable, other measures are required. The residents should wear brightly-colored, reflective identification shirts. Slippers and shoes should be checked on a regular basis to ensure stability. The resident may require constant supervision to avoid falls when walking on floors that are polished and wet. Doors to the nursing station and storage rooms should always be closed, as open doors are a magnet to the wanderer. Regularly scheduled, supervised walks should be part of their daily program.

Can anything be done to stop her from wandering into other residents' rooms?
A large brightly colored disk with Mrs E.'s name was placed on her door, and she was trained to direct her attention to it. Each time a staff member accompanied her to her room they pointed out the disk. When she was found in other residents' rooms the staff showed her that there was no disk on the door. After several weeks, this simple behavioral intervention reduced her tendency to wander into other rooms.

Can wandering ever become a serious problem?
Mrs. E.'s wandering began to escalate again over a period of several months. She became increasingly agitated and anxious, and paced the halls in a frantic manner. The time spent wandering increased dramatically until she spent all her waking hours pacing. She appeared exhausted, dehydrated, and had lost 15 lbs in an 8 week interval.

What can be done to manage wandering when it becomes a threat to health?
Because Mrs. E. was only sleeping 2–3 hours a night, a benzodiazepine was started. Oxazepam 15mg was chosen because of its relatively short half-life. Although her sleep improved slightly, her wandering continued unchanged. She was drowsier during the day which led her to stumble several times. The oxazepam was therefore discontinued and an antipsychotic was started. Quetiapine was chosen because it is quite sedating. Her wandering continued unchanged, but her falls became more frequent as a result of drug-induced orthostatic hypotension. The antipsychotic was discontinued and an antidepressant was started. Trazodone was chosen because of its sedating effects and relatively low incidence of other side-effects. The wandering and agitation showed a gradual but significant reduction over a period of weeks, and she stopped losing weight.

This case demonstrates how pharmacological intervention is potentially problematic in residents such as Mrs. E. Medications, that were meant to decrease the wandering, all had serious side-effects which placed her at greater risk for falling. Because Mrs. E.'s wandering had increased dramatically over a short period of time, it was considered a possible behavioral manifestation of depression, requiring treatment with an antidepressant. In general, pharmacological intervention should be avoided in wanderers. When indicated, however, it should be initiated and monitored closely for side effects.

Case Illustration: Dementia, Shouting, and "Sundowning"

Mrs. F., an 87-year-old resident, had a longstanding history of memory loss and disorientation that led to placement in a nursing home. She required a lot of assistance with activities of daily living. Mrs. F. spent most of the day standing in front of the nursing station shouting, "Nurse, where am I?" She would become increasingly agitated at night and spent several hours screaming, "Help, help!" after being put to bed. Her shouting disturbed the other residents and irritated the staff because of its repetitive nature.

Comment

What specific behavioral disturbances does this resident display?
There are many causes for shouting and screaming in dementia. Pain, loneliness, and sensory over-stimulation are common causes. Mrs. F. had a long history of being disoriented, and expressed her fear and frustration about not recognizing where she was by shouting. The repetitive nature of the shouting was interpreted as evidence of *perseveration*, the pathological repetition of speech or actions caused by damage to specific areas of the brain. Her shouting and agitation increased markedly at night, a behavioral phenomenon known as "sundowning." The decreased sensory stimulation (less lighting, noise, and activity) increased her disorientation in the evenings and resulted in an increase in her agitation as well.

How can shouting be managed?
The staff were reminded that Mrs. F.'s shouting was perseverative and related to her underlying brain disease. It was not manipulative, and would therefore require some tolerance on the part of the staff. To manage her disorientation, a bulletin board was placed in her room with the date, the name of the nursing home, and her name in large letters. A bold-faced clock was placed in her room to orient her to the time of day. The staff also scheduled regular brief interactions with her each hour, aimed at reorientation and providing empathic support. When she would call out between these scheduled interactions she was reminded that a staff member would see her at "the regularly appointed time."

Are there any techniques to manage sundowning?
Mrs. F.'s daytime schedule was modified to assist her to become more active and avoid afternoon naps. She was allowed to remain near the nursing station and encouraged to watch television or listen to the radio until it was time for sleep. A radio playing soft music was also placed in her room. These interventions reduced her repetitive verbalizations during the day, but she continued to shout immediately after being put to bed. A benzodiazepine, lorazepam 0.5 mg, was given half an hour before bedtime and was effective in decreasing her shouting at night. An alternative to the benzodiazepine is trazodone, which is not addictive, does not cause tolerance, and may have less of an effect on memory. However, trazodone can cause day-time drowsiness and orthostatic hypotension.

To facilitate accurate and reliable assessment of behavioral change, there are now many available rating scales which are easy and quick to use, and which may even reduce the time needed for documentation. Examples include the BEHAVE-AD, the Neuropsychiatric Inventory (which has a version specifically for nursing homes) and the Cohen-Mansfield Agitation Inventory. The use of such scales in nursing homes is highly recommended.

Case Illustration: Dementia, Depression, and Paranoia

Mr. G. was a 76-year-old married gentleman with a long history of numerous strokes and progressive intellectual decline. His wife reluctantly placed him in a nursing home when he became incontinent of urine. On admission he presented as a pleasant somewhat withdrawn gentleman who tended to isolate himself in his room. His speech was vague and fragmented. His wife visited daily, and Mr. G. was always tearful after each visit. One month after his admission his wife became ill and was hospitalized. Mr. G. became more withdrawn and spent more time in bed. His appetite decreased and he lost weight. Occasionally staff found him crying in his room, but when questioned, he denied crying or feeling depressed. He became more suspicious of the staff, and would barricade his door with furniture at night.

Comment

Is this resident depressed, or is he just adjusting to his recent admission?
On admission Mr. G. was noted to be somewhat withdrawn, but seemed to make a fair adjustment to the home. It is not uncommon for residents with dementia to be tearful following family visits, a pattern which may persist for many months after admission. His behavior changed dramatically, however, when his wife's visits stopped. He was more tearful, had decreased energy, was more withdrawn, and began to eat poorly. All these features make the diagnosis of depression likely. The denial of depression may have been related to his difficulty understanding and expressing himself, a common problem in diagnosing depression in residents with dementia. For Mr. G., the denial may also have been related to another feature of his illness, the paranoia. Psychiatric consultation revealed that Mr. G. believed that he was in jail, and that his wife had been executed by the nursing home staff. He barricaded his room to protect himself from attack.

How are depression and paranoia managed in residents with dementia?
Management begins with the recognition that residents with dementia are even more likely to develop depression as cognitively intact residents. One cannot assume that depression in a patient with dementia however, is the same as a young cognitively intact adult. There are specifiers in the DSM-IV-TR for Dementia with depressed mood. Additionally, there are proposed criteria for the diagnosis of depression in dementia as noted previously. Although in Mr. G.'s case there appeared to be an obvious precipitant (i.e., his wife's hospitalization) it was still important to review his medical status for other conditions that can precipitate depression (e.g., another small stroke).

Most research for the treatment of depression has studied nondemented subjects. There are a small number of studies about the treatment of depression in dementia which suggest antidepressant and nonpharmacological approaches can be helpful. Treatment for Mr. G. began with the prescription of an antidepressant and an antipsychotic. The antipsychotic was essential because the paranoia and fear were interfering with his care, making it impossible for the staff to intervene with psychological, social, or recreational therapies.

A family meeting was arranged, in which Mr. G.'s children were asked to increase the frequency of their visits while their mother was in hospital. The staff attempted to get Mr. G. to speak to his wife on the telephone, but he refused insisting that it was just a trick to confuse him. After about 10 days on the antipsychotic he appeared less suspicious, and began to weep openly for his wife. The staff met with him for regularly scheduled sessions during which they explained his wife was ill and in hospital. They continuously repeated empathic comments such as, "It must be very difficult for you to be *here* in the *nursing home*, while your wife is *sick* in *hospital*." The staff began to gradually integrate him into ward activities. Over the next four weeks, he became less tearful, less withdrawn, and started eating more. He no longer thought his wife had been killed, but stated that he thought she had died.

The management and outcome of this case demonstrate several important principles. Pharmacological intervention was an essential prerequisite for the implementation of other dimensions of the multi-modal management approach. As soon as possible, family intervention was requested. Psychotherapeutic interventions were frequent but brief because of the resident's inability to tolerate lengthy interactions. Psychotherapy provided support and validated his feelings about his wife. He was gradually integrated into the ward activities.

The biopsychosocial approach to Mr. G.'s problems was effective in treating his depressive symptomatology and reducing his fear and paranoia. Despite the improvement in his emotional state Mr. G. continued to believe incorrectly that his wife had died. This firmly-held, fixed belief was less distressing to him than his earlier belief that she had been killed, but was still clearly delusional in nature. The underlying dementia may have contributed to the development of this psychotic symptom, and may help to explain why it persisted even after treatment.)

Case Illustration: Apathy

Mrs. A. was an 81-year-old woman with advanced dementia who was bedridden and severely apathetic. She no longer fed herself nor responded to staff attempts to get her to eat or drink. After intravenous rehydration, the family was asked to consent to placement of a PEG tube to allow ongoing feeding. The family was concerned about the invasive nature of this treatment, but was strongly committed to finding a way to allow her to continue to receive nutrition. A trial of a psychostimulant, methylphenidate 5 mg twice daily, was successful in treating the apathy enough so that she was able to be fed, and she ultimately lived another two years without requiring invasive treatments for feeding. The family was pleased with this outcome.

Comment

What are the treatment goals for apathy?
Clearly the answer to this question will depend on the patient and his or her circumstances, but in general an improvement in functioning, with a view toward optimizing quality of life, is the goal.

What are the treatment options?
Treating any underlying causes, such as depression, or medical illness, is crucial. Providing stimulation, and rewarding activity, is also essential. Often finding a role for the resident can be very helpful, as can the use of a highly structured routine. Medications such as the amphetamines, methylphenidate, or dopaminergic drugs such as amantadine, may also help, however their use has not been well studied yet, and they do have potential side effects.

HERMAN®

10-11

"He's getting better. He can remember everything now except getting married."

References

1. Molloy, D.W. (1999). Standardized Mini Mental State Examination. Troy, Ontario: New Grange Press.
2. Olin, J.N., Schneider, L.S., Katz, I.R., Meyers, B.S., Alexopoulos, G.S., Breitner, J.C. et al. (2002). Provisional diagnostic criteria for depression of Alzheimer disease. American Journal of Geriatric Psychiatry, 10:125–128.
3. Canadian Coalition for Senior's Mental Health (CCSMH). (2006). Assessment and Treatment of Mental Health Issues in Long Term Care Homes. Toronto, CCSMH. Available at http://www.ccsmh.ca.
4. International Psychogeriatric Association. (2002). Behavioral and Psychological Symptoms of Dementia (BPSD) Educational Pack. Northfield, IL: Author.
5. Sink, K.M., Holden, K.F., Yaffe, K. (2005) Pharmacological treatment of neuropsychiatric symptoms of dementia: A review of the evidence. Journal of the American Medical Association, 293:596–608.
6. American Geriatrics Society and American Association for Geriatric Psychiatry. (2003). Consensus statement on improving the quality of mental health care in U.S. nursing homes: Management of depression and behavioral symptoms associated with dementia. Journal of the American Geriatrics Society, 51:1287–1298

Suggested Reading

1. Livingston, G., Johnston, K., Katona, C., Paton, J., Lyketsos, C.G., and Old Age Task Force of the World Federation of Biological Psychiatry. (2005). Systematic review of psychological approaches to the management of neuropsychiatric symptoms of dementia. American Journal of Psychiatry, 162:1996–2021.
2. Landreville, P., Bédard, A., Verreault, R., Desrosiers, J., Champoux, N., Monette, J., & Voyer, P. (2006). Nonpharmacological interventions for aggressive behavior in older adults living in long-term care facilities. International Psychogeriatrics, 18:47–73.
These two papers are excellent comprehensive reviews on the available nonpharmacological approaches to treat behavioral and psychological symptoms of dementia.

Dementia – Family Information Sheet*

- The dementias are a group of illnesses that cause people to have problems with their ability to remember things.
- Besides memory, people with dementia may also have problems with keeping track of time, concentrating, and speaking. They may also have difficulty with judgment and decision-making.
- As the illness progresses, the person's ability to perform everyday activities such as dressing, grooming, feeding, and toileting becomes impaired.
- People with dementia may develop a variety of emotional problems including depression, anxiety, angry and sometimes aggressive outbursts, suspiciousness, and hallucinations.
- The most common cause of dementia is Alzheimer's disease, which is a progressive illness. The cause of Alzheimer's disease is still unknown, although there are many theories. In some cases genetic factors appear to play a role.
- There are a large number of less common causes of dementia including vascular dementia (dementia caused by strokes), dementia with Lewy bodies, frontotemporal dementia, dementia with Parkinson's disease, etc. Dementia may also occasionally be caused by some medications, thyroid disease, and vitamin deficiencies.
- The person with dementia in a long-term care facility will require a variety of approaches to help them with their everyday activities (feeding, dressing, toileting, etc.), keeping them appropriately active and stimulated (e.g., exercise, craft groups), and medically healthy.
- While there is no cure for Alzheimer's disease yet, there are medications that may modestly improve abilities and possibly slow the progression of the illness.
- From time-to-time people with dementia may also require special treatment for problems like depression, anxiety, and aggression which may interfere with their care, decrease the quality of their lives, and cause problems for the staff and other residents. These treatments might include making changes to their rooms and their nursing care, and the use of medication such as antidepressants and antipsychotics.
- Caring for a relative with dementia is extremely stressful even when they have been placed in a long-term care facility. If you find yourself having problems with depression, anxiety, poor sleep, or guilty feelings you should approach a staff member (e.g., a social worker) and/or visit your family doctor.
- There is a rich source of information on dementia that is readily available through the local Alzheimer Society in your area, or international organizations such as Alzheimer's Disease International (www.alz.co.uk). There are also a variety of excellent well-written books for families (for example, Nancy L. Mace and Peter V. Rabins. (1991). The 36 Hour Day, Revised Edition. Baltimore: Johns Hopkins University Press).

* From *Practical Psychiatry in the Long-Term Care Home: A Handbook for Staff* (D.K. Conn et al., Eds.). ISBN 978 0-88937-341-9.

4 Delirium

Barbara Schogt and David Myran

Key Points

- Delirium is a biologically based syndrome characterized by a rapid onset, a fluctuating course, and global cognitive impairment.
- Delirium is produced when one or more biological factors stress brain function to the point where decompensation occurs.
- If a resident's behavior and/or cognitive status undergo a sudden change, consider delirium after eliminating obvious physiological factors such as pain, thirst, or hunger.
- Demented individuals are particularly vulnerable to delirium. Any sudden deterioration in a demented resident may represent a delirium superimposed on dementia.
- If the biological factors underlying the delirium can be corrected, recovery from the delirium is usually rapid and complete, although some symptoms may linger for months, especially in the elderly.
- As medications are so often implicated in delirium, all nonessential medications should be discontinued, especially in the absence of other etiological possibilities.
- Delirious residents are often very frightened. They should be approached in a calm, reassuring manner and cared for in a restful, familiar environment.
- Psychoactive drugs may be required to manage the disruptive and violent behavior that sometimes occurs.
- Transfer to a general hospital may have to be considered.

People suffering from an acute physical illness sometimes experience a mental disturbance characterized by inattention and wandering of the mind. These people seem to be in a world of their own, often unable to tell whether it is night or day, what meal they have just had, and sometimes even where they are. Such people can be in a state of frenzied excitement, perhaps as a result of hallucinations, and then several hours later become withdrawn and stuporous. They may mistake familiar caregivers for hostile strangers or misidentify strangers as long-lost relatives.

These symptoms are the result of an acute disturbance of brain function precipitated by physical illness. Biological factors related to that underlying physical condition are sufficient to disrupt the brain's usual equilibrium. The resulting symptoms constitute the syndrome of delirium.

Delirium has been best studied in the general hospital where there is a concentration of acutely and critically ill people with very high rates of delirium. Yet even in this setting, delirium is often missed. Less is known about delirium in long-term care settings. Although residents in these settings are for the most part neither critically nor acutely ill, they are nevertheless at high risk for developing delirium. They are old, often frail and demented, and on many medications that may have to be juggled repeatedly in an effort to maintain a fragile homeostasis.

There are a number of reasons why it is important for those working in long-term care settings to be familiar with the identification and management of delirium:

Delirium Is Common

The elderly are more likely than younger people to have multiple illnesses and to be on many different medications. They are also more likely to be demented and to have limited cognitive reserves. These factors make them vulnerable to delirium.

Delirium Is Serious

Unrecognized and untreated, the underlying disease processes that give rise to delirium can lead to serious illness or even death. In the elderly, delirium may be the first and only evidence of an acute medical problem. For example, all the usual signs and symptoms of myocardial infarction may be absent in an elderly person. Only a sudden change in the person's mental status (i.e., delirium) points to the need for medical investigation. In the course of that investigation the silent myocardial infarction may be identified.

Delirium Gives Rise to Behavior Problems

Delirium can be extremely frightening for both residents and staff. Although delirious individuals may be withdrawn and drowsy to the point of stupor, they can become agitated and sometimes violent. This behavior can pose a risk to staff, other residents and to the delirious person himself.

Delirium Is Often Reversible

If properly identified and managed, delirium is often fully reversible. With the correction of underlying medical problems, the symptoms of delirium usually resolve and the resident is restored to baseline levels of functioning. There is perhaps no other behavioral disturbance that is so dramatic, challenging, and treatable.

Symptoms of Delirium

Delirium is a syndrome. A syndrome is a cluster of signs and symptoms that tend to occur together in such a way as to produce a recognizable and discrete diagnostic entity. Before Lipowski's work in 1980, there was a great deal of disagreement about the definition of delirium. This hampered identification and treatment of the disorder as well as research and education. Since the advent of the DSM, delirium has been defined more rigorously [1]. The DSM-IV-TR criteria for delirium are listed in **Table 1**.

Delirium is a disturbance of consciousness. It affects the individual's ability to focus, maintain, and shift attention. This experience may be somewhat familiar, albeit in mild form, to anyone who has struggled with a complex task while suffering extreme fatigue. The mind has a tendency to wander until it is jogged abruptly and with considerable effort, back to the task at hand. While in such a state, people often startle easily and may become very irritable.

Because consciousness is disturbed in delirium, thinking is affected. Speech may become rambling, slurred, and incoherent. Memory impairment, especially in the area of recent memory, is often evident. If people cannot focus their attention, it is obvious that they will also have difficulty with recall of recent events. Delirious individuals frequently experience disorientation, especially to time, but also to place. Day and night, past and present are blurred together as the delirious individual drifts between fantasy and reality. Hallucinations and other perceptual disturbances may occur. Because sensory information is misinterpreted and difficult to integrate, delirious individuals may develop delusional explanations to account for their bewildering experiences.

Table 1 Diagnostic Criteria for Delirium

A. Disturbance of consciousness (i.e., reduced clarity of awareness of the environment) with reduced ability to focus, sustain, or shift attention.

B. A change in condition (such as memory deficit, disorientation, language disturbance) or the development of a perceptual disturbance that is not better accounted for by a preexisting, established, or evolving dementia.

C. The disturbance develops over a short period of time (usually hours to days) and tends to fluctuate during the course of the day.

D. There is evidence from the history, physical examination, or laboratory findings that the disturbance is caused by the direct physiological consequences of a general medical condition.

Adapted from DSM-IV-TR, American Psychiatric Association, 2000.

Another characteristic feature of delirium is that, unlike most psychiatric disorders, it usually develops acutely in a period of hours to days, with a sudden, significant decline in level of functioning. The delirious individual's mental status can fluctuate markedly over the course of a single day from apparently normal during so-called "lucid intervals," to stupor, or frenzied hyperactivity. The disturbances in activity level and the sleep–wake cycle can be particularly troublesome in an institutional setting.

By definition, delirium is caused by an underlying medical problem. Evidence pointing to physiological disturbance might be present in the history, on physical examination or is identified using routine diagnostic techniques. Identifying the *presence* of physiological disturbance, while an important part of making a diagnosis of delirium, must not be confused with the task of finding out the *cause* of that disturbance. Nearly every physical illness, many different medications, as well as withdrawal syndromes can produce delirium in elderly people. Not until the underlying medical diagnosis is established and the appropriate treatment implemented will the symptoms of delirium begin to resolve.

Mental Status in Delirium

There is no unique mental status picture in delirium. Different residents present with different abnormalities and even the same resident can display enormous variation over the course of an episode of delirium. Certain general observations, nevertheless, can be made regarding the mental status in delirium.

Appearance

A sudden dramatic change in the appearance of a resident can be an important clue in the diagnosis of delirium. The individual who is ordinarily appropriately dressed may suddenly appear disheveled and inappropriately or partially attired. Make-up may be poorly applied, buttons and flies undone, hair uncombed, and dentures left by the bedside.

Psychomotor Behavior

As already noted, delirious individuals have difficulty attending to external stimuli. At times they appear to "tune out," look apathetic, and be unaware of what is happening around them. They may sit or lie listlessly for hours at a time. Conversely, a delirious person may become hyperalert, responding to all stimuli but without being able to do so in a selective manner. Such hypervigilant residents have a tense, even hounded look. Their eyes dart around the room and they jump at the slightest noise. They are often as unable to attend to a conversation as the listless residents. Moreover, because the world stops making sense to them, they may become very fearful and agitated. Lipowski points out that individuals with angry outbursts and an exaggerated fear response are the ones likely to be noticed and to receive staff attention, while those who are quietly delirious may remain unattended and untreated.

Delirious residents may be seen picking at things on their clothes and bedding or pointing at things in a distressed fashion. This is evidence that they are responding to internal stimuli (see "Perceptual Abnormalities" below).

Affect

The affect displayed by the delirious resident is labile, characterized by rapid shifts and variability. The individual may appear anxious, apathetic, excited, or depressed. Sudden unprovoked outbursts of anger, sometimes associated with violence toward self or others, may occur. These exaggerated and unpredictable emotional responses can make management difficult.

Thought Process and Content

Thinking is fragmented and disorganized with rapid shifts from topic to topic. Delirious residents often experience the world around them as hostile and threatening. Delusions, frequently present, can give rise to anger or fear. The delusions of delirium tend to be simple and transient, changing rapidly in response to environmental stimuli. Most of them are thought to arise out of the perceptual distortions described below. With blurring of the distinction between fantasy and reality, the resident may confabulate in response to questions, weaving elaborate tales around events that may never have taken place. Occasionally there is a preoccupation with sexual themes resulting in disinhibited behavior.

Perceptual Abnormalities

Perceptual abnormalities, very common in delirium, usually arise when the individual misinterprets ordinary environmental stimuli. These illusions are frequently visual but may occur in other sensory modalities. Familiar objects and faces become distorted and frightening. A housecoat flung over a chair takes on a life of its own. Voices and ordinary noises can sound unusually grating, or muffled and remote.

Delirious individuals exist in a twilight state drifting in and out of sleep. It is difficult to distinguish dreams from reality in what becomes for them a "living nightmare." Not surprisingly, many develop delusional explanations for these terrifying experiences. Innocuous sounds in the hall become evidence of attacking soldiers, perhaps recalling a childhood trauma. Familiar caregivers are seen as impostors. Much of the violence in delirium is a defensive lashing-out at perceived attackers.

Cognition

Assessment of cognitive functions may not be possible if the resident is too agitated or stuporous to participate in a focused task. Where possible, testing can help confirm the diagnostic impression formed on the basis of the rest of the mental status.

Because of disturbed consciousness and attentional deficits, the cognitive functioning of delirious residents is globally impaired. Word-finding difficulties and problems with articulation reflect difficulties with language and speech. There is usually disorientation to time, including time of day and often to place as well. Disorientation to people is also common, while disorientation to self is rare. The resident will perform poorly on tests of recent memory although long-term memory is usually intact. Praxis is affected resulting in difficulty with constructional tasks. Insight is almost always impaired. Faulty judgment may lead residents to act impulsively and even dangerously.

Identifying Early Delirium in a Long-Term Care Setting

While most psychiatric disorders develop gradually, delirium does so in hours to days. Even before florid symptoms are present, staff who know the resident will often have a sense that the resident is not him- or herself. The resident too may voice concerns that something is wrong without being able to easily identify what it is. Staff can respond by increasing their level of observation. A mental status screening done at this time might reveal deficits not previously present. Even if the mental status examination is normal or unchanged, it provides a recent baseline against which any subsequent deterioration can be measured. Worsening sleep, increasing restlessness, irritability, nightmares, and daytime sleepiness are subtle warning signs that may appear before the delirium progresses to its full-blown state. Several scales have been developed to assist staff in identifying possible cases of delirium. These include the Confusion Assessment Method (CAM) [2] – see Appendix 1 – as recommended in the Canadian Guidelines for the Assessment and Treatment of Delirium [3] and the Delirium Rating Scale (DRS) [4].

Implications of the Fluctuating Course of Delirium

Even when delirium is well established, its clinical picture can be very puzzling to those not familiar with its fluctuating course. The fluctuations, although not universally present, can be quite dramatic. During lucid intervals the resident appears normal, although cognitive deficits can be demonstrated on mental status screening.

Agitation, if present, often occurs at night when the resident is most likely to misinterpret visual stimuli and when opportunities for reassurance and reorientation are less readily available. Symptoms reported during the night-shift might not be present or as obvious the next morning. These symptoms are sometimes dismissed as transient or attributed to "a bad night," until the larger picture of deteriorating functioning emerges more clearly. This points to the importance of keeping delirium in mind whenever a resident displays a new behavioral disturbance.

The fluctuation of symptoms also has important implications for management. An individual who is calm and apparently "normal" after a stormy night cannot be assumed to have recovered from the delirium. The possibility of reemergence of agitation and disruptive behavior, especially the following night, should be considered when planning staffing needs. A sustained period of return to baseline mental status is necessary before staff can safely relax their vigilance.

Differentiating Delirium from Other Disorders

There are a number of conditions commonly encountered in the long-term care setting that may be confused with delirium:

Acute Physical Discomfort

Residents unable to put physical distress into words, perhaps as a result of dementia or stroke, may present with a sudden onset of severe agitation resembling delirium. Obvious sources of discomfort such as thirst, hunger, and pain (e.g., from a fracture or urinary retention) must be considered and ruled out. Unlike the more persistent symptoms of delirium, those caused by acute physical discomfort are usually relieved as soon as the physical problem is addressed.

It should be kept in mind that for those delirious residents who are also impaired in their ability to tell staff about physical symptoms, unrecognized pain may exacerbate the fear and agitation of delirium.

Dementia

Given the high prevalence of dementia among nursing home residents, it is important that staff in these settings be able to differentiate between delirium and dementia. This differentiation is complicated by the fact that those with cognitive reserves limited by dementia are more vulnerable to developing delirium than the general population. Delirium is therefore frequently superimposed on dementia.

In dementia, residents are normally alert and relatively stable from day to day. The demented resident does decline, but the progression of the illness is usually very gradual. The demented resident does not show dramatic fluctuations in mental status over the course of a single day, although some residents may become more impaired and agitated in the late afternoon and evening ("sundowning"). Residents with dementia alone are less likely to experience perceptual distortions and difficulties with sleep. The memory problems in dementia are primary rather than secondary to attentional difficulties as in delirium.

A longitudinal knowledge of the resident and his baseline mental status are crucial to recognizing delirium when it is superimposed on dementia. A sudden change in the mental status of a demented resident may indicate the onset of delirium and should always prompt further investigation.

Depression and Mania

Although apathetic delirious individuals can sometimes appear depressed, depression has a much more gradual onset and is not usually associated with global cognitive impairment. A recent history of dysphoric mood and a past history of depression are also more suggestive of depression than delirium. The importance of past history underscores the need for a thorough intake history when a resident enters the nursing home.

Mania is sometimes difficult to differentiate from agitated delirium, especially since mania can also develop quickly. The absence of global cognitive impairment, and the presence of a past history of mania helps establish this diagnosis.

Paranoid Disorders and Schizophrenia

Residents with paranoid disorders or schizophrenia may have delusions and hallucinations resembling those in delirium. These disorders generally have a more gradual onset, are not characterized by a fluctuating course or global cognitive impairment, and are often associated with a past history of psychiatric disability. The delusions in these disorders tend to be more complex and stable than those in delirium. The hallucinations in schizophrenia are often auditory while delirium is typically characterized by visual hallucinations.

Investigating Delirium

By definition, delirium has a physiological basis. There are a myriad of diverse biological factors that can stress brain function to the point of decompensation and ensuing delirium. Delirium in the elderly is often complex and produced by many different factors acting simultaneously. Sometimes the physical causes are known or easily identified, but often, delirium is the first and only sign that something is wrong. If so, a thorough search into possible etiological factors must follow. Some of the causes of delirium are listed in **Table 2**. At first glance, the list in this table may look overwhelming. Although the investigation of many of these conditions is beyond the scope of the long-term care setting and would require transfer to a general hospital, certain principles can guide the preliminary investigation.

A thorough review of the resident's medical history will reveal areas of particular vulnerability. The resident may have a history of recurrent urinary tract infections, unstable diabetes, or partially compensated congestive heart failure. When a newly admitted resident develops delirium shortly after admission, a withdrawal state must always be suspected. Less commonly, newly admitted residents become delirious when they begin to take prescribed medications regularly after a period of noncompliance at home.

In the absence of such clues, it is useful to keep in mind that "common things are common." Toxic states induced by medication and infection are particularly likely to be

Table 2 Common Causes of Delirium

Category	Examples
Intracranial problems	Strokes, vasculitis, post-ictal states, meningitis, space-occupying lesions such as tumors and subdural hematomas
Systemic illness	Cardiovascular disease such as myocardial infarction and congestive heart failure, renal or hepatic failure, respiratory insufficiency, anemia, diabetes, and other endocrine disorders
Infection	Generalized sepsis, pneumonia, urinary tract infections, meningitis
Toxic/metabolic	Medications, alcohol, electrolyte problems, acid-base disturbances, and hypoxia
Deficiency states	Folate, thiamine, and iron deficiency
Trauma	Head injury, surgery, burns

Table 3 Medications that Can Cause Delirium

Category	Examples
Analgesics	Salicylates, opiates (e.g., codeine)
Anticonvulsants	Barbiturates, carbamazepine, phenytoin
Antihistamines/decongestants	Many over-the-counter preparations
Antiparkinsonians	Amantadine, benztropine, levodopa
Cardiac medications	Digitalis, antiarrhythmics, antihypertensives
Gastrointestinal medications	Antidiarrheal agents, antinauseants, antispasmodics, cimetidine, and to a lesser extent ranitidine
Psychoactive medications	Antidepressants, antipsychotics, lithium, benzodiazepines, and other sedative hypnotics
Other	Antineoplastic agents, anesthetics, antidiabetic agents, some antibiotics

contributing factors in delirium. A detailed review of medications includes looking at the chronology of changes in dose and the introduction of new medications while correlating these with the behavioral changes. The resident should be taken off all nonessential drugs. Numerous different medications can act or interact with other medication to produce delirium. **Table 3** lists some categories of medication frequently implicated. Especially prominent are drugs that have anticholinergic effects. These include many over-the-counter hypnotics, antihistamines, psychoactive drugs such as antipsychotics and antidepressants, and certain antiparkinsonian agents (e.g., amantadine). Even eyedrops containing

Table 4 Baseline Laboratory Investigations

- Complete blood count with differential
- Erythrocyte sedimentation rate
- Blood chemistry: electrolytes, blood urea nitrogen, creatinine, glucose, calcium, phosphate, liver enzymes
- Urinalysis
- Electrocardiogram
- Chest X-ray if indicated

anticholinergic agents can be absorbed systemically and have been implicated in delirium. Many residents are on more than one medication with anticholinergic effects. Often some of these medications can be discontinued or replaced with a less anticholinergic substitute (see Chapter 11, Psychopharmacology). Other commonly used medications that frequently produce delirium are benzodiazepines, digoxin, corticosteroids, and cimetidine.

The resident may be able to identify symptoms of physical illness if interviewed during a lucid interval. A complete physical examination is essential, although it may be difficult to perform if the resident is uncooperative.

Baseline laboratory investigations such as those listed in **Table 4** should be done.

Watching Closely for Delirium

The following residents should be watched especially closely for delirium:

- Residents who have just been admitted from the community or from a hospital are particularly vulnerable. Unsuspected alcohol or benzodiazepine dependence may be unmasked and result in withdrawal syndromes.
- Residents who are on new medications or on higher dosages of their regular medications may become delirious.
- Any acutely ill resident can develop delirium. In this situation, even though the resident's underlying illness is known, awareness that the resident may become behaviorally unstable can guide the level of observation and other aspects of the management plan.
- Residents who have had a previous episode of delirium are especially likely to respond to future biological stressors with delirium.

Managing Delirium

While the team investigates and implements treatment for the underlying physical causes of the delirium, the affected resident remains in an altered mental state. Helping the resident through this turbulent period is sometimes very challenging. Several general principles can be followed.

Approaching the Delirious Resident

Imagine yourself drifting off to sleep, only just aware of the sounds in the room receding. A sudden clatter shocks you out of your slumber. Was the clatter part of your dream or did something fall in the next room? Heart racing, your mind still suspended, it takes you a moment to reorient yourself. The delirious resident is trapped in this twilight state. Reorientation if it happens at all is short-lived. Little wonder a delirious person may perceive your approach as an attack, and lash out in self-defense.

When entering the room it is best to get a sense of the resident's mental status before any physical contact takes place. Speaking clearly, slowly and in a direct manner, staff can introduce themselves, gently orient the resident and explain in simple terms the purpose of the visit (e.g., taking vital signs). It may become obvious at this point that the resident is too agitated to be touched, while at other times approach is possible. Abrupt movements and loud noises should be avoided wherever possible.

While in the resident's presence, staff and visitors should avoid holding discussions among themselves as these are likely to be misinterpreted. Even a stuporous resident is often able to hear everything that is said. There is sometimes an unfortunate tendency to talk about people who look "out of it" as if they are not present. Residents can be deeply hurt by things they were not meant to hear and remember these comments long after the delirium has resolved.

"Going crazy" is something everyone fears: in delirium that fear becomes a reality. The delirious resident derives great benefit from a simple explanation of what is happening. It can be reassuring to hear that a medical problem is causing a disturbance in the way the brain works and that the frightening symptoms will eventually go away. This information is best conveyed during lucid intervals and should be repeated later in the course of the delirium as the resident's ability to retain the information may be impaired.

In the course of an episode of delirium, many decisions have to be made regarding investigation and treatment. Although the resident's status is affected by delirium, it does not automatically follow that the resident is incompetent to give informed consent regarding proposed interventions. Guidelines for assessing decision-making ability and, where necessary, putting substitute decision makers in place are discussed in Chapter 20, Legal and Ethical Dimensions.

Optimizing the Resident's Environment

Environmental factors can contribute to the onset of delirium and seriously aggravate its symptoms. Change is bad for delirious residents. It will cause further disorientation and increase the resident's sense of a world out of control. Whenever possible, room changes should be avoided and staff continuity maintained. Familiar faces, voices, and objects are reassuring and reorienting. As in dementia, clocks and calendars are helpful.

The level of sensory input has to be monitored carefully. Too much light and noise and too many people create panic. It may be necessary to limit the number of people in the room at any one time and the number of different visitors who can come on a particular day. Sensory deprivation, however, can also exacerbate the resident's fears. Adequate but not glaring lighting and regular human contact are optimal.

Supportive Measures and Ongoing Monitoring

Adequate intake of fluid and nutrition must be maintained. Inactive residents should be mobilized to prevent pressure sores and deep vein thromboses. Hyperactive residents have to be protected against injuries and exhaustion. Constant observation is sometimes required.

Delirious residents are medically ill and may require frequent monitoring of vital signs, laboratory tests, and treatment interventions. The importance of any procedure must always be weighed against the risk of further aggravating an already agitated resident. Ideally, flexibility should be preserved so that necessary interactions take place when the resident is relatively calm.

Involving the Family

Relatives need to be given an explanation and ongoing reassurance that the puzzling and frightening changes taking place in the resident arise out of physical problems. Coping with the hostile, bizarre, or embarrassing behaviors of their family member is often painful and difficult (see Information Sheet for Families).

Psychoactive Medications

Psychoactive medications can help manage the behavioral disturbance accompanying delirium. In most cases of delirium, haloperidol, an antipsychotic medication with minimal anticholinergic effects, is the treatment of choice for agitation and behavioral disturbance. Further advantages of haloperidol include its ability to be administered intramuscularly or intravenously (off label) as well as orally, and that it is relatively less likely to cause sedation and hypotension [5]. If haloperidol is used in older adults the dosage should be very low e.g., 0.25–0.5 mg daily or twice per day in most cases. Atypical antipsychotics such as risperidone and olanzapine are being investigated in the management of delirium [6]. The atypical antipsychotics are potentially useful in cases of delirium in residents with Parkinson's disease or Lewy body dementia, as they are less likely than haloperidol to cause extrapyramidal side effects.

It should be stressed that medications used for symptom control do not treat the underlying medical problems that are causing delirium. An exception to this rule occurs in delirium secondary to withdrawal from alcohol, barbiturates, or benzodiazepines. In these cases, the treatment of choice is a benzodiazepine, not only to alleviate the symptoms of delirium but also to correct the underlying medical problem of withdrawal. Based on a review of the recent literature, the Canadian Guidelines for the Assessment and Treatment of Delirium recommend using a shorter acting benzodiazepine, such as lorazepam, for the

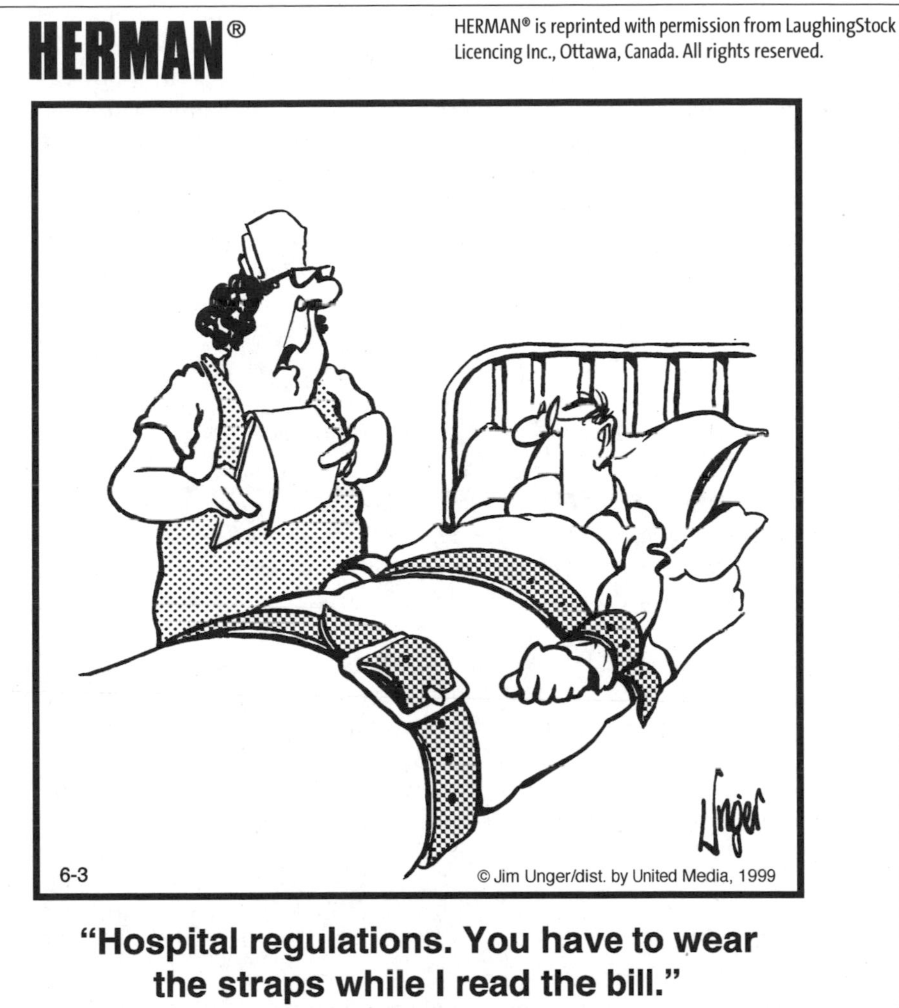

treatment of withdrawal [3]. Lorazepam has better IM bioavailability than do the long-acting benzodiazepines and the risk of oversedation is reduced.

It may be possible to predict the need for medication early in the course of delirium and avoid a crisis. If a resident is highly agitated on the night the delirium begins, it is likely that the behavior will recur and possibly escalate on subsequent nights. In this case, the use of a regular dose of an antipsychotic given early in the evening, before the agitation begins, is far more effective than trying to administer an as needed (p.r.n.) dose to a frenzied resident at 11:30 pm.

Psychoactive medications should be discontinued when the delirium has resolved so that side effects associated with the long-term use of these drugs are avoided.

Physical restraints should be used only as a last resort as the experience of being held down will only add to the delirious resident's terror. Staff should be familiar with the restraints policy of their institution, or in settings with a "no restraint" policy, what protocol to follow when behavior resulting from delirium puts the resident or others at risk. Whenever residents are physically restrained, a specific protocol should be followed to monitor the resident's status and to ensure that there is adequate circulation, and mobilization of restrained limbs. A more appropriate means of achieving behavioral control, usually through the use of psychotropic medications, should be initiated at the same time. Careful charting of the team's actions and the reasons for these actions is recommended. Restraints are never a substitute for constant observation. A literature review found little evidence that restraints prevent injury and in addition suggested that restraint-reduction programs have not resulted in increased falls or injuries [6].

Transfer

At some point in the course of treatment, transfer to a general hospital may have to be considered. Sometimes the etiology of the delirium remains obscure despite adequate initial investigation and management. The resident's condition may deteriorate and require investigation and treatment beyond the scope of a long-term care facility. Occasionally transfer is necessary when the resident's behavior exceeds the bounds of what the setting can manage.

It is important to involve family, and where possible the resident in this decision since not transferring the resident may lead to deterioration or even death within days or weeks. In some cases the decision to transfer for further investigation has to be weighed against the difficulty the delirious resident will experience in relocating to a new environment. The resident's overall prognosis and expected quality of life can also be a factor in the decision, especially since delirium is extremely common in the terminally ill.

The Recovery Phase

The prognosis of delirium varies from rapid and complete recovery to death. Clearly, the outcome depends on the nature of the underlying medical problems. Evidence suggests that with early identification and treatment of these problems there is a better prognosis for recovery from the symptoms of delirium.

Although the duration of an episode of delirium is usually measured in days to weeks, it is not uncommon for an individual to take much longer to reintegrate. This is especially true for the elderly. Symptoms of cognitive impairment sometimes linger for months before a new baseline is established. Serial mental status examinations may show a very gradual improvement with an eventual return to the premorbid level of functioning. Some residents may be left with permanent deficits [5]. Staff and family sometimes assume that there has been complete recovery once the more florid symptoms of delirium have resolved. This can lead to unrealistic expectations being placed on the resident. Yet staff should not conclude prematurely that the resident has become demented as gradual improvement can continue for months.

The resident's memory of what took place during the delirium is usually incomplete. Many will say it was like a bad dream. Recovering residents may need opportunities to discuss the experience and express their feelings about it. Particularly in cases where aggressive and sexually disinhibited behavior has occurred, the resident may be deeply ashamed. If residents do not remember these disruptive incidents, it serves no purpose to remind them. Fears regarding the chances of a recurrence of the delirium may also have to be addressed.

Case Illustration

Mrs. H., a 76-year-old widow, had always been pleasant and cooperative with staff. She showed signs of mild memory impairment. She had a number of medical problems, all of which were well controlled, including diabetes mellitus, hypertension, osteoarthritis, and hypothyroidism. She used a walker because of osteoarthritis in her hips. Much of her time was spent socializing with other residents and she attended crafts programs regularly.

Over a period of several days, the staff noted changes in Mrs. H. At first these were quite subtle. While she slept well, she complained of restlessness. She refused to go to her usual activities and stayed in her room instead. She reacted with completely uncharacteristic irritability when asked if she was feeling well. She did not think it was anyone's business how she was feeling.

On the third night her sleep was disrupted and she became agitated. She screamed that she had seen a man in her room. She had thrown a glass of water at him to chase him away. The clothes on the chair in the corner were wet. Staff were able to settle her but noted that she still looked frightened and wary, her eyes darting around the now well-lit room. She mistook staff for her deceased mother. The resident appeared improved in the morning but over the course of the day she developed a fever and began to complain of shortness of breath. She no longer recognized staff and at one point believed she was on a boat cruise. Nursing staff put Mrs. H. on close observation and called her physician. On the basis of her assessment, the physician suspected that the resident had pneumonia.

Mrs. H. was transferred to a general hospital where she was assessed in the emergency room and found to be hypoxic. She was admitted with a diagnosis of pneumonia and started on oxygen and intravenous antibiotics. She became less short of breath and appeared to be settling. That night however, shouts were heard coming from her room. Nurses found Mrs. H. brandishing her I.V. pole. She had pulled out the I.V. believing it to be a snake attacking her. Several nurses were required to restrain Mrs. H. The physician who reassessed her placed her on a low dose of haloperidol (0.5 mg p.o. b.i.d.) and constant observation.

Her family, visiting the next morning, was shocked that Mrs. H. could not recognize them and kept shouting, "Stop staring at me." Later in the day though, she was observed to be more herself. She was taken out of the posey restraint and ambulated. The next two days were uneventful. Mrs. H. was taken off of constant observation. She remained distractible and had no understanding of why she was in hospital. She had some awareness that she had been through a very frightening time but had difficulty believing the accounts of her condition and behavior over the previous days. She alternated between disbelief and embarrassment.

When Mrs. H. was well enough to return to the nursing home, staff noted she was not as bright as she had been prior to the illness. She worried about her concentration and memory. Repeatedly she asked

the staff and her family if she might be suffering from Alzheimer's disease. She seemed less confident, requiring more reassurance and guidance from staff. Her relatives wondered whether she needed to be transferred to a unit where she could have more supervision.
The staff reassured the family that the resident appeared to be improving slowly and that it was premature to make any changes until her recovery reached a plateau. After five months the resident appeared to be almost back to her usual self.

Comment

This case illustrates a situation encountered frequently in residents who have mild cognitive impairment that pre-dates the onset of their delirium. The first manifestation of a serious physical illness may be mental status changes rather than the more usual physical signs and symptoms. Even after Mrs. H. has recovered from the acute phase of the delirium, subtle deficits in her mental status and functioning linger for many months. Staff are able to reassure Mrs. H. and her relatives because they are familiar with the protracted course that an episode of delirium can have in this population, and because in monitoring Mrs. H.'s mental status carefully, they are able to document a gradual improvement in her condition.

Case Illustration

Mr. W. was an 87-year-old man with mild dementia. He had been through a difficult period of adjustment since his admission to the nursing home several months earlier. He was critical of staff, impatient with his roommate, and plagued by insomnia.
One night at 3:00 a.m., he woke up, put his clothes on over his pajamas, and went to the dining room for breakfast. When staff tried to orient him he exploded in anger and accused them of trying to make him look like a fool. He refused to go back to bed and paced the halls until morning. Staff who changed his sheets noticed that, for the first time since admission, he had been incontinent of urine.
On reviewing his chart, the team noted that he had been started on oxazepam 30 mg q.h.s. for insomnia 5 days earlier. Mr. W. was not very cooperative with a physical examination and refused to answer mental status questions, complaining bitterly that this was an infringement of his rights.
The oxazepam was discontinued. Two weeks later, however, Mr. W. had deteriorated further. He appeared dishevelled, swore at staff, and shook his fist at them whenever they tried to approach him. During the afternoon he slept for hours snoring loudly and moaning restlessly in his sleep. At night he paced the halls and refused to go into his room demanding that cleaning staff get rid of the bugs in his room.
Prior to the delirium, Mr. W. had been physically healthy. Although assessment had been difficult since the delirium had started, a fairly complete physical examination and baseline laboratory tests did not reveal any abnormalities.
The team called Mr. W.'s daughter who lived in another city to report their concern about him and to discuss their decision to transfer him to a general hospital. During this conversation it emerged that three weeks earlier, the daughter, concerned about her father's insomnia, had left him some of the pills

she used for the same problem. Fourteen tablets of flurazepam were recovered from Mr. W.'s room. A week later, Mr. W. began to improve. He was soon back to his premorbid level of functioning.

Comment

Medications are a very common cause of delirium in the elderly. In those cases where there is no apparent physical illness to account for the mental status changes, it is especially important to review the medications carefully. Mr. W.'s case also points to the need to keep in mind the possibility of self-medication with substances ranging from alcohol and over-the-counter medications, to prescription drugs obtained outside the institution.

References

1. American Psychiatric Association. (2000). Diagnostic and statistical manual of mental disorders (4th Ed. – Text Revision). Washington, DC: American Psychiatric Association.
2. Inouye, S.K., van Dyck, C.H., Alessi, C.A., Balkin, S., Siegal, A.P., & Horwitz, R.I. (1990). Clarifying confusion: The confusion assessment method. Annals of Internal Medicine, 113:941–948.
3. Canadian Coalition for Seniors' Mental Health (CCSMH). (2006). National Guidelines for Seniors' Mental Health: The Assessment and Treatment of Delirium. Toronto: CCSMH. Available at www.ccsmh.ca.
4. Trzepacz, P.T., Baker, R.W., Greenhouse, J. (1988). A symptom rating scale for delirium. Psychiatry Research, 23:89–97.
5. American Psychiatric Association. (1999). Practice guideline for the treatment of patients with delirium. American Journal of Psychiatry, 156:5, May, Supplement.
6. Frank, C., Hodgetts, G., Puxty, J. (1996). Safety and efficacy of physical restraints for the elderly. Canadian Family Physician, 42:2402–2409.

Suggested Readings

1. Canadian Coalition for Seniors' Mental Health (CCSMH). (2006). National Guidelines for Seniors' Mental Health: The Assessment and Treatment of Delirium. Toronto: CCSMH. Available at www.ccsmh.ca.
   Highly practical guidelines developed by a multidisciplinary team of experts based on an exhaustive literature review.
2. Lipowski, Z.J. (1980). Delirium: Acute brain failure in man. Springfield, IL: Charles C. Thomas.
   Groundbreaking work that led to better identification and treatment of delirium. Full of rich clinical detail.
3. Fawdry, K. & Berry, M.L. (1989). The Nurse's role: Fear of senility in managing reversible confusion. Journal of Gerontological Nursing, 15(4):17–21.
   This paper is a sensitive exploration of managing delirium and its sequelae from a nursing perspective.
4. Lipowski, Z.J. (1982). Differentiating delirium from dementia in the elderly. Clinical Gerontologist, 1(1):3–10.
   This paper provides a useful guide to a difficult diagnostic area.

4. Lipowski, Z.J. (1989). Delirium in the elderly patient. New England Journal of Medicine, 320:578–582.
A comprehensive overview of delirium in the elderly.
5. American Psychiatric Association. (1999). Practice guideline for the treatment of patients with delirium. American Journal of Psychiatry 156:5, May, Supplement.
A useful review of current evidence and recommendations regarding the diagnosis and management of delirium.

Appendix 1: Confusion Assessment Method (CAM)[1]

Acute onset

1. Is there evidence of an acute change in mental status from the patient's baseline?

*Inattention**

2. A. Did the patient have difficulty focusing attention, for example, being easily distractible, or having difficulty keeping track of what was being said?
   - Not present at any time during interview
   - Present at some time during interview, but in mild form
   - Present at some time during interview, in marked form
   - Uncertain

   B. (If present or abnormal) Did this behavior fluctuate during the interview, that is, tend to come and go or increase and decrease in severity?
   - Yes
   - No
   - Uncertain
   - Not applicable

   C. (If present or abnormal) Please describe this behavior:

Disorganized thinking

3. Was the patient's thinking disorganized or incoherent, such as rambling or irrelevant conversation, unclear or illogical flow of ideas, or unpredictable switching from subject to subject?

Altered level of consciousness

4. Overall, how would you rate this patient's level of consciousness?
   - Alert (normal)
   - Vigilant (hyperalert, overly sensitive to environmental stimuli, startled very easily)
   - Lethargic (drowsy, easily aroused)
   - Stupor (difficult to arouse)
   - Coma (unrousable)
   - Uncertain

Disorientation

5. Was the patient disorientated at any time during the interview, such as thinking that he or she was somewhere other than the hospital, using the wrong bed, or misjudging the time of day?

1 Reproduced from Inouye et al. (1990). Clarifying confusion: The confusion assessment method. Annals of Internal Medicine, 113:941–948, with permission of the American College of Physicians.

* The questions listed under this topic are repeated for each topic where applicable.

Memory impairment

6. Did the patient demonstrate any memory problems during the interview, such as inability to remember events in the hospital or difficulty remembering instructions?

Perceptual disturbances

7. Did the patient have any evidence of perceptual disturbances, for example, hallucinations, illusions, or misinterpretations (such as thinking something was moving when it was not)?

Psychomotor agitation

8. Part 1. At any time during the interview, did the patient have an unusually increased level of motor activity, such as restlessness, picking at bedclothes, tapping fingers, or making frequent sudden changes of position?

Psychomotor retardation

8. Part 2. At any time during the interview, did the patient have an unusually depressed level of motor activity, such as sluggishness, staring into space, staying in one position for a long time, or moving very slowly?

Altered sleep-wake cycle

9. Did the patient have evidence of disturbance of the sleep-wake cycle, such as excessive daytime sleepiness with insomnia at night?

Note: A diagnosis of delirium requires the presence of acute onset/fluctuating course, inattention and *either* disorganized thinking *or* an altered level of consciousness.

Delirium – Family Information Sheet*

You have learned that a member of your family is suffering from delirium. The information below is intended to address some of the questions you might have about this condition.

What is Delirium? Delirium is a disorder that can be recognized by the sudden onset of a significant change in thinking and behavior. It is caused by the presence of one or more medical problems, such as an infection or a reaction to a new medication. The medical problem, even though it may be anywhere in the body, disrupts the brain's ability to function. As a result, people with delirium have great difficulty focusing their attention. Sleeping patterns are disrupted. At any time of the day or night a person with delirium can rapidly go from being drowsy and difficult to awaken to being very agitated and fearful. Because their thoughts are drifting and disorganized, delirious people cannot always distinguish between fantasy and reality. They often become confused about the time and the date, and may not know where they are. They may mistake you for someone else or not recognize you at all. They may lose their usual social graces and may even remove their clothing or become sexually inappropriate. When delirious people lash out it is because they are frightened and trying to defend themselves. They may feel that everything around them is dangerous and unfamiliar.

What are Staff Doing to Help? There are two approaches to helping a delirious person: (1) The staff try to find out what medical condition is causing the delirium. Their investigations may include a physical examination, laboratory tests, and a review of medications. If the condition that is causing the delirium is already known, and if it is treatable, staff will begin the appropriate treatment. (2) Much can be done to help the delirious person feel safer and more comfortable. In a gentle, steady tone, caregivers will explain who they are and what they are going to do. They will remind the person where they are and what time it is. They will provide the necessary care and ensure that fluid intake is adequate. Medication may be started to calm the person and to reduce the strange and terrifying thoughts. Medication can also help to prevent the person from striking out when they are frightened. Staff may limit visiting if they feel that the delirious person is getting too agitated by the visits.

How Can We Help? Your relative may be soothed and supported by your presence. Try to keep things "low-key." Avoid abrupt movements or loud noises as these are startling and extremely unpleasant for delirious individuals. If your relative becomes agitated, he or she may behave in ways that are very painful to you. Although it may be difficult for you not to take this personally, the behavior should be understood as arising from abnormal brain functioning. It is best not to criticize or argue as this will often make the agitation worse.

What Can We Expect? If the medical problem that caused the delirium can be treated, the symptoms will gradually resolve. Usually people return to normal and regain their previous level of functioning in a matter of weeks. It may take longer for elderly people to recover

* From *Practical Psychiatry in the Long-Term Care Home: A Handbook for Staff* (D.K. Conn et al., Eds.). ISBN 978-0-88937-341-9. © 2007 Hogrefe & Huber Publishers.

and on occasion they don't make a full recovery. People may remember nothing from the time they were delirious. It does not help to remind them. If they do have memories, these may be frightening, painful, or embarrassing. Along with staff, you can help your relative make some sense of the experience they have just been through.

5 Mood and Anxiety Disorders

David K. Conn and Alanna Kaye

Key Points

- Depression can be subdivided into major depression, dysthymic disorder, adjustment disorder with depressed mood, and mood disorder due to a general medical condition.
- If there is a history of mania or hypomania a diagnosis of bipolar affective disorder is made.
- The most common anxiety disorders in the elderly are GAD and phobias. Anxiety and mood disorders often coexist.
- Diagnosis may be difficult in the elderly. Neurological and other medical illnesses can mimic depression. Elderly individuals with a depressive illness tend to complain less frequently of actually experiencing a depressed mood.
- Many medical illnesses and medications can precipitate depression, mania, and anxiety.
- Major depression represents a final common pathway, that is, a nonspecific response to a variety of biological, psychological, and/or social factors.
- Treatment approaches for depression should therefore include medication, psychotherapy, and social modalities as indicated. Treatment is often highly effective and therefore rewarding for all involved.
- Treatments for anxiety disorders include medication, psychotherapy, and behavior therapy.

"Coming in here is the last stop, it's the end of the road . . ."
A nursing home resident

The focus of this chapter will be the mood disorders, including depression and mania, and anxiety disorders. A basic overview of each group of disorders is provided with special consideration of how these illnesses affect elderly residents of long-term care facilities.

Depression

When an elderly person enters an institution, there is invariably some degree of sadness. Of course not everyone who feels sad suffers from a depressive illness. The term "depression" is used in a variety of situations to denote either a feeling, a mood, a symptom, a reaction, or an illness. The terms "clinical depression" or "major depression" refer to a depressive illness. It is important that staff are alert to the possibility that a resident may be suffering from major depression as this is an eminently treatable condition. Without treatment there may be considerable suffering with a decreased level of physical and cognitive functioning and, in severe cases, a potential risk of suicide. **Table 1** outlines the criteria used to make a diagnosis of major depressive episode as listed in the Diagnostic and Statistical Manual of Mental Disorders, DSM-IV-TR [1].

Table 1 DSM-IV-TR Diagnosis of Major Depression

At least five of the following symptoms have been present nearly every day, for most of the day, during the same 2-week period and represent a change from previous functioning; at least one of the symptoms is either (1) depressed mood or (2) loss of interest or pleasure.

1. Depressed mood, either subjective or reported by others
2. Markedly diminished interest or pleasure
3. Significant change in weight or appetite
4. Insomnia or hypersomnia
5. Psychomotor agitation or retardation
6. Fatigue or loss of energy
7. Feelings of worthlessness or excess of inappropriate guilt
8. Diminished ability to think or concentrate or indecisiveness
9. Recurrent thoughts of death or suicidal ideation

Symptoms cause significant distress or impairment in daily activities, social life, or other important areas of functioning.
Symptoms are not due to the direct effects of a substance (e.g., drugs of abuse or medication) or a general medical condition.

Adapted from DSM-IV-TR, American Psychiatric Association, 2000.

Symptoms and Signs in a Clinically Depressed Patient

Although residents may report a persistently depressed mood, it is not infrequent for depressed people to minimize or even deny the presence of depressive feelings. Other feelings such as nervousness or irritability may be reported. Frequently there is marked change in behavior with a loss of motivation and interest in usual activities. The person may withdraw from social interactions, slow down almost to the point of immobility, or conversely become highly agitated, anxious, and restless. Some of the classical symptoms of a depressive illness, such as changes in sleep, appetite, weight, and energy can also be caused by physical illness. It is therefore critically important, although often especially difficult in the elderly, to differentiate between symptoms attributable to a physical illness and those caused by depression. In the elderly, depressive thinking may be the best clue to the presence of underlying depression, especially if this presents a distinct change. The person may view themselves, the world and the future in totally negative terms, feeling hopeless, helpless and worthless, often with associated feelings of guilt and self-blame. When the depression is severe, the person may dwell on thoughts of death and develop suicidal ideation. It is widely recommended that residents of LTC homes be screened for depression both in the early postadmission phase and subsequently at regular intervals [2]. A number of screening tools for depression are available including the Geriatric Depression Scale (GDS) [3]. Other tools include the Cornell Scale for Depression in Dementia (CSDD) and the Centre for Epidemiological Studies of Depression Scale (CES-D) [4, 5]. The original GDS has 30 true–false questions (see Chapter 2, Appendix 2) but shorter versions with 15, 10, or 4 questions are available. The Cornell Scale is particularly useful in assessing individuals with significant cognitive impairment.

Other Forms of Depression Besides Major Depression

There are several other forms of depression. The term "dysthymic disorder" is used to describe a more chronic and usually less severe form of depression that may persist for many years. It is not clear whether this disorder is related to major depression or whether it is a separate entity related in part to an individual's personality structure. Transient depressions can occur following a major life event and are referred to as adjustment disorders with depressed mood. This is common in newly admitted nursing home residents. Although not in the DSM-IV-TR, the term "existential depression" is sometimes used to describe individuals suffering from a depression related to difficult life events. If an "organic" factor, for example, a stroke is judged to be the cause of a depression, a diagnosis of mood disorder due to a generalized medical condition (stroke) is made. A bipolar affective disorder is diagnosed if the individual has a history of mania or hypomania. When symptoms of depression are present it is important to try to establish a diagnosis of the type of depression in order to determine the most appropriate management strategies.

Depression in the Elderly

There is debate about whether depression in the elderly is distinct from depression in younger adults. Although more research is needed it appears that depression in the elderly is characterized by less frequent complaints of depressed mood, more cognitive symptoms and signs, more hypochondriasis, less guilt, and more frequent completed suicide. It is important to stress that the elderly often do not openly describe feelings of sadness or depression.

Epidemiology of Depression in the Elderly

There is considerable debate as to whether the elderly are more at risk for major depression than younger adults. When strict definitions of major depression are applied, the prevalence appears to be between 2% and 4% in the general population. Community studies report depressive symptoms in 10% to 15% of the general population. Comparisons of the elderly with younger adults show that teenagers and younger adults may have the highest levels of reported symptoms. However, 20% or 30% of medically ill patients and an even higher percentage of patients and residents in long-term care report significant depressive symptoms. The prevalence of depression in nursing home residents appears to be 15 to 20% for major depression, 25 to 40% for minor depressions, with an even higher percentage experiencing significant sadness or unhappiness [6, 7]. The mortality rate of the institutionalized elderly rises when depression is present although this is partly explainable by the effects of associated medical illness, functional disability and impaired cognitive status. A study of patients in a chronic care hospital in Toronto found that 35% of patients able to complete rating scales had scores in the depressed range [8]. Interestingly, in the latter study feelings of sadness were equally present in both depressed and nondepressed institutionalized patients. In two-thirds of the medical patients who were found to be depressed their depression had been previously unrecognized. This finding highlights the need for greater awareness of the high prevalence of depression in institutionalized geriatric patients with chronic medical illness.

Differential Diagnosis

Psychiatric Disorders

As mentioned above, if depression is present, the differential diagnosis includes major depression, bipolar affective disorder, adjustment disorder with depressed mood, dysthymic disorder, or mood disorder due to a general medical condition. It is important to differentiate the depressive disorders from other conditions that resemble depression: anxiety disorders such as agoraphobia, panic disorder, generalized anxiety disorder, or post-traumatic stress disorder, and other psychiatric disorders such as paranoid disorders and hypochondriasis which can present with depressive features or may coexist with a depressive disorder.

Grief

A grief reaction following the loss of a spouse or other relative can often present with depressive symptoms and may progress to a significant depressive illness. In the acute phases it can be difficult to differentiate grief from depression. The process of grief is discussed later in this chapter.

Physical Illness

Various physical illnesses, whose main symptoms are weakness, lethargy, or pain can resemble depression. A good example is the post-viral syndrome in which the individual is overwhelmed with fatigue and is unable to perform the normal activities of daily living. If the clinician is unsure whether to attribute certain symptoms to depression or underlying physical illness, the "inclusive" approach ensures that depression is diagnosed and treated. When using the "inclusive" approach if doubt exists the symptom is attributed to depression. The rationale of the inclusive approach is that the benefits of alleviating possible depression outweigh the risks of unnecessary treatment in cases where in fact there is no depression.

Neurological Disorders

The majority of patients in the nursing home setting will have some form of underlying brain disease that can mimic depression. Patients with Parkinson's disease look and sound depressed. They typically have a blank emotionless facial expression and their speech is monotonous and barely audible. Damage to many different areas of the brain may result in dysprosody, which is an inability to communicate one's emotional state through voice pitch, voice inflection, posture, and mimicry. Consequently, patients with dysprosody may sound depressed when they are not, or may actually be depressed but unable to adequately express their feelings.

Other patients with brain lesions can present with pathological crying or emotional lability which can be mistaken for depression. These patients complain that they cannot control their emotions. They will cry spontaneously or in response to any emotional thought or feeling. Some patients with frontal lobe damage or subcortical dementia present with apathy and psychomotor retardation.

It should be noted that, although the above conditions can mimic depression, depression may coexist with any of these diagnoses. Depression is especially common following stroke and in Parkinson's disease.

Other Presentations of Depression

Masked Depression

The term “masked” depression refers to a depressive illness characterized primarily by physical complaints such as headache or abdominal pain. Residents with masked depression usually report vegetative signs of depression, negative depressive cognitions, anxiety, and agitation. When confronted with the suggestion that they might be depressed, however, they typically deny it and focus entirely on their physical symptoms. Masked depression frequently responds well to antidepressants.

Dementia Syndrome of Depression (Pseudodementia)

Some patients with a picture of dementia actually have a depressive illness. Treatment leads not only to an improvement in depression but also restores normal cognitive functioning. Clues to this particular presentation include patients who highlight their failures, worry about their memory, have a short rapidly progressive history of cognitive impairment, perform inconsistently on testing, and have an equal impairment of recent and remote memory. Most clinicians find this to be a rare syndrome, the more common presentation being a coexisting depression and dementia. The syndrome may in fact be an early warning, signaling the beginning of a dementia process.

Delusional Depression

Severe forms of depression can be associated with delusions that are typically somatic or persecutory. These delusions are usually mood-congruent, that is, the content is consistent with depressive themes of guilt, disease, death, nihilism, or deserved punishment. Associated features include ruminations and agitation. Residents with delusional depression often require transfer to a psychiatric unit for optimal care.

Depression and Physical Illness

Physical illness is another contributing factor to the development of depression in the elderly. There are four possible relationships between medical illness and depression:

- Depression may be a presenting complaint related to an underlying and as yet undiagnosed medical disorder, such as carcinoma.
- Physical symptoms may at times arise from an underlying depression in which there is virtually no complaint of a depressed mood (e.g., masked depression, often presenting as headache or other pain).
- Depression and physical illness may occur together and be directly related.
- Depression and physical illness may coexist but be essentially unrelated.

Table 2 lists some of the medical illnesses and medications that are frequently associated with depression.

Table 2 Medical Illnesses and Medications often Associated with Depression

Neurological
– Stroke
– Parkinson's disease
– Hydrocephalus
– Multiple sclerosis
– Cerebral neoplasms
– Head-injury
Endocrine
– Hypothyroidism
– Hyperthyroidism
– Cushing's syndrome
– Addison's disease
Collagen-vascular diseases
Carcinoma-lymphoma
Viral illness
– Hepatitis
– Influenza
– Mononucleosis
Medications
– Methyldopa
– Propranolol
– Corticosteroids
– L-dopa
– Cimetidine
– Barbiturates

Causes of Depression

Various biological, psychological, and social factors have been proposed as causative agents in depression. The development of depression resulting from several contributing factors has been termed a "Final Common Pathway."

Biological

Possible biological etiologies include a genetic vulnerability, a functional deficiency of monoamine neurotransmitters such as norepinephrine and serotonin, circadian rhythm desynchronization, specific relationships to medical illnesses (e.g., strokes), and abnormal neuroendocrine functions. These potential biological etiologies may overlap and be interrelated.

Psychosocial

A variety of psychological factors have been described in the precipitation of depression. As mentioned above, the elderly often experience multiple losses which can in turn contribute to the development of depression. The loss of loved ones, in particular, leads to grief which can develop into a full blown major depression. A history of earlier losses predisposes an individual to the later development of depression. Erikson conceptualized the psychology of later life as a conflict of "integrity versus despair" [9]. He pointed out that as older persons try to come to terms with their life, there is either an acceptance and ultimately a sense of integrity, or despair about lost opportunities. Cognitive theories of depression assign a central role to dysfunctional or negative thoughts. Behavioral theories suggest that depression results from a social skills deficit which prevents individuals from receiving positive reinforcement from important others in their environment. Social factors contributing to the development of depression include lack of family support, lack of friends, and deprivation such as poverty.

Factors in Long-Term Care

Loss is an important factor in the development of depressive feelings. Many elderly people experience the move into an institution as the loss of home, independence, control over decision-making, freedom, and privacy. Sadness in response to this situation is normal. These feelings are exacerbated by other losses that occur in association with institutionalization. Often there has been the loss of a spouse or other close relatives and friends, as well as a developing illness or disability. Sensory deprivation from failing hearing or eyesight may result in feelings of isolation from the world. The degree to which the elderly person has been able to participate in the choice of institution and in the process of moving affects the transition process. If individuals have the cognitive and emotional capacity to participate in the process and have had the opportunity to orient themselves to the institution before they move in, then they may feel more in control of the situation. Perceiving oneself as being in control reduces or allays feelings of helplessness and depression.

Assessment

In view of the multiple causes of depression described above, good management starts with a comprehensive assessment, which would include a full history and examination. It is important to rule out underlying medical conditions. It is also important to ask about hopelessness and suicidal ideation or behavior (see Chapter 6). Investigations may include laboratory and other diagnostic tests, psychological assessments, and review of the social and/or physical environment.

It may be important to obtain a past history of treatment response. The goal of the assessment is to arrive at a diagnosis and differential diagnosis, informed by appropriate diagnostic criteria.

Managing Residents with Depression

Individuals with major depression often respond best to a combination of medication and psychotherapy or other psychosocial interventions. As the cases below will illustrate, a variety of interventions may be necessary.

Appropriate antidepressants for the elderly include the selective serotonin reuptake inhibitors (SSRIs) (e.g., citalopram and sertraline) and most clinicians now use the SSRIs as first line therapy. Other options include venlafaxine, mirtazapine, and bupropion. Mirtazapine is relatively sedating and often helps sleep, whereas Bupropion is generally more activating. Tricyclic antidepressants (e.g., nortriptyline, desipramine) are used on occasion. The choice of medication is usually made by taking into account target symptoms, potential drug-drug interactions, and likely side effects. Clinicians should start at half of the dose recommended for younger adults and ensure that therapeutic doses are reached as quickly as possible. Residents should be monitored regularly after starting treatment. Residents who start on serotonergic antidepressants (e.g., SSRIs or venlafaxine) should be monitored for common side effects such as nausea and diarrhea, as well as less common ones, such as hyponatremia (leading to fatigue, malaise, delirium) or serotonin syndrome (with agitation, tachycardia, tremor, hyperreflexia). Venlafaxine can cause increased blood pressure. There is an increased risk of seizures with higher dosages of bupropion and weight gain is more common with mirtazapine.

Antidepressants usually take several weeks to work but once they do the response to treatment is often dramatic. The severely agitated or psychotic patient with depression may require antipsychotic medication. The role of medications in the management of depression is discussed in Chapter 11.

For the seriously depressed patient who is unresponsive to medication and/or whose life may be endangered, a trial of electroconvulsive therapy (ECT) may be indicated. Unilateral ECT administered to the nondominant hemisphere causes less post-ictal confusion than bilateral ECT. There is still some debate regarding the efficacy of bilateral versus unilateral ECT, with some evidence that a greater percentage of patients respond to bilateral treatment. Patients requiring ECT usually require transfer to a psychiatric inpatient unit.

Supportive psychotherapy and more specific approaches such as cognitive behavior therapy and reminiscence therapy can be of particular benefit to the depressed resident. Group therapies and activities can also be helpful, although it may be difficult to get the seriously depressed resident to participate. Individual psychotherapeutic techniques are discussed in Chapter 14 and group psychotherapy in Chapter 15.

Patients with less severe forms of depression, such as an adjustment disorder with depressed mood, generally do not respond well to antidepressants. These individuals usually require support, time, and sometimes psychotherapy or other psychosocial interventions to help in the recovery process. In the nursing home situation, the most likely time for an adjustment reaction is the period following admission. It is important during this time to let the resident know that the staff understand this kind of reaction. The resident should be encouraged to form new relationships and to participate, where possible, in programs such as structured recreational activities.

Grief

The process of grief after the death of a loved one varies considerably. If death occurs after a lengthy illness during which the process of dying has been evident, the family has the opportunity to begin grieving prior to the death. In these instances of anticipatory grief, death may be accepted as an inevitable part of life or even as a timely release for the dying. In situations of sudden death or where levels of denial are high, the grief process cannot begin until the individual has died.

Parkes [10] describes four stages of grief:

1. Initial numbness
2. Protest and searching
3. Disorganization and despair
4. Acceptance and reorganization of a new life

The initial stages of numbness can last from days to weeks. The person may deny all feelings and feel as through in a dream. This state may be interspersed with overwhelming feelings of distress and episodes of crying.

During the stage of protest and searching, the person feels anxious and pines. He/she is in a state of high physiological arousal with uncomfortable physical sensations such as tightness in the chest, hollowness in the stomach, and generalized weakness. The strong desire for contact with the lost person commonly results in illusions or, on occasion, hallucinations in which the grieving person imagines he sees or hears the deceased.

The stage of disorganization and despair is characterized by apathy, aimlessness, and feelings of hopelessness. It is difficult to establish plans or new goals. Symptoms of depression such as insomnia, loss of appetite, and energy are common. If severe and persistent, the symptoms may require treatment with antidepressant medication.

Although there is rarely a clear ending to the process of grief, most individuals eventually reach a point of acceptance where they can begin to live life and experience pleasure again. Nevertheless, anniversaries, birthdays, and holidays often precipitate exacerbations of grief feelings.

Many people need support and assistance during the process of grieving. This support most often comes from relatives and friends but health professionals and clergy can also be of assistance. At times it is helpful to simply spend time with the individual: listening, accepting, reassuring, and gently encouraging. It is considered to be important for the bereaved to go through the pain of grief and to express all their feelings about the deceased, a process referred to as "grief work." For some, widow's or widower's support groups are invaluable.

Grief can become complicated and atypical when, for example, the person withdraws totally, feels excessively guilty or angry, experiences severe anxiety or panic attacks, or shows no signs of grief whatsoever. In these cases a referral to a psychiatrist is advisable as it is important to rule out an underlying major depression or other psychiatric illness.

Mania (Bipolar Affective Disorder)

The cardinal symptoms of mania are listed in **Table 3**. The person with mania is generally agitated, euphoric, or cantankerous and irritable, and is often awake much of the night.

A significant proportion of elderly patients, especially males, with late-onset bipolar affective disorder have evidence of an organic brain disorder or history of a neurological insult. A variety of medical illnesses and drugs are believed to precipitate secondary mania. These are listed in **Table 4**. It is probable that those who develop secondary mania have an underlying vulnerability to mood disorders. Sometimes individuals can display features of both depression and mania, termed a "mixed bipolar disorder."

Managing Residents with Mania

Residents with severe mania can be very difficult to manage in the nursing home setting. Less severe mania (hypomania) however is usually manageable without transfer. Treat-

Table 3 DSM-IV-TR Diagnosis of Manic Episode

A distinct period of abnormally and persistently elevated, expansive, or irritable mood lasting at least one week. During the period of mood disturbance, three (or more) of the following symptoms have persisted (four if the mood is only irritable) and have been present to a significant degree:

1. Inflated self-esteem or grandiosity
2. Decreased need for sleep, e.g., feels rested after only 3 hours of sleep.
3. More talkative than usual or pressure to keep talking
4. Flight of ideas or subjective experience that thoughts are racing
5. Distractibility, i.e., attention too easily drawn to unimportant or irrelevant external stimuli
6. Increase in goal-directed activity or psychomotor agitation
7. Excessive involvement in pleasurable activities that have high potential for painful results

Symptoms do not meet criteria for Mixed Episodes.
Mood disturbance is sufficiently severe to cause marked impairment in occupational functioning or in usual social activities or relationships with others, or to necessitate hospitalization to prevent harm to self or others, or there are psychotic features. Symptoms are not due to the direct effects of a substance (e.g., drugs of abuse or medication) or a general medical condition.

Adapted from DSM-IV-TR, American Psychiatric Association, 2000.

ment generally involves lithium carbonate, valproic acid, or carbamazepine, in combination with an atypical antipsychotic for treatment of agitation and insomnia. The elderly appear to require lower levels of lithium to control their affective illness. Lithium levels of 0.4 to 0.8 mEq/l will generally be sufficient but treatment must be individualized. Lithium levels should be monitored carefully as the elderly are much more susceptible to lithium toxicity and it appears that some elderly patients can develop toxicity at relatively low levels, e.g., 1.0 mEq/l. The cognitively impaired elderly are especially vulnerable to developing neurotoxicity. Valproic acid or carbamazepine may be used instead of lithium if the patient is unable to tolerate lithium or if lithium proves to be ineffective. Long-term treatment of bipolar disorder includes mood stabilizers and/or atypical antipsychotics.

Although pharmacological approaches are most critical in the care of the bipolar resident, psychosocial interventions are also important. During a

Table 4 Medical Illnesses and Medications Associated with Mania

Medical illnesses
- CNS stroke/cerebral neoplasms (esp. right hemisphere)
- Multiple sclerosis
- Encephalitis
- Syphilis
- Head injury
- Hyperthyroidism
- Uremia
- Hemodialysis

Medications
- Corticosteroids
- Thyroxin
- Levodopa
- Bromocriptine
- Sympathomimetics
- Amphetamines
- Cimetidine

manic or hypomanic episode setting limits regarding inappropriate behaviors and trying to reduce excessive environmental stimulation are necessary. Many individuals with bipolar disorder are ambivalent about taking mood stabilizers and tend to reduce or stop the medication, claiming that they feel better without pills. Psychotherapy, especially during periods of stability, can help to enhance the therapeutic alliance, which in turn may help to increase compliance with medication. Family counseling and education regarding the illness is also important.

Anxiety Disorders

How Common are Anxiety Disorders in the Elderly?

The Epidemiological Catchment area (ECA) study reported a 5.5% prevalence rate of all anxiety disorders in individuals over age 65, 3.6% for men and 6.8% for women [11]. The most common form of anxiety was phobic disorder (4.8%). A review of random-sample community surveys concluded that generalized anxiety disorder and phobias account for most anxiety in late life [13]. A study of elderly residents of nursing homes and congregate housing found that the prevalence of generalized anxiety or panic disorder was 3.5% [12]. Another 13.2% reported symptoms of anxiety, which were not sufficient to qualify for a specific diagnosis.

Table 5 DSM-IV-TR Criteria for Generalized Anxiety Disorder

Excessive anxiety and worry about a number of events or activities, occurring more days than not for at least 6 months. The person finds it difficult to control the worry.

The anxiety and worry are associated with 3 or more of the following 6 symptoms:

1. Restlessness or feeling keyed up or on edge
2. Being easily fatigued
3. Difficulty concentrating or mind going blank
4. Irritability
5. Muscle tension
6. Sleep disturbance

The focus of the anxiety and worry is not confined to features of another Axis I mental disorder
Clinically significant distress or impairment of functioning
Not due to a medication, drug, or medical condition and does not occur exclusively during a mood or psychotic disorder

Adapted from DSM-IV-TR, American Psychiatric Association, 2000.

Clinical Presentation of Anxiety Disorders

Anxiety disorders include generalized anxiety disorder (GAD), panic disorder, social phobia, specific phobia, obsessive compulsive disorder, post-traumatic stress disorder, and anxiety disorder due to a generalized medical condition. GAD is characterized by excessive worry, often about insignificant matters. The anxiety and worry are excessively intense and out of proportion to circumstances. The DSM-IV-TR criteria for GAD are listed in **Table 5**. Many individuals with GAD also experience somatic symptoms, which may include dry mouth, sweating, diarrhea, urinary frequency, headaches, dizziness, palpitations, tremor, and a subjective sense of shortness of breath.

It is not unusual for substance disorders, such as alcohol abuse or dependence, benzodiazepine abuse or dependence, and nicotine dependence to accompany GAD. Symptoms of anxiety and anxiety disorders often coexist with other psychiatric disorders, for example depressive disorders. Medical conditions and medications which may precipitate an anxiety disorder are listed in **Table 6**.

Panic disorder is characterized by recurrent, unexpected panic attacks. DSM-IV-TR criteria for a panic attack are listed in **Table 7**. These attacks are accompanied by one month or more of persistent concern about having additional panic attacks, worries about the seriousness of the attacks, or significant behavioral changes related to the attacks. Some individuals are plagued by anticipatory anxiety based on a concern or dread about the development of further attacks. Because the panic attacks may be associated with particular situations, avoidance of those situations is common. Patients can become phobic and avoid crowds as well as situations from

Table 6 Medical Illness and Medications Associated with Anxiety

Cardiovascular disorders
- Congestive heart failure
- Arrhythmias
- Myocardial infarction/angina
- Mitral valve prolapse
- Syncope

Respiratory disorders
- Chronic obstructive pulmonary disease
- Hypoxia
- Pulmonary embolus
- Asthma
- Pulmonary edema

Endocrine disorders
- Hyperthyroidism/hypothyroidism
- Cushing's disease
- Hypoglycemia
- Hypocalcemia/hypercalcemia
- Pheochromocytoma
- Carcinoid syndrome
- Insulinoma

Neurologic disorders
- CNS infections
- Parkinson's disease
- Focal seizures
- Postconcussion syndrome
- Multiple sclerosis

Drugs
- Anticholinergic toxicity
- Digitalis toxicity
- Excessive thyroid supplementation
- Stimulants
  - Amphetamines
  - Methylphenidate
  - Caffeine
- Sympathomimetics
  - Decongestants
  - Bronchodilators
- Antidepressants

Other
- Neuroleptic-induced akathisia
- Withdrawal
  - Alcohol
  - Sedative-hypnotics
- Chronic pain syndromes

Table 7 DSM-IV-TR Criteria for a Panic Attack

A discrete period of intense fear or discomfort, in which four (or more) of the following symptoms developed abruptly and reached a peak within 10 minutes.

1. Palpitations, pounding heart, or accelerated heart rate
2. Sweating
3. Trembling or shaking
4. Sensations of shortness of breath or smothering
5. Feeling of choking
6. Chest pain or discomfort
7. Nausea or abdominal distress
8. Feeling dizzy, unsteady, lightheaded, or faint
9. Derealization (feelings of unreality) or depersonalization (being detached from oneself)
10. Fear of losing control or going crazy
11. Fear of dying
12. Paresthesias (numbness or tingling sensations)
13. Chills or hot flushes

Adapted from DSM-IV-TR, American Psychiatric Association, 2000.

which they feel it is difficult to escape. This is called agoraphobia and often severely restricts the activities of the person. Such individuals may become housebound and need companions in order to perform everyday activities. Many elderly individuals who develop agoraphobia do not have a history of panic attacks. The onset is often precipitated by a traumatic event.

A phobia is defined as an excessive or persistent fear of a specific situation or of a clearly identifiable object, that is out of proportion to the inherent danger. This fear cannot be explained or reasoned away. Phobic individuals have no voluntary control over their fear and tend to avoid the feared situation or object in order to control the fear. Individuals with social phobia are fearful of interactions with other people or performance situations, such as public speaking. They fear that they might act in ways that will be embarrassing or humiliating. Other specific phobias include certain animals or insects, heights, storms, medical procedures, and being in specific situations, such as elevators, airplanes, bridges, and tunnels. A common phobia in the elderly is a fear of falling which often develops in individuals who have had a traumatic injury caused by a previous fall.

Obsessive compulsive disorder (OCD) is an anxiety disorder in which the manifestations are either obsessions and/or compulsions which cause significant distress or dysfunction. Obsessions are thoughts which are defined as recurrent, persistent ideas, images, or impulses that are experienced as intrusive and inappropriate and that cause marked anxiety or distress. Compulsions are behaviors or mental acts that are repetitive, purposeful and intentional, and performed in response to an obsession or to prevent a more dreaded event or situation. The thoughts or behaviors that cause distress are resisted, at least initially, and are recognized as senseless. Anxiety is a central feature of OCD and the repetitive behaviors or mental acts are often an attempt to counteract the distress associated with obsessions. The most common compulsions involve washing and cleaning, counting, checking, and requesting or demanding assurances.

In post-traumatic stress disorder (PTSD), the individual has been exposed to an event which involves death, serious injury or threat to the physical integrity of the self or others and which evokes a response of intense fear, helplessness or horror. Typical events include military combat, concentration camp experience, violent assault, or automobile accidents. The response consists of persistent reexperiencing of the event, persistent avoidance of associated stimuli, and persistent symptoms of increased arousal. The reexperiencing may include intrusive recollection of the event, dreams, flashbacks, and intense distress with exposure to reminders of the event. Thoughts, feelings, or other reminders of the event may be avoided and accompanied by partial amnesia, withdrawal, and restriction of emotions. Symptoms of increased arousal may include irritability, sleep disturbance, poor concentration, hypervigilance, and an exaggerated startle response. PTSD can be categorized as either acute, chronic, or delayed. Associated features of PTSD may include survivor guilt, self-destructive or impulsive behavior, dissociative symptoms, somatic distress, decreased ability to regulate and tolerate feelings, and social withdrawal.

It is not unusual for individuals to have short-lived episodes of anxiety related to a specific life event. If the anxiety does not meet criteria for an anxiety disorder, then an adjustment disorder can be diagnosed. A typical example would be the development of anxiety following admission to a nursing home. Residents with dementia may become acutely anxious and agitated in stressful situations – sometimes termed a "catastrophic reaction."

Managing Residents with Anxiety Disorders

The first step is to consider the differential diagnosis of the anxiety symptoms and make a specific psychiatric diagnosis when appropriate. It is important to eliminate or modify any medications which may be causing or exacerbating the anxiety. It is also important to eliminate or minimize the use of any substances which are anxiogenic, such as caffeine. The clinician should treat any concurrent psychiatric disorder such as major depression and any underlying associated medical disorders.

Depending on the type of anxiety disorder, various pharmacological treatments may be indicated. It is preferable, however, to attempt nonpharmacological approaches first. These may include psychotherapy or behavior therapy. Behavior therapy may include relaxation techniques such as progressive relaxation or systematic desensitization. Desensitization is particularly helpful for the treatment of phobias and consists of gradually exposing the patient to a series of stimuli whereby each successive stimulation is closer to the object of the phobia. As the individual tolerates increased intensity of the exposure, the anxieties gradually diminish. Exposure therapy is the treatment of choice for agoraphobia without panic.

The use of benzodiazepines, preferably on a short-term basis, may be helpful (see Chapter 11). Antidepressants (e.g., SSRIs) are often effective in the treatment of GAD, panic disorders, PTSD, and OCD. Although considerable concern is often raised regarding the use of benzodiazepines, they can also be helpful for some individuals with chronic anxiety and some individuals appear to benefit from low dose benzodiazepines without developing tolerance. Finally, buspirone, which is a nonbenzodiazepine anti-anxiety agent, may be of some benefit, although it has not been well studied in the elderly with anxiety disorders.

Case Illustration: Masked Depression, Responsive to Treatment

Mrs. A, an 82-year-old retired school teacher, began to deteriorate shortly after admission. She had been a widow for 8 years, and had one daughter. She withdrew from social contacts and described severe headaches, constipation, and pain in her abdomen. A full medical workup was negative. She completely denied any feelings of depression, saying that she "wasn't crazy," and found it difficult to describe any emotions. She was, however, distressed and felt that she should be left alone to die. Her appetite was decreased and she had lost 8 pounds over a two-month period. Her sleep was broken and restless. She was able to give a clear account of her life and had evidently always been a fiercely independent woman who hated to rely on others. She confided that she had never wanted to go into a nursing home, but that she could no longer manage at home and refused to be a burden to her daughter. She nevertheless complained that her daughter was only visiting twice a week.

The difficulty in assessing Mrs. A, was determining whether her symptoms represented an adjustment disorder with depressed mood or a major depression. She was started on an antidepressant, citalopram, with the dose increasing to 20 mg per day, and was seen for a half hour of supportive psychotherapy each week. After approximately 15 days of treatment, she noted that her headaches had diminished. She was feeling less worried and was surprised that her appetite was picking up. She gradually began to talk to some of the other residents and noted that her sleep was improving. She started to attend the exercise group and the arts and crafts programs. Within a month her daughter felt that her mother was back to her usual self.

Comment

Can patients who deny being depressed actually suffer from a depressive illness? Elderly patients often are reluctant to admit to psychological or emotional distress, considering this to be a stigma and a sign of weakness. As a result, "masked depression" whose primary presenting symptom is physical pain, is relatively common in elderly patients. It is extremely important, therefore, for staff to be vigilant to the possibility of an underlying depressive illness.

Case Illustration: Depression, Paranoid Delusions, and Dementia

Mr. L., a 90-year-old widower, was admitted to a home for the aged following his second wife's death. He had always been an active, social man who now thought that the home would give him the opportunity to continue his social activities. He had no children from his first marriage, but had become extremely close to his stepsons. Some time before this, Mr. L. learned that one of his stepsons was in hospital following a stroke. His status and prognosis was unclear at that time. Mr. L. responded to the news by becoming increasingly agitated and seeking staff out incessantly with many somatic complaints. He was eating poorly, lost 2 kilograms within a week, and had difficulty falling asleep. In time, he began expressing fears that his food was being poisoned by certain staff members who had joined together in a plot to kill him. Antidepressants and antipsychotic medication were not effective in reducing the psychotic symptoms. He was then transferred to an inpatient psychiatric unit and he ultimately required of course of nine ECT treatments. He recovered significantly from the psychotic symptoms and returned to the home.

Mr. L, however, never completely regained his previous level of independence and remained fearful, requiring direction and reassurance that staff would always be available to him. Despite his fear of falling, he did go to the main dining room or would sit for brief periods in the lobby, a pastime he had previously enjoyed. Within three months, the staff noticed that he was becoming more agitated and refusing to go off the floor, except with his stepson who had recovered by this time. His delusions of being plotted against resurfaced. Medications were used unsuccessfully in an attempt to decrease the agitation, delusions, and depressive symptoms of sleeplessness and weight loss. He began to voice feelings of helplessness and hopelessness in the face of the onslaught of his "attackers." He became suicidal wanting to kill himself but unable to think of means to accomplish this. Another inpatient admission was arranged. As his delusions now encompassed the hospital staff so that he refused to agree to the admission, it became necessary to certify him.

He was beginning to show signs of memory loss, and word-finding difficulties which contributed to his sense of suspiciousness. The inpatient staff, after much deliberation, felt that Mr. L.'s depressive episodes were a response to his chronic delusions and increasing dementia. Mr. L. now saw the whole world as threatening and malevolent. His medications when carefully titrated, were effective in decreasing some of the agitation associated with the delusions.

After Mr. L. returned to the nursing home, staff witnessed his increasing dependence, continued fear of being poisoned, and increasing memory loss. The agitation decreased further as he became more debilitated but the delusions remained fixed. The staff, who once considered themselves to be his friends, had to contend with his repeated accusations of poisoning and "torturing." They were able to understand his illness, however, and continued to give him ongoing supportive care.

Comment

Why were Mr. L.'s symptoms so persistent? In addition to depression, Mr. L also had paranoid delusions and dementia. His deteriorating cognitive state compounded the other problems and, because of a low tolerance to antipsychotic medications, it was not possible to use an adequate dosage. In addition, persistent paranoid symptoms are notoriously difficult to treat. It is difficult for staff to accept that there are some individuals with psychiatric problems whose symptoms are essentially incurable. In spite of this, the care and support offered to Mr. L was crucial and did make his difficult existence somewhat more tolerable. Techniques such as reassurance, frequent interactions, and a gentle, nonconfrontational approach are often effective in decreasing fear and promoting trust.

Case Illustration: Chronic Depression and Somatization

Mrs. B., an 80-year-old divorced woman, was admitted to a nursing home when she could no longer manage on her own effectively. Although she was only mildly cognitively impaired, she had several physical ailments including heart disease, numerous past surgical procedures, arthritis, and mild diabetes. She was placed on a minimal care floor since she was capable of doing most of her care herself.

Mrs. B. described herself as having been an outgoing and happy person. She was proud of her roles as hairdresser to "the Queen of Rumania." She fell in love at the age of 21 and married her "one true love." Five years later her life was shattered with the onset of the World War II. Her husband was taken away and subsequently died, her daughter was "shot in (her) arms," and she was in prison camps for close to 5 years. During this time, she described horrific conditions and experiences including experiments without anesthesia, beatings, and deaths of friends and family. She managed to survive, met her second husband, and settled in Israel. She subsequently gave birth to two children who both died of TB. Unable to cope, she and her husband emigrated to Canada. After several years she discovered that her husband was having an affair. She left him and lived on her own until admission to the nursing home.

Not long after her admission, staff became aware of her excessive demands and reacted to her imperious attitude toward them. Interviews revealed chronic depression related to her past experiences and grief over the many losses she had faced. She tended to focus on somatic concerns, describing in detail her various maladies, pains, and sleeplessness. An antidepressant was started at night in order to ameliorate her sleeping difficulties and improve her mood. A nurse-clinical specialist saw her on a weekly basis for the next 3 years. Staff meetings were held weekly for 6 weeks for the nurses to examine the reasons for her behavior and to facilitate care planning. A strong supportive component was necessary throughout the sessions since her unabating demands, attitude of entitlement, and derogatory personal comments tried the patience of staff working with her.

Over time, the staff realized that Mrs. B.'s demands represented her "need to be treated as a somebody." The somatic complaints were her way of communicating psychic pain. Her treatment became a delicate balance between investigating her complaints, treating her symptoms when indicated, and reassuring her when no changes to her mental status were apparent. She tended to interpret decreased interventions as a lack of caring and would hurl intense accusations at medical and nursing staff that they were not "doing anything," until they relented. The myriad of medications, tests and surgeries she had undergone in the past were a testimony to her strength and ability to get what she perceived she needed. Dilemmas arose frequently over whether a new or intensified symptom warranted further investigation. The staff became attuned to her and were able to discern minute changes in behavior which were often correlated with actual changes in her physical status.

As the staff grew to know and understand Mrs. B, they were less likely to take her suspicious accusations personally and they used humor as a method of interacting with her. Her time was more structured and her routines became more predictable. Although her moods and corresponding demands fluctuated, she was finally able to form attachments, go on outings, and participate in programs. At times she was able to describe her accomplishments with a sense of self-worth. When she died 7 years after admission, staff were able to discuss the pride they felt in caring for this warm but difficult woman.

Comment

How can Mrs. B's difficulties be explained? Mrs. B had a history of numerous psychic traumas and losses. It was difficult to fully comprehend the psychological effects of these events. At times Mrs. B seemed to exaggerate her symptoms and even embellish her history, which staff found difficult to understand. Because of deprivation during her life, she used physical symptoms as a way of gratifying her dependency needs. Her more rewarding relationships were ultimately with health care professionals. As the staff grew to understand Mrs. B, their tolerance of her behavior increased and they were able to provide her with the care she desired.

Case Illustration: Depression and Cancer

Mr. A., a 78-year-old married man, decided to live in the same nursing home as his wife, an Alzheimer's victim, and moved in several months following her institutionalization. He was a warm, quiet man who generally kept to himself and would rarely venture off the floor except for meals and short visits with his wife. About a year after his admission, staff became concerned about his lack of motivation, increased isolation, sudden weight loss, and tearfulness. The psychiatric team was called in to assess the possibility of an acute depression. An interview revealed a tall emaciated-looking man who was able to engage quickly and openly. He described past episodes of depressive and psychotic-like symptoms in his earlier years, which had been treated effectively with perphenazine 4 mg per day. He had been on this medication for many years and had refused to have it discontinued. He was tearful when describing his experience of having a wife who was dementing. He reported a decrease in appetite, energy, and sleep, poor concentration and pains in the upper left abdominal quadrant. The psychiatric team recommended investigation of his pain, and sertraline 25 mg daily. A nurse-clinician began weekly supportive psychotherapy sessions aimed at helping him cope with his current life situation.

A week later, Mr. A. described a "miraculous cure" after taking the sertraline. He stated that his sleep, appetite, and mood had improved significantly. The miracle was short-lived, however, and by the next week he began to apologize, saying "I know you and the doctor are trying to help me but I don't think the pill is working." The dosage of the antidepressant was increased. In the meantime, investigations of the left-sided pain proved negative. Since Mr. A. continued to lose strength and weight and was not responding well to antidepressants, he was transferred to a psychiatry inpatient unit. Despite pharmacotherapy, milieu therapy, and interactional therapy, he became increasingly focused on the pain. He was adamant that there was something physically wrong and that his depression was related to the pain he was experiencing.

Teasing out organic pain from psychic pain was difficult. Mr. A.'s lack of progress and the nagging possibility of a malignancy prompted reinvestigation. This time, CT scan of the abdomen revealed a pancreatic tumor. Mr. A, his family, and the staff experienced mixed emotions as a result of the diagnosis – sadness at the prognosis but relief that there was a physical reason for the pain and depression. Mr. A. was more at peace now that at last his pain was "heard" and knowing there would be a response to relieve this suffering.

Comment

When should it be suspected that "somatic" symptoms are due to physical illness? The term "somatic" should be used with caution as it can lull us into a false sense that we can "explain away" certain physical complaints. Physical causes should always be ruled out. However, practical problems include the cost and risks associated with over-investigation and the fact that some diseases such as carcinoma can be difficult to identify in the early stages. It is important to remember that physical illnesses often present initially with emotional symptoms.

Case Illustration: Bipolar Affective Disorder, Dementia

Mrs. C. was an 89-year-old woman with a 52-year history of mood disorder. She had had several psychiatric admissions in the past requiring treatment with ECT for depression. Over the 4 years prior to admission, she had become increasingly cognitively impaired and had been diagnosed as having Alzheimer's disease. At the time of her admission to the nursing home, she scored 13/30 on the Folstein Mini-Mental State Exam (MMSE). She continued to have frequent episodes of mood change. Although she was significantly demented, the character of these mood shifts was clearly that of a bipolar disorder. When she was manic she was irritable and abusive towards nursing staff particularly during the night. She would perseverate on themes related to sex and money and insisted on telling all visitors to the unit that she had absolutely no interest in sex. She was managed with lithium levels ranging from 0.4 to 0.6 mEq/l. On one occasion her lithium level increased to a level of 0.9 mEq/l and she became quite withdrawn and delirious. A lowering of her level resulted in a reduction of her confusion.

Comment

What approaches should be taken in the management of the manic patient? Pharmacological management is critical and it is particularly important to ensure that the resident receives enough medication to promote adequate sleep. The patient with mania is easily over-stimulated and it is important, therefore, to try to reduce excessive sensory stimulation. Some behaviors may be quite bizarre. For example, one nursing home resident would, when manic, empty all of the local newspaper boxes and deliver "free" newspapers to the residents in the institution. In general, a clear setting of limits is necessary to manage the disruptive behaviors of the manic resident. This may require the involvement of the nursing home administrator. Although generally not a major issue in the nursing home setting, it should be noted that residents with mania often have poor judgment and may be incompetent to manage their own financial affairs. Once the acute manic episode has been brought under control it is important to monitor the lithium levels closely and to find an optimal level for the individual resident.

References

1. The American Psychiatric Association (2000). Diagnostic and Statistical Manual of Mental Disorders (4th Ed. – Text Revision). Washington, DC: The American Psychiatric Association.
2. Canadian Coalition for Seniors' Mental Health (CCSMH). (2006). National Guidelines for Seniors' Mental Health: The Assessment and Treatment of Mental Health Issues in LTC Homes. Toronto: CCSMH. Available at www.ccsmh.ca
3. Yesavage, J.A., Brink, T.L., Rose, T.L., Lum, O., Huang, V., Adey, M., Leirer, V.O. (1983). Development and validation of a geriatric depression screening scale: A preliminary report. Journal of Psychiatric Research, 17(1):37–49.
4. Alexopoulos, G.S., Abrams, R.C., Young, R.C., Shamoian, C.A. (1988). Use of the Cornell scale in nondemented patients. Journal of the American Geriatric Society, 36(3):230–236.
5. Radloff, L.S. (1977). The CES-D scale: A self-report depression scale for research in the general population. Applied Psychological Measurement, 1:385–401.
6. Katz, I.R., Lesher, E., Kleban, M., Jethanandani, V., Parmelee, P. (1989). Clinical features of depression in the nursing home. International Psychogeriatrics, 1:5–15.
7. Ames, D. (1991). Epidemiological studies of depression among the elderly in residential and nursing homes. International Journal of Geriatric Psychiatry, 6:347–354.
8. Sadavoy, J., Smith, I., Conn, D.K., Richards, B. (1990). Depression in geriatric patients with chronic medical illness. International Journal of Geriatric Psychiatry, 5:187–192.
9. Erikson, E.H. (1959). Identity and the life-cycle. Psychological Issues, Monograph 1. New York: International Universities Press.
10. Parkes, C.M. (1972). Bereavement. New York: International Universities Press.
11. Reiger, D.A., Boyd, J.H., Burke, J.D., et al. (1988). One-month prevalence of mental disorders in the United States. Archives of General Psychiatry, 45:977–986.
12. Parmelee, P.A., Katz, I.R., Lawton, M.P. (1993). Anxiety and its association with depression among institutionalized elderly. American Journal of Geriatric Psychiatry, 1:46–58.
13. Flint, A.J. (1994). Epidemiology and comorbidity of anxiety disorders in the elderly. American Journal of Psychiatry, 151:640–649.

Suggested Readings

1. Rubinstein, R.L., Lawton, M.P. (Eds.). (1997). Depression in long term and residential care: Advances in research and treatment. New York: Springer Verlag.
An excellent multiauthored text focusing exclusively on depression in the long-term care setting.
2. Schneider, L.S., Reynolds, C. F., Lebowitz, B.D., Friedhoff, A.J. (1994). Diagnosis and treatment of depression in late life: Results of the NIH consensus development conference. Washington, DC: American Psychiatric Press.
Very useful multiauthored text focusing on depression in the elderly. Well referenced.
3. Canadian Coalition for Seniors' Mental Health (CCSMH). (2006). National Guidelines for Seniors' Mental Health: The Assessment and Treatment of Mental Health Issues in LTC Homes. Toronto: CCSMH. Available at www.ccsmh.ca
4. American Geriatrics Society, American Association for Geriatric Psychiatry (AGS/AAGP). (2003). Consensus statement of improving the quality of mental health care in U.S. nursing homes: Management of depression and behavioral symptoms associated with dementia. Journal of the American Geriatrics Society, 51(9):1287–1298.
5. American Medical Directors Association (AMDA). (2003). Depression: Clinical practice guidelines. Columbia, MD: AMDA.

Depression – Family Information Sheet*

What Is Clinical Depression? Depression is an illness, not just a feeling of sadness or being "down in the dumps." When depression is severe and persistent enough to require treatment, it is called "clinical" or "major" depression. Depression affects feelings, thoughts, physical health, and behavior. A person suffering from a major depressive episode reports at least 5 symptoms which are present almost every day for a minimum of two weeks. These include: (1) loss of interest in things that are usually enjoyed (2) feeling sad, blue, or down in the dumps (3) feeling slowed down or restless and unable to sit still (4) feeling worthless or guilty (5) increased or decreased appetite or weight (6) thoughts of death or suicide (7) problems concentrating, thinking, remembering, or making decisions (8) trouble sleeping or sleeping too much and (9) loss of energy or feeling tired all of the time. Other symptoms sometimes include being anxious or worried, feeling pessimistic or hopeless, having headaches or other pain, digestive problems, and decreased interest in sex. The term dysthymia is used to describe a long-term, usually less severe form of depression present for at least two years.

What Is the Cause of Depression? Depression rarely has a single cause and often develops as a result of a combination of physical changes in the brain or body, internal psychological changes, and changes in the person's environment or social situation. Certain life situations, such as extraordinary stress or grief in response to a loss, may bring on a depression. Some individuals have a chemical imbalance in their brain which makes them susceptible to depression. A family history of depression and genetic factors may also contribute. Depression can also develop when a person has another medical or psychiatric illness, is taking certain medications or over uses drugs or alcohol. People who are persistently unhappy with their life situation or disappointed with relationships sometimes become clinically depressed.

How Is a Diagnosis of Depression Made? The diagnosis is made clinically, meaning that it is based on a history and examination. We do not have a blood test or brain scan for depression. We must always rule out the possibility of an underlying undiagnosed medical illness and other psychiatric conditions which might be contributing to the problem. Family members can often help a great deal by providing extra details regarding the history of such illnesses.

What Kinds of Treatment Are Available for Depression? The most effective treatment usually involves a combination of medication and psychotherapy. The most commonly used antidepressants are called selective serotonin reuptake inhibitors (SSRIs), although other kinds are sometimes prescribed. (Ask for the family information sheet on antidepressants.) There are also different types of psychotherapy, such as cognitive behavioral therapy which focuses on helping the person deal with excessive negative thinking, supportive psychotherapy, and interpersonal psychotherapy where the primary focus is on improving relationships.

* From *Practical Psychiatry in the Long-Term Care Home: A Handbook for Staff* (D.K. Conn et al., Eds.). ISBN 978-0-88937-341-9. © 2007 Hogrefe & Huber Publishers.

How Can Family Members Help? (1) Sometimes family members can provide valuable information with regard to a relative's recent or previous history. (2) Spending time with your loved one, offering encouragement, support and on occasion humor is very important. Realize though, that depression is an illness and recovery is more complicated than just "pulling up your socks," or trying harder. (3) If your relative ever tells you that he or she has lost the will to go on living or wants to die, it is important to inform the staff. (4) If your relative is reluctant to take the prescribed medication, it is most important that you encourage him or her to take the pills regularly.

For more information there are several excellent Web sites such as The National Institute of Mental Health (http://www.nimh.nih.gov/) and Dr. Ivan Goldberg's Depression Central (http://www.psycom.net/depression.central.html).

6 The Suicidal Resident

David K. Conn and Alanna Kaye

Key Points

- Team members should be vigilant with regard to the potential occurrence of suicidal behaviors.
- Where the potential for suicide is considered to be high, active interventions should be made to minimize the risk and identify and treat any associated psychiatric illness.
- It should be recognized that it is not possible to eliminate all self-destructive behaviors, and that not all suicides are preventable.
- There is increasing awareness of the possibility of "rational" suicide and of the possibility that in some situations, especially in terminal illness or chronic illness with very poor quality of life, decisions by competent patients to refuse treatment or nutrition may have to be respected. Ruling out depression in these instances is a therapeutic priority.

"The thought of suicide is a great consolation:
by means of it one gets successfully through many a bad night."
F. Nietzsche

This chapter will focus on the assessment and management of the suicidal resident. The term suicide is generally used to refer to the act of taking one's own life deliberately and intentionally. Self-destructive behavior is a very complex phenomenon, however, and several distinctions must be made:

- A completed suicide refers to a death resulting from deliberately self-inflicted causes.
- A suicide attempt refers to self-inflicted injury that does not result in death. Because in many suicide attempts there is no intention to cause death, but rather a desire to communicate to others feelings such as despair or anger, the term self-harm is preferred by many over the term suicide attempt.

Suicidal behavior may manifest itself as an acute violent act, but frequently more chronic and passive forms are seen. Reckless behavior, refusal to adhere to prescribed diets and medications or to continue life-sustaining treatments such as dialysis are examples of less active forms of self-destructive behavior. We will initially review active suicidal behavior and conclude with a discussion of more chronic passive suicidal behavior which is not infrequent in the long-term care setting.

Suicidal Behavior in the Elderly

The elderly have the highest completed suicide rates of any age group. For example, in the United States this group comprises approximately 13% of the population and accounts for 20% of all reported suicides. Moreover, suicide may be under-reported in the elderly, as the cause of death can be attributed to medical illness more easily than in the young. The high suicide rate in the elderly is predominantly due to extremely high rates among white elderly males. Despite the high rate of completed suicide, suicide attempts occur less often than in the younger population. This points to the fact that suicidal acts among the elderly are more likely to be lethal.

The Long-Term Setting

The rate of suicide in nursing homes and other long-term care facilities has not been well investigated. A 2-year study of all completed suicides in Los Angeles county by Litman and Farberow did not reveal the rate of suicide in institutions to be much higher than that in the community [1]. Out of a total of over 2,000 suicides 20 occurred in "nursing convalescent units." The mean age of these patients was 76 years. The primary medical diagnosis included diabetes, cardiac disorders, cancer, multiple sclerosis, and atherosclerosis. Nursing staff had noted severe depression in most of these suicidal patients and the majority of the patients had communicated something about their suicidal intention. Death was most likely to occur from the ingestion of pills that had been saved up or smuggled in or from self-inflicted lacerations. During the survey some informants raised the philosophical/ethical problem of why there should be any sanction against suicide in patients who were old, ill with incurable diseases, suffering from loneliness and abandonment, and conscious of being a drain on the resources of their families. It was noted that many of these patients had been chronically suicidal. Nevertheless, despite the fact that nearly all patients in such settings share to some extent the pattern of chronic illness and isolation, suicide was in fact quite rare. The authors suggested that the patients who committed suicide were characterized by a special inability to adjust to the nursing home environment. The little data that is available suggests that the rates of completed suicide in elderly long-term care residents are lower than their counterparts in the community. This may be related to the increased supervision and decreased access to potentially lethal means which is provided by a long-term care facility.

Theories of Suicidal Behavior

Sociocultural Theories

Durkheim's work, published in 1897, is still relevant today and suggests that the nature and extent of one's involvement in society is important in determining the vulnerability to suicide [2]. He used the term "egoistic suicide" to describe suicide in individuals who lacked a sense of belonging and were not well integrated into the society. These ideas clearly have relevance in the nursing home setting because many individuals feel abandoned by and removed from society when they are placed in an institution. This emphasizes the need to create a community atmosphere in the long-term care setting in order to counter the social withdrawal and isolation of residents.

Sociocultural theories also emphasize the importance of a rapidly changing society as a result of technological advances, urbanization, and "Westernization." Durkheim referred to suicide resulting from crises in the collective societal order as "anomic suicide." Suicides rates tend to be highest in urban industrialized countries where a negative stereotypical view of the elderly ("ageism") is prevalent, and where youth, beauty, productivity, progress, speed, and independence are highly valued.

Psychological Theories

Suicide often follows an "acute suicidal crisis," characterized by a period of hopelessness. The suicidal act is at times regarded as a form of communication to another person (a cry for help, an act of aggression or both).

Freud viewed suicide as aggression turned against the self, rather than expressed externally toward a person with whom the victim has a close but ambivalent relationship [3]. It may be precipitated by loss and feelings of abandonment and rejection associated with the loss. Again, this is clearly relevant in the long-term care resident. Bibring and Seligman emphasize the role of helplessness [4, 5]. Feelings of helplessness are common in the elderly, especially the depressed elderly and result from the belief of individuals that they cannot control aspects of their lives.

Miller [6] notes that lying dormant within everyone is an extremely personal equation that determines the point at which the quality of one's life would be so poor that one would no longer wish to live. He termed this point the "line of unbearability" and we are not normally aware of it until we are actually confronted by an intolerable situation. At that time those who have the ability to maintain some hope will cry out for help, whereas those who are completely hopeless will attempt to kill themselves.

Biological Theories

Depression is very common but not universal in suicidal people. Depressed individuals typically perceive themselves as useless, worthless, and may have profound feelings of low self-esteem and self-hatred. Suicide may be seen as a preferred solution and an honorable way out. A number of studies have identified an underlying abnormality of neurotransmitter function in suicidal patients, which may be age-sensitive.

The Relationship Between Medical Illness and Suicide

A high percentage of patients who have committed suicide also have active medical illnesses. Disorders that have been found to have a high association with suicide include pulmonary disease associated with severe shortness of breath, rheumatoid arthritis, chronic renal failure being treated with dialysis, and peptic ulcer. In patients with cancer or incurable diseases there are several critical periods particularly while the diagnosis and prognosis are still being determined and during the phase when the true nature of the condition becomes apparent.

Assessment

Identifying Suicidal Potential

One of the most valuable resources for determining suicide potential is the staff who work day to day with the resident. Their intuitive "knowledge" that something is wrong, in the experience of the authors, has proven to be an excellent guide to further assessment and management. Acting on staff's observations that a resident is "different" or causing "worry," a major depression and/or suicidal potential have often been discovered and managed. Without these perceptions of the staff, successful management would not be possible. Finally, since suicidal ideation may represent a response to psychosis or major depression, a complete assessment is indicated in order to identify any treatable psychiatric illness. Guidelines for the assessment of suicide risk and prevention of suicide in older adults were released in Canada in 2006 [7].

It is important for staff to document clearly all relevant information (see assessment checklist). Direct observations and quotes are particularly useful in determining suicide potential as there is less opportunity for misinterpretation of the data.

Detecting Whether a Resident Is Suicidal

It is not always clear when someone is contemplating suicide. In certain cases, if impulsive behavior or cognitive impairment is a factor, there may be no warning signs.

Behavioral, situational, or verbal cues may be encountered. Behavioral cues include putting affairs in order or giving away possessions, increasing isolation, and alcohol or drug abuse. Recent losses such as loss of health, independence, cognitive capacity, family or friends are situational factors that can precipitate suicide. Responses to these life crises vary with previous coping styles and abilities as well as with the degree of available support systems. Grief and mourning, especially when support systems are diminished, may contribute to the development of suicidal ideation.

Today's elderly belong to a generation that emphasized survival, rigid gender roles, and conformity. Little importance was attached to psychological awareness and the value of communication. Thus, the ability to recognize psychological distress and to communicate it verbally may be limited in this population. Spontaneous, direct expression of suicidal intent is less frequently encountered than are indirect veiled references. It is therefore crucial for staff working with the elderly to be aware of this factor during interactions. Phrases such as, "There's nothing left for me," "I can't take it anymore," or saying, "good-bye" to a staff person when "good-night" would be more appropriate, may convey an underlying message of desperation, isolation, and a feeling of being trapped. Directing conversation toward expression of these feelings promotes a sense of caring and trust. The assessment of suicidal ideation can then be facilitated.

When Residents Say They "Just Want to Die"

Are they suicidal? Not necessarily. It is important to distinguish between active and passive suicidal ideation. Active suicidal thoughts are present in individuals who discuss or demonstrate specific plans and intent to end their lives. Motivation to take control of their current situation is evident. For example, a mobile man who has decided that life is not worth living states, "I can't live this way any more. I'm going to stand in the road to get hit by a car." Clearly, there are plans, intent, motivation, and an ability to actually make an attempt.

The intent behind passive thoughts is more difficult to determine. During an interaction, the resident may say, "I want do die." When this statement is pursued more fully, the resident may voice active suicidal thoughts. Frequently, a true wish to die may exist, but moral or religious beliefs preclude active steps to accomplish this goal. Residents who appear to have "given up" may be among these individuals (see section on Chronic or Passive Suicide). Residents who reveal a wish to die may require a mechanism to express their feelings of despair, depression, hopelessness, or helplessness without any actual intent for self-harm.

Questioning Residents About Suicide

Does asking residents whether they are suicidal give them an idea or encourage them to think these thoughts? Although this is a common concern, asking directly about suicidal thoughts does not increase the risk of suicidal ideation or behavior. Generally, if an individual has decided definitively to commit suicide, he will attempt to do so despite any and all attempts to intervene. For some individuals, the opportunity to talk about the depth of their psychic pain may decrease the likelihood of an attempt. The act of asking these specific and sensitive questions conveys caring, acceptance and gives the individual permission to speak, all of which are essential to decreasing the sense of isolation and pain associated with suicidal thoughts.

Asking specific questions about suicidal thought or intent can be difficult and may produce anxiety in the caregiver during assessment. Phrases such as "Have you ever felt life was not worth living?" or "Have you been thinking about ending your life?" can soften the tone of discussion and convey acceptance of the topic, thereby opening the door to further exploration directed at issues such as: whether a plan of action has been considered; if so, what this might be; do they intend to follow through with their plan; when would this occur; do they feel there may be other options other than suicide to deal with their current situation?

Through these questions the level of suicide risk can be determined. For example, a vague, guarded response such as "Who knows?" or a question such as "Why are you asking me?" may indicate a higher risk than a direct answer. Verbalizing observations, e.g., "I notice this is a hard question for you to answer." can act as a catalyst for further discussion.

Invariably, our own thoughts, attitudes, and judgment about suicide play a part in the interview process. It is crucial, therefore, that the interviewer be aware of his/her own feelings in order to minimize the effect on the discussion. When someone expresses suicidal thoughts it raises a myriad of reactions within the listener that can include anger, fear, vulnerability, guilt, helplessness, and denial. These reactions may be reflected in the way interviewers phrase their questions. For example, discomfort with the issue is revealed in questions such as "Just a routine question, you're not thinking of suicide are you?" It is clear from this question that the interviewer wants the answer to be "No," could not tolerate an honest answer and is therefore, creating an unwitting block to an open discussion of suicidal thoughts. Confronting the issue in an accepting, honest and gentle manner creates a climate in which painful issues can be revealed and discussed.

Assessing Potential Risk

While all expressions of self-harm require active exploration and intervention, the likelihood of death by suicide may be somewhat lower in an institutional setting than in the community. As previously stated, this may be due to the presence of staff and the decreased access by residents to a means of inflicting self-harm. Nevertheless, attempts are sometimes made.

Predicting risk in individual remains difficult. There are, however, certain factors that have been associated statistically with a greater potential for suicide. These factors are listed in **Table 1** along with the behavioral cues already mentioned in previous sections.

The first part of the assessment checklist reflects the extent to which the resident has developed a plan. For example, if a bedbound resident states that he is planning on ending his life by going to the roof of the building and jumping off, there is less of a possibility of completion than if he had stated he was going to starve himself to death. Thus, careful attention must be directed toward exploring the details of the plan.

The second and third parts of the checklist identify the behaviors and life situations which contribute to the likelihood of suicide. Potential risk tends to increase with the intention to die, the specificity of the plan, availability of means, greater physical illness, resolving depression (which adds an energy to complete the act), and impulsivity either as a characterological trait or resulting from brain damage.

Management

Several principles guide the care of the suicidal resident. Safety, dignity, and promoting the trust within the relationship are primary considerations when determining a plan of care. Listed below are general guidelines for management.

On an immediate level, it is imperative for the staff to remove any potentially dangerous objects, i.e., medications, sharps, glass, ropes, belts. This is usually done by two staff members conducting a room search. Explanations to the resident regarding concerns for his/her safety must be provided to promote a sense of trust and to reduce the risk of the resident perceiving the search as punitive. If possible, permission and cooperation from the resident to perform the search should be obtained. Careful documentation in the chart of actions taken, the reason why, personnel present, and the whereabouts of the resident's property is mandatory for legal reasons.

Close observation of the resident is important. Individuals at high risk require constant observation, while lower-risk residents can be maintained on frequent checks (every 15 to 30 minutes). Realistically. this may not always to possible. Adequate staffing is rarely available with current constraints in budgets. Other options may include utilizing resources such as volunteers, family members, program workers. Rotating the nursing team to maintain frequent checks may be possible. This would require the staff to take turns staying with the resident for specified lengths of time throughout the shift. If family members can afford the cost of a sitter, this may be a short-term adjunct to professional observation. There are, however, pitfalls to this option. Once the crisis has passed, discontinuing a sitter may be problematic since residents can become very attached to the sitter and enjoy the one-to-one contact. The decision to obtain constant care must be made after carefully weighing the risks and benefits.

Table 1 Assessing Suicidal Behavior

I. Suicidal intent
- Verbalizes suicidal thoughts
- Describes suicidal intent
- Can outline a concrete realistic plan
- Methods are available
- Physical ability to carry out threat

II. Behavior
- Gives guarded answers to questions
- Diverts interviewer off topic
- Increasing withdrawal
- Depressed affect
- Resolving depression
- Sudden interest/disinterest in religion
- Gives away possessions
- Puts affairs in order
- Drug/alcohol abuse

III. Risk Factors
- Male
- White
- Low self-esteem
- Family history of suicide
- Support systems: decreased or none existent
- Decline in physical status
- Decline in cognitive status
- Impulsivity
- History of suicide attempts or violence
- Recent loss or change in life
- Substance abuse

Where the situation is acute, access to a psychiatrist and/or psychiatric nurse specialist may be helpful. Since current research suggests that psychiatric illness, generally major depressive disorder, are most commonly associated with the presence of suicidal ideation/intent, definitive assessment and treatment becomes necessary. There may also be circumstances which necessitate transfer of a resident to an acute care facility for psychiatric assessment and treatment. It is these authors' experience, however, that the majority of cases can be managed on their own units. Access by the long-term care facility to psychiatric services has proven to be beneficial to staff and residents, providing both support and assistance in diagnosis and management, while the residents are maintained in their own environment. Maintaining continuity of care is especially important since relocation of a frail and/or demented individual can produce catastrophic reactions, increase fear, and possibly worsen the risk of suicide.

Working with the residents to structure their day can help to build contact, self-esteem, and trust, as well as decrease the sense of isolation. Predictable, consistent routines provide a sense of stability and are reassuring to those whose inner life is chaotic. Setting aside a few minutes each day to talk with the resident about concerns and fears, as well as achievements, assists in providing some of this structure and promotes the rapport. Staff should try to foster hope and help residents to develop or regain a sense of meaning and purpose in life.

The degree of risk and a clear management plan should be determined and documented. The efficacy of the management plan must be evaluated in an ongoing manner and adjusted to accommodate the resident's changing needs.

Case Illustrations

The following case illustrations underscore a number of different factors that can contribute to suicide potential. It should be noted that in clinical practice and in our case histories these factors tend to overlap.

Case Illustration: Depression

Mr. W., a 72-year-old married man, was admitted to a long-term care facility one year after suffering a stroke. He had residual left-sided hemiparesis and contracture of his left hip. Although he had some cognitive deficits in the areas of memory, word-finding, and judgment, as well as problems with impulsivity, he was well able to communicate his thoughts verbally and understand staff's responses to him. Staff requested assistance for his extreme combativeness, especially during care or feeding.

Examination revealed a large man, curled up in bed, moving about restlessly and complaining of pain in his left hip. He was able to respond to questions about his life before the stroke. He had been a truck driver and spoke with great pride of "never (having) had an accident." In his spare time, he went to taverns with his friends or went up north with his wife in their trailer. He described himself as somewhat "wild" in his earlier years. He then spoke poignantly of how the stroke had affected him and the many losses with which he grappled. Mr. W. was, at times, aware of his aggressive behavior stating that he become impatient during care, at which time his awareness of his physical deficits and dependency on others was heightened. He described some decrease in appetite and difficulty falling asleep. He had little interest or enjoyment in anything. It was determined that Mr. W. was suffering from a major depression as a result of the stroke and his response to his many losses.

The management plan included investigation of his hip pain and an antidepressants (sertraline) to address the depression and agitation. Nursing measures included approaching him from his left side, and using two staff members to do his care. This lessened the chances of being hurt when he would strike out with his right arm. Adjusting the times of his a.m. care to later in the morning, when he was less agitated, proved to be beneficial in decreasing some of the aggression. Whenever possible, the assistance of male staff was enlisted as Mr. W. seemed to relate better to men. The anger and aggression began to decrease. Three months later, however, the aggression escalated again, but this time Mr. W. began talking about ending his life. He wrapped the telephone cord around his neck, attempted to drink a bottle of mouthwash and later tried to climb out through the bottom of his bed in order to "fall and break my head or my hip and die."

Comment

What kind of management would be appropriate? He was assessed by the psychiatrist, who increased the antidepressant and added a neuroleptic, risperidone, to decrease the intensity of agitation. Although Mr. W.'s statement of intent, his planning, and impulsivity placed him at a high level of risk, the chances of a completed suicide were lessened by his compromised mobility. Staff removed all objects from his room, used paper plates, plastic utensils, and remained with him while he ate. A system of frequent observations was instituted by rotating staff to check on his activities every half hour. Firm limit setting was adopted, as his insight and judgment were impaired. These external limits added structure and provided Mr. W. with realistic feedback on the impact of his behavior on others.

Although Mr. W.'s depression and behavioral difficulties improved, the possibility of further self-harm remained. Staff continued their efforts to offer support to Mr. W. but his cognitive deficits and the importance of mobility and independence to his self-esteem impeded his ability to work through, and accept his devastating losses. As a result, continued use of the antidepressant and neuroleptic remained an important part of his management.

Case Illustration: Dementia

Mr. A., an 80-year-old widower, was admitted to a nursing home as a result of declining physical health and difficulty managing at home. He had always been a deeply religious man who took great pleasure in teaching his students about the complexities of the Bible. His daughter reported to the staff that at one point prior to admission, her father had said he would kill himself if he ever had to live in a nursing home. The staff grew to like Mr. A.'s quiet, gentle ways with everyone around him.

Three months after admission staff were making early morning rounds and noticed that Mr. A.'s sheets were wet. Thinking that Mr. A. had been incontinent, staff began to change the sheets. To their horror, the sheet was not wet from urine, but blood from a stabwound next to the right carotid artery. They found a pair of small, steel surgical-type scissors among the sheets. Appropriate steps were taken to care for him through the night and a psychiatric consultation was requested. During the interview, it was apparent that Mr. A. was grossly cognitively impaired. Although unaware of his whereabouts, the day, the month, or the year, he was able to remember the stabbing but could not relate why is had occurred. Painfully slowed in his responses, he was able to relate his thoughts about aging via Bible stories and eventually was able to state that he had been incontinent of urine for the first time several days previ-

ously. Although Mr. A.'s primary diagnosis was dementia, a major depression could not be ruled out. An antidepressant was started in an attempt to elevate his mood and activate him.
Mr. A. did not make any subsequent suicide attempts. Despite treatment with antidepressants and the staff's provision of support and contact Mr. A. continued to withdraw as the dementia progressed. He died 5 months following the suicide attempt.

Comment

How can we understand Mr. A.'s suicide attempt? It is most likely that the insight into his increasing disabilities coupled with the decrease in impulse control resulting from his dementia precipitated Mr. A.'s suicide attempt. His profound shame may have had some effect in preventing any further attempts. The caregiving team met for several weeks to resolve their own feelings arising from this episode. The questions "Where there warning signs?" or "Was this preventable?" arose and professional guilt was addressed in these sessions. In a supportive atmosphere, the staff became more comfortable with the knowledge that, at times, there may be no warning preceding a suicide attempt.

Case Illustration: Personality Disorder

Mr. X., an 85-year-old widowed man, was admitted to a nursing home as a result of increasing debilitation secondary to Parkinson's disease. He was a man who had never formed close relationships but did marry and have one child. Both his wife and child were killed in concentration camps during the Holocaust. He had been interred in both German and Russian war camps and had attempted to hang himself during that period. A prominent editor of political newspapers, he had always been a very independent, strong-willed man who scorned emotional ties as a sign of weakness. He had a long history of alcoholism and occasional violence. He spoke of hunting the officer responsible for his wife's death and murdering him. He also admitted to three other suicide attempts. On one occasion he had evidently shot himself, narrowly missing his heart.
Despite taking pride in his intelligence, he had poor self-esteem. He frequently became angry and demeaning to the staff trying to care for him.
His frequent references to suicide, coupled with his history and continued alcohol consumption, led to psychiatric evaluation. Clinical depression was ruled out at this time but the risk of suicide was apparent as he would often threaten to walk out into the snow in order to freeze to death. He experienced life as a burden and was aware of his progressing Parkinsonism and failing cognitive abilities. Mr. X. had no family support or religious affiliation. He had always been fairly suspicious and guarded in nature but these feelings were greatly intensified by paranoia associated with his Parkinson's disease. The staff had become the objects of his paranoid delusions and he would frequently lash out at them with his cane when he became angry.
The management plan attempted to address his sense of isolation and impulsivity as well as the emotions of those caring for him. The psychiatric nurse clinician met with him individually several times per week. Low doses of olanzapine were used to attempt to control the impulsivity, with careful monitoring due to his Parkinson's disease. He would not stop drinking and found elaborate ways of obtaining alcohol

until staff began to dispense modest amounts at the nursing station. Volunteers were used to provide contacts and would engage him in chess games and political discussions. Threats of suicide occurred episodically but his explosiveness and paranoia continued to increase. He became unrelenting in his pursuit of one particular staff member, not unlike his hunt for the Nazi officer. Mr. X.'s accusatory, threatening manner evoked fear, hurt, and anger in the staff. The situation gradually escalated as staff and Mr. X. began to react to each other's intense emotions.

Comment

What issues were the staff struggling with? Staff meetings were held to provide support and explore the reasons for some of Mr. X.'s behavior. Staff reported a number of concerns, including a sense that this behavior was purposeful and the staff's bewilderment as to how they may have contributed to his wrath, discomfort with the chronic risk of suicide, the feelings of helplessness and inadequacy, and difficulties ensuring safety for Mr. X, other residents, and the staff, The length of time needed to resolve these issued speaks to the complexity of the case and the intensity of emotions aroused.

As the months passed, Mr. X. never attempted suicide but succumbed gradually to the effects of end-stage Parkinson's disease. Following Mr. X.'s transfer to another floor for medical reasons, staff were able to obtain some distance from their experience of caring for Mr. X. and ultimately to view their role with some measure of satisfaction. They had been able to provide as much care as humanly possible under extremely stressful conditions. The perseverance of the staff and their ability to provide some continuity in his life likely played a role in Mr. X. never having carried out his threat to end his life.

Case Illustration: Dependency

Mrs. B., an 83-year-old widow, had lived in a nursing home since the death of her husband several years previously. She had a history of episodes of depression which were treated with antidepressants. She had always been a very dependent woman, unable to tolerate being alone for any length of time. She frequently sought out the staff for reassurance that they liked and cared for her. Frequent weepy periods were precipitated by perceived insults and rejection by other residents. Although she had many friends in the community who visited her frequently, she often felt slighted and said that they did not include her often enough in their gatherings. Problems with room-mates were frequent as she found fault with everyone. On one occasion following a particularly vocal argument with a room-mate, she announced to the staff that she planned to kill herself and then became very guarded, refusing to answer when questioned about her plans. She simply stated she wanted to change room because she "couldn't live like this any more."

Comment

What did assessment reveal? Clear evidence of a major depressive disorder was not found during psychiatric evaluation. Her agitation and her lack of awareness of how her behavior was affecting staff were more prominent. She was, in many ways, attempting to gratify her needs in the only way she knew how

– to become helpless, weepy, and threaten self-harm. She was indeed very distressed and agitated over her current plight but settled with assurance that staff would help her. Suicide precautions were instituted. She refused, however, to remain on the floor for observation.

How could staff respond? Contact was increased through regularly scheduled interview times. She gradually became less agitated, weepy, and clingy as she began to realize that staff would respond to her distress. In turn, the staff began to understand her need to feel special and that this need might be met by providing her with a single room in addition to the increased support and structure. Once this move was accomplished, Mrs. B. settled and made no further threats to end her life. Crucial to this case was the staff's ability to look beyond the obvious demands. Staff's ability to tolerate her clinginess and address her need to feel wanted and special, allowed Mrs. B.'s relationships to evolve without anger and rejection.

Case Illustration: Terminal Illness

Mrs. D., a 74-year-old widow, was admitted to a palliative care unit with a diagnosis of metastatic cancer. Over the course of the first week, staff became aware of her apparent inability to "connect" with anyone. One day, staff overheard her ask her son to bring in her sleeping pills from home as she was having difficulty falling asleep. She was also noted to have alluded to the fact that she wanted to die. The next day another staff member saw bottles of medication in her purse. These incidents led to a psychiatric assessment regarding the question of suicide. During the initial interview, Mrs. D. spoke openly about these incidents, denying intent to attempt suicide and dismissing the team's concerns about her as "unnecessary." She gave an impression of politely complying with the interview in order to finish with us as soon as possible and graciously rejected any offers of support. She did, however, make a promise not to attempt to end her life. She was able to talk about how the cancer had "taken over" her life and what this meant to her. A fiercely independent woman, she could not easily accept anyone or anything having control over her. The implications of hospitalization were clearly troublesome to her. Having some control over when and how she would die seemed to be connected to her need for independence.

Comment

How did the team approach this dilemma? Despite assurances from her that she would not end her life, the unit team's discomfort remained very high. They had difficulty resolving the ethical issues of autonomy versus paternalism inherent in the act of removing the bedside medications (see Chapter 16). The team also felt that if they did take them, she might perceive this act as a breach of trust which would then impede any chance of making a therapeutic connection with her. The psychiatric team also struggled with these questions and met with Mrs. D. daily for 4 days. On the fourth day, a decision was made to remove the medications. The goal of this decision was to communicate that her distress was heard and taken seriously. In an attempt to promote her relationship with the unit staff, the psychiatric team decided to do the search. Persistent, gentle persuasion finally yielded permission from Mrs. D. to search her belongings with her assistance and all potentially harmful objects were removed. This act seemed to be catalyst for Mrs. D. to then "connect" with many of the staff members. She was subsequently able to work through and resolve important issues with her children before her death 6 weeks later.

Staff Considerations

Dealing with suicidal residents in a long-term care facility is a great challenge for caregivers. As the 8-year-old son of one of the authors stated, "Suicide is not a nice thing for anybody." Our own emotional responses can be varied and intense. Anxiety, fear, anger, and guilt are commonly experienced. Medicolegal, moral, religious, and ethical issues frequently surface. Emotions within caregiving teams may manifest themselves at the bedside as anger, over-solicitousness, protectiveness, or avoidance of the resident. Realistically, there are limits to what can be done to prevent suicide and it may occur regardless of precautions. Sometimes there are no warning signs at all. These factors contribute to the caregivers' sense of helplessness and frustration.

Frequent supportive meetings are important not only for staff to plan care, but to air thoughts and feelings about the situation. Creating a climate in which staff's opinions are accepted and valued is an integral component to the supportive nature of those meetings. These sessions facilitate open and honest discussion and give rise to creative solutions to circumvent problems associated with budget restraints and limited resources. It is important to balance the focus of these meetings so that positive achievements are recognized and intense emotions are dealt with as well. As staff work through these complex issues, a greater comfort and level of confidence are achieved and transmitted to residents. Thus, the key to effective management of suicidal residents involves the support of both staff and residents. Rosowsky [8] described the need for support of both clinical staff and administration following the death of a nursing home resident who shot himself.

Chronic or Passive Suicide

The concept of suicide can be extended to include individuals who undertake passive measures to shorten their lives. Indirect self-destructive behavior, can be defined as "an act of omission or commission that causes self-harm leading indirectly, over time, to the patient's death" [9]. This includes such behaviors as refusing to eat, refusing to take medications, drinking excessively, delaying or refusing treatment of medical conditions, and taking unnecessary risks. Such patients should be carefully assessed from a psychiatric standpoint to consider the possibility of an associated depression or other psychiatric disorder. These cases often present difficult ethical and medicolegal dilemmas.

Suicidal Behavior in the Terminally Ill

The term "rational" suicide has been used to describe the behavior of individuals who make a personal decision to end their lives, in the absence of mental disease and often in association with terminal or chronic medical illness. There is increasing recognition that for an individual with severe chronic pain, that is untreatable and unbearable, or for individuals with terminal illness the decision to end their lives can be considered rational.

Discussion around this issue dates back to the Greeks but its acceptance runs contrary to traditional Judeo-Christian thinking.

A recent review of six cases of terminally ill suicidal patients showed that their suicidal behavior was associated with depression that appeared to respond to treatment [10]. In studies of cancer patients, pain and suicidal ideation has been associated, however, a co-existing major depression was generally present [11]. The authors suggested that suicidal behavior in this population should be evaluated and treated as it would be in physically healthy patients and should not be viewed as an inevitable result of serious physical disease. Nevertheless, some health professionals believe that suicide is a reasonable alternative for the terminally ill. One study of 32 cases of patients with cancer in a Veteran's Administration hospital who committed suicide revealed a particularly high suicidal potential among elderly men with throat cancer, younger men with Hodgkin's disease or Leukemia, or persons of any age with cancer associated with heightened stress, severe anxiety, or low tolerance for pain [12].

Indirect Self-Destructive Behavior in the Institutionalized Elderly

Passive suicidal, or indirect self-destructive behavior in the institutionalized elderly was studied by Mishara and Kastenbaum [13]. They found that self-injurious behaviors occurred at least once in 43% of men and 21% of women during a 1-week observation period. Their definition of self-injurious behavior was rather broad, however, and included behavior such as falling out of wheelchairs, injury from careless cigarette smoking, scalding oneself with hot water, eating foreign objects, injury from fighting or pushing, injury from being tripped over, striking solid objects, refusing medication, and refusing to eat. In a controlled study of the introduction of milieu techniques, they showed a decrease in such behaviors through the use of both a token economy program that rewarded individuals for engaging in desirable behaviors and an enrichment program involving increased activities, social stimulation, and increased opportunity to make decisions regarding their own care.

At a workshop held in 1994, the data regarding these behaviors in long-term care was reviewed, and a plan identifying future research questions was developed. Issues requiring further study included the relationship between self-destructive behaviors and the need to exert control over one's life, the identification of long-term care residents who are at risk, and increasing our understanding of the range of self-injurious behaviors, with the goal of developing preventative measures [9]. One difficult question is how professionals can learn to differentiate between behaviors which are essentially signals of distress, as opposed to legitimate preferences for terminating treatment.

Case Illustration: "Rational" Passive Suicide

Mrs. E., a 72-year-old widow, was referred for psychiatric consultation because she had threatened to discontinue her peritoneal renal dialysis. She was on a continuing care floor of a geriatric hospital having developed acute renal failure at the time of moving into a residential setting 6 months earlier. She travelled by taxi to the general hospital about 5 miles away for dialysis 3 times per week, which she found to be an exhausting process. Shortly after her own illness her husband was discovered to have metastatic carcinoma and died 3 months later. Psychiatric consultation was requested some weeks after his death because Mrs. E. said that she was seriously considering discontinuing her dialysis. She also made it clear that if her already failing vision worsened she would certainly opt to discontinue her dialysis.

Mrs. E. had no children although she had a niece and several nephews with whom she was close. At the time of initial evaluation she was actively grieving her husband's death. She appeared fatigued and unable to experience any pleasure. She found dialysis to be an uncomfortable and exhausting process. She was clearly depressed about her situation, although it was unclear whether she was indeed suffering from a "clinical depression." Because a major depression could not be ruled out, an antidepressant was started but despite adequate dosage, the medication appeared to have no impact on her state of mind. Mrs. E. was asked to postpone her decision with regard to dialysis because of the fact that she was actively grieving for her husband. Although she agreed to this, she began to talk with increasing determination about discontinuing the dialysis. The attending team discussed the situation and had mixed feelings about her decision. Although the issue of her competence to make this decision was raised because she showed signs of cognitive impairment, it was concluded that she was competent to make the decision. Several weeks later she made it clear to the attending physician and team that she would not go to the general hospital the following day for her dialysis. To everyone's consternation her condition deteriorated that same day and she slipped into a semicomatose state. Medical examinations showed signs of mild congestive heart failure but did not reveal a cause for her loss of consciousness. She died peacefully that same evening.

Comment

Did Mrs. E. will herself to die? It has been suggested that individuals may have a degree of control over the timing of their deaths, and there is some literature to suggest that severe emotional reactions can precipitate cardiac arrhythmia and death (e.g., voodoo deaths). In this case, Mrs. E.'s apparent decision that she was going to die and the decline in her condition, which occurred at exactly the time that she had made her decision, seemed to be more than a mere coincidence.

Should she have been treated more vigorously for depression?

It was not clear that she was suffering from a major depression. The use of the antidepressant in this case was an attempt to rule out a clinical depression and also to reassure staff that everything possible was being done. When depression is suspected there is always a question of how vigorous the treatment should be. In this case pursuing aggressive measures such as ECT made no clinical sense.

Was Mrs. E. competent to make the decision?

Mrs. E. was at times somewhat vague and confused with regard to details. When it came to a discussion around her dialysis and her overall view of her life, however, she was consistent and able to give a clear explanation of her feelings. She believed she had lived an active and full life and that the quality of her life at present was virtually zero. Following her husband's death she believed her major role in life was over. In spite of feeling strongly about her relatives she did not feel the same kind of obligation towards them as some parents might feel toward their children. The determination of competence is often difficult (see Chapter 16) but in this case there was little doubt that she was competent to make this decision.

Was the team's attitude towards this issue important to Mrs. E.?
Mrs. E. seemed acutely aware of the fact that her decision was controversial. She asked on a number of occasions for team members, to whom she had became attached, to understand her position and to support her. It seemed important to her for the team members to accept her decision and recognize the courage that had been required to make it.

How does the team deal with its feelings?
Because of the differences among team members with regard to questions of life and death there will be varying degrees of disagreement that may engender heated debate and even hostility. It is important that team members have discussions among themselves both in small groups and as a whole team. All members of the team should get an opportunity to express their beliefs. It may be helpful to invite a consultant or an ethics committee (if available) to review the situation and discuss it in an group forum. It is important that medicolegal issued be clarified as they can increase the level of anxiety among team members.

References

1. Litman, R.E., Farberow, N.L. (1970). Suicide prevention in hospitals. In E.S. Shneidman, N.L. Farberow, R.E. Litman (Eds.), The psychology of suicide. New York: Science House.
2. Durkheim, E. (1951). Suicide. New York: Free Press (originally published in 1897).
3. Freud, S. (1955). Mourning and melancholia. In J. Strachey (Ed.), The standard edition of the complete works of Sigmund Freud. London: Hogarth Press (originally published in 1917).
4. Bibring, E. (1953). The mechanism of depression. In P. Greenacres (Ed.), Affective Disorders. New York: International Universities Press.
5. Seligman, M.E.P. (1975). Helplessness. San Francisco: W.H. Freeman.
6. Miller, M. (1979). Suicide after sixty: The final alternative. New York: Springer-Verlag.
7. Canadian Coalition for Seniors Mental Health. (2006). National guidelines for seniors mental health: The assessment of suicide risk and prevention of suicide. Toronto: CCSMH. Available at www.ccsmh.ca.
8. Rosowsky, E. (1993). Suicidal behavior in the nursing home and a postsuicide intervention. American Journal of Psychotherapy, 47:127–142.
9. Conwell, Y., Pearson, J., DeRenzo, E. (1996). Indirect self-destructive behavior among elderly patients in nursing homes: A research agenda. American Journal of Geriatric Psychiatry, 4(2): 152–163.
10. Brown, J.H., Henteleff, P., Barakat, S., et al. (1986). Is it normal for terminally ill patients to desire death? American Journal of Psychiatry, 143:208–211.
11. Leibenluft, E., Goldberg, R.L. (1988). The suicidal, terminally ill patient with depression. Psychosomatics, 29:379–386.
12. Farberow, N.L., Shneidman, E.S., Leonard, C.V. (1970). Suicide among patients with malignant

neoplasms. In E.S. Shneidman, N.L. Farberow, R.E. Litman (Eds.), The psychology of suicide. New York: Science House.
13. Mishara, B.L., Kastenbaum, R. (1973). Self-injurious behavior and environmental change in the institutionalized elderly. International Journal of Aging and Human Development, 4:133–145.

Suggested Readings

1. Osgood, N.J., Brant, B.A., Lipman, A. (1991). Suicide among the elderly in long-term care facilities. New York: Greenwood Press.
   A useful overview of issues related to suicide in long-term care facilities. Includes the results of a large scale study of the prevalence of suicide in U.S. institutions.
2. McIntosh, J.L., Santos, J.F., Hubbard, R.W., Overholser, J.C. (1994). Elder suicide: Research, theory and treatment. Washington, DC: American Psychological Association.
   A comprehensive review which includes sections on prevalence, theories, assessment, treatment, and prevention.
3. Heisel, M.J., Flett, G.L. (2006). The development and initial validation of the Geriatric Suicide Ideation Scale. American Journal of Geriatric Psychiatry, 14:742–751.
   Describes a new scale to evaluate risk of suicide in older adults.

7 The Suspicious Resident

Barbara Schogt

Key Points

- Suspiciousness occurs on a "trust" continuum from excessive trust to psychotic mistrust.
- Suspiciousness is common among the elderly, especially in long-term care settings. Risk factors include cognitive and sensory impairment.
- Suspiciousness is a symptom, NOT a diagnosis or illness. It can occur as a symptom in a wide range of psychiatric and medical disorders.
- Environmental, psychosocial, and biological strategies are used to manage suspiciousness.
- A comprehensive approach to identifying and managing the underlying illness should always take place in conjunction with efforts to achieve symptom control.

We all make assumptions about the extent to which we can trust those around us. These assumptions usually have some basis in fact. Our behavior is influenced by prior experience and by knowing how others have fared under similar circumstances. Thus, we decide when and where it is safe to leave the car unlocked, how much personal information to disclose to a new friend, and on whom to count in times of crisis.

Some degree of suspiciousness is necessary in any society. Individuals who are too trusting will encounter problems. At the other end of the spectrum, excessive mistrust also results in a wide range of difficulties both for suspicious individuals and for those with whom they interact.

Excessively suspicious individuals perceive the world as a very hostile place, populated by people who are selfish, uncaring, and possibly motivated to do harm. When suspicious people encounter misfortune or make mistakes, they tend to blame others. They are extremely sensitive to real and imagined slights, criticisms, and injustices. In its most extreme form, suspiciousness reaches psychotic proportions. The individual loses touch with reality and begins to believe in, and act upon, imaginary ideas called delusions (see Chapter 2, The Mental Status Examination). The delusions can take many forms but common themes are those of being persecuted, harmed, or robbed.

It is not uncommon for suspicious people to feel that they have been singled out as targets for persecution because they are important and special. Grandiosity is thus closely related to suspiciousness and the two symptoms are often encountered together.

Paranoia is often used interchangeably with suspiciousness and persecutory ideation. The term, which comes from the Greek and means "beside the mind," was originally used to describe any delusional state. This has resulted in confusion about what is described by this term. To avoid ambiguity, paranoia will not be used as a synonym for suspiciousness in this chapter.

In order to better understand suspicious individuals, it is useful to trace the development of their suspiciousness from a psychological perspective. A synthesis of elements from prevailing psychodynamic models suggests that some vulnerable individuals are unable to tolerate their need for others. Fearing rejection, they develop an attitude of hostility to protect themselves from feeling needy and inadequate so that "I love you" and "I need you" become, "I hate you because I need you." Rather than experiencing this anger as originating within themselves, suspicious people perceive it as coming from those around them. Thus, "I hate you" becomes, "You hate me." Grandiosity and feeling special further protect such individuals from an intolerable awareness of their underlying feelings, needs, and vulnerabilities: "You hate me because I am special." This psychological process occurs at an unconscious level beyond the person's awareness and control. The resulting symptoms of suspiciousness and grandiosity serve a protective function. This point will be discussed again later as it has important implications for management.

Suspiciousness in Long-Term Care Settings

There are several reasons why a chapter of this book is devoted to the problem of suspiciousness:

Suspiciousness Is Common in the Elderly

In a community sample of almost 1420 elderly people done in 1998, 6.3% were found to have paranoid ideation [1]. Sensory and cognitive impairment are associated with an increased risk of suspiciousness. Impairments such as these make it more difficult for people to comprehend what is happening around them and result in misperceptions that can lead to persecutory ideation.

Rates of cognitive impairment and hearing loss are extremely high among institutionalized elderly. It is therefore reasonable to assume that suspiciousness will occur at least as frequently in long-term care settings as it does in the community.

Residential Settings Can Bring out Suspiciousness

Living within the highly structured setting of the long-term care facility requires a considerable capacity to adapt to new circumstances, develop relationships, and cooperate with others.

Many very suspicious and even psychotic people lead a very isolated existence in the general community. Symptoms may not come to light until such individuals are forced into closer contact with people. Only under the stress of institutionalization will their inability to trust and failure to adapt emerge as problematic to others. For suspicious individuals, the move often represents a realization of their fears of being assaulted and imprisoned by strangers.

Others, who may not have been suspicious in the past, are limited in their capacity to adapt by sensory and cognitive difficulties. These individuals may also decompensate under the stress of moving from their familiar environment into a residential setting. Suspiciousness is a common response in these situations.

Suspiciousness Often Indicates the Presence of a Psychiatric Disorder

Suspiciousness, like fever, is a symptom and not an illness. Its presence indicates a need for a full assessment in order to establish an underlying diagnosis. There is a wide range of psychiatric disorders in the elderly in which suspiciousness may be one of the symptoms (see **Table 1**). Some of these disorders are covered in greater detail in other chapters of this book (see Chapters 3, 4, 5, and 8). A brief description of how suspiciousness manifests itself in different syndromes is given here, since understanding and managing the symptom of suspiciousness will differ depending on the underlying diagnosis.

Table 1 Disorders in which Suspiciousness Can Occur

- Dementia
- Delirium
- Delusional syndrome due to a physical condition
- Schizophrenia and late-onset schizophrenia
- Delusional (paranoid) disorder
- Mood disorder
- Paranoid personality disorder
- Suspiciousness in the absence of a psychiatric disorder

Dementia

It is not unusual for individuals in the early and middle stages of dementia to accuse others of causing or contributing to the chaos for which they cannot account in any other way. They sometimes blame people for stealing the things they misplace or for purposefully tricking and shaming them. The accusations can be very painful for family, friends, roommates, and staff as they struggle to cope with the gradual loss of the person they once knew. The suspicions and persecutory delusions in dementia are usually quite simple. They are an attempt by the resident to make sense of an increasingly incomprehensible world and to preserve self-esteem.

Delirium

Because delirium affects attention, level of consciousness, thinking and perception, delirious people perceive the world as if in a dream. The dream is usually a nightmare. The terrifying suspicions and delusions of delirium tend to be fleeting, poorly organized, and associated with perceptual disturbances such as illusions and hallucinations (see Chapter 2, The Mental Status Examination).

Delusional Syndrome from Medical Disorder

In this disorder, delusions, usually persecutory, are the predominant finding. The global cognitive impairment seen in dementia and delirium is absent. The disorder is due to a specific biological factor such as medication or a brain lesion. In the elderly, this disorder is sometimes seen in the context of Parkinson's disease or after strokes. The delusions are variable in nature, ranging from simple ideas to highly organized, complex delusional systems.

Schizophrenia

Schizophrenia, a psychotic illness, typically starts in late adolescence or young adulthood. It is characterized by disturbances in many areas of mental functioning, although the clinical picture is quite variable. Thinking, perception, behavior, motivation, and emotional life are all affected. The illness is associated with varying degrees of impaired functioning in the areas of work, relationships, and self-care.

Delusions in schizophrenia often have a persecutory component. They can be elaborate and quite bizarre. Simpler delusions where people are spying on or planning to harm the affected individual are also common. Certain delusions occur in schizophrenia far more often than in other psychotic disorders. These include the belief that one's thoughts are being broadcast from inside one's mind to the outside world, and the idea that thoughts are being controlled, inserted into or taken out of one's mind. The delusions of schizophrenia may be accompanied by hallucinations, most often auditory.

From the histories of elderly patients with long-standing schizophrenia, it is usually clear that they have been struggling with their symptoms for many years. Even when active symptoms are present, patients and their families have to some extent grown accustomed to coping with what is by then a familiar illness picture. Patients who have had treatment for their schizophrenia may be suffering from movement disorders associated with the long-term use of antipsychotic medication. Needless to say, adapting to new physical or cognitive disabilities in late life and adjusting to the long-term care setting present special challenges for this population. These life-crises may be associated with exacerbations in the symptoms of the schizophrenic illness.

Late-Onset Schizophrenia

A significant minority of schizophrenic illnesses begin in middle age and even in late-life. Because schizophrenia has a high prevalence, this minority represents a sizable group of individuals in any population. A panel of experts who met to review the literature on this subject concluded that this important condition needs further study now that the syndrome of late-onset schizophrenia has finally been described in unambiguous terms [2]. Individuals who develop the disorder probably share a genetic predisposition with those who suffer from early-onset schizophrenia. Unlike schizophrenia of earlier onset, the late-onset condition is more common in women.

Late-onset schizophrenia is clinically similar to schizophrenia that starts in early adulthood. Delusions are often persecutory and can be elaborate or bizarre. Hallucinations may be present. As in younger patients, the illness may be associated with deterioration in many aspects of living including self-care and social functioning. This decline is not associated with clinical or brain-imaging evidence of a progressive dementing disorder. Social withdrawal or isolation may be present although individuals living with this condition in the community may emerge to report "evidence" of persecution or harassment to police and other local authorities. Sensory impairment, if present, can exacerbate persecutory ideation and lead to further isolation.

The recognition that schizophrenia-like illnesses can arise at any age has significant implications for long-term care settings. Symptoms may arise for the first time in the institution. More often though, individuals with late-onset schizophrenia enter institutions when physical illness or the onset of cognitive impairment separate from the schizophrenia forces them to give up their independence. In either case, the condition presents diagnostic challenges. Assessment, investigations, and, where available, brain imaging are recommended to identify coexisting illnesses [2]. Sensory impairments should be ruled out.

Management of late-onset schizophrenia in the long-term care setting may be difficult for the reasons outlined in this chapter. Problems that arise are similar to those of patients who suffer from persecutory ideation for other reasons. As in early-onset schizophrenia, antipsychotic medications are the treatment of choice for late-onset schizophrenia. Dosages must be modified for the elderly (see Chapter 11, Principles of Geriatric Psychopharmacology).

Delusional (Paranoid) Disorder

This relatively uncommon disorder is characterized by the presence of a persistent, usually well-organized delusion. Although most often persecutory, various delusional themes can occur. The elderly sometimes develop delusional jealousy becoming convinced, without due cause, that their spouses are unfaithful. The onset of the disorder may coincide with a loss of sexual functioning resulting, for example, from prostate surgery. Other individuals develop a delusional conviction that someone, perhaps an important person, is in love with them. In the somatic type of delusional disorder, individuals believe that they emit a foul odor or are infested with vermin.

Hallucinations are not prominent in delusional disorder. Unlike in schizophrenia, there is little or no impairment in areas of the individual's life not involved in the delusion. The symptoms may be similar to those in the delusional syndrome due to a medical disorder, but no specific biological factor is identified.

Mood Disorder

Persecutory delusions can occur in both depression and mania. When they do, the suspicions are usually consistent with the predominant mood. Severely depressed individuals can develop a conviction that they are being punished and persecuted or that their imagined poverty results from their having led bad, sinful lives. The irritability and the grandiose themes seen in mania may be associated with beliefs that others are envious and wish to do them harm. The suspiciousness almost always resolves with treatment of the underlying mood disorder but may be hard to manage in the acute phase.

Paranoid Personality Disorder

People with this problem have a life-long history of difficulty with trust and intimacy. They tend to be aloof, suspicious loners who are quick to take offense and bear grudges. In old age, they become increasingly reclusive and eccentric. They are vulnerable to psychosis when under stress, and have great difficulty adapting to institutional settings.

Suspiciousness in the Absence of a Psychiatric Disorder

The possibility that suspiciousness is justified should be explored before concluding that it is a manifestation of illness. Stealing does occur in institutional settings from time to time and life in a small community can foster intrigue, the formation of cliques and the subsequent isolation or even persecution of certain individuals.

Behavior seen as excessively suspicious in one culture may be normal or prudent in another. Sometimes the safest place to store money may well be under the mattress and there are societies in which officials cannot be trusted to tell the truth. As already noted, (see Chapter 2, The Mental Status Examination), it is important to keep an open mind when evaluating the ideas and behaviors of others, particularly when their life experiences are significantly divergent from those of the predominant cultural group.

Suspiciousness Can Give Rise to Serious Management Problems

Although reclusive behavior is not necessarily problematic, suspiciousness contributes to many serious difficulties within institutional settings. Failure to comply with investigation and management of medical disorders and to accept help with self-care or activities of daily living can result in significant risk to suspicious individuals.

The potential for violence must always be kept in mind. It is natural for people to respond to perceived attack with defensive behavior or even counterattack. Suspicious individuals may lash out against those they suspect of wanting to harm them. From their perspective, they are acting in self-defense and the attacks are justified. The violence may be random or directed at specific persons involved in the delusions. Verbal attacks can include threats of violence and highly personal comments regarding the physical characteristics, sexuality, status, or racial background of others. Suspicious people can be physically violent, especially if they are agitated and psychotic (suffering from delusions and hallucinations).

Management of Suspiciousness: General Principles

There are some general principles that can be applied to the management of suspicious individuals. The approaches outlined focus on managing suspiciousness as a symptom. A comprehensive approach to the suspicious resident must also involve an attempt to identify and treat any underlying medical and psychiatric problems. The overall management plan should be based on the history, mental status, physical examination, and appropriate laboratory investigations. Management strategies are divided into environmental, psychosocial, and biological.

Environmental Strategies

Optimizing the Level of Stimulation

Modifying the environment in order to minimize the potential for misinterpretation by the suspicious resident is particularly important when dealing with disorders such as delirium and dementia that affect the capacity to integrate sensory information.

Whenever possible, agitated individuals should be brought to a quiet area where sensory stimuli are kept to a minimum. The number of people in the room with the resident at any one time may have to be restricted. Adequate but not glaring lighting decreases the risk of visual illusions. Abrupt movements and sudden loud noises such as those from telephones, buzzers, intercoms, and slamming doors can be very alarming to agitated suspicious residents.

Removing Dangerous Objects

Sometimes, environmental modifications are necessary to reduce the risk of violence. This involves removing objects that can be used as weapons such as glass, knives, vases, and small lamps. Canes can be used to trip and hit staff or other residents. Replacing the cane temporarily with a walker can be an effective safety measure. Room searches are indicated when residents say they are hiding weapons or when staff have reason to believe that there may be danger. The question of room searches is discussed further in Chapter 6, The Suicidal Resident. Whenever such interventions are made, staff should follow the institution's protocol. Time should be taken to prepare the resident and explain that the aim of the search is to promote safety, not to be punitive.

Reducing Contact Between the Resident and Individuals at Risk

When the resident's delusions involve one particular person, placing that person at risk, it is wise to limit contact between the resident and that individual as much as possible. Changes in room-mates and staff assignments are sometimes warranted. Unfortunately, there is a possibility that the delusions will extend to incorporate the new room-mates and staff.

Physical Restraint

Under extreme circumstances, it may be necessary to use physical restraint in order to isolate a suspicious resident who has become aggressive. This is justifiable from an ethical perspective only in crisis situations, when there is an imminent risk of violence by the resident to self or others. In addition to weighing ethical considerations, staff should be familiar with the legislation in their jurisdiction. Ideally an institutional protocol should be in place. (See Chapter 20, Legal and Ethical Dimensions). In institutions with a "no restraints" policy, an alternative strategy should be in place to manage violent situations.

Physical restraint should be undertaken with adequate personnel under the guidance of one staff member assigned to coordinate the procedure. Frequent if not constant observation of the restrained individual is recommended along with detailed documentation in the chart of the reasons for and the consequences of the intervention. Physical restraint is a temporary crisis measure kept in place only until a more effective management strategy can be implemented.

Sometimes psychotic individuals respond favorably to being restrained since the imposition of external controls can be reassuring when internal controls have been lost. In many other cases, however, the restraints serve as further proof for suspicious individuals that others are out to harm them. Seeing an agitated person placed in restraints is also extremely frightening for other residents, who may then require extra support.

Barricades

Suspicious residents occasionally barricade themselves in their rooms and cannot be persuaded to come out by staff or family. Although such residents may allow medications and food to be passed to them, they cannot be adequately supervised. Their deteriorating hygiene can eventually pose a public health risk to an entire unit. If the risks become too great, forceful intervention is necessary. Because removal of the barricade can be physically difficult and will certainly be frightening to the resident who already perceives himself as being under siege, no action should be taken without careful planning and adequate staff resources.

Psychosocial Strategies

There are a number of general guidelines to follow when interacting with suspicious residents.

Maintaining a Natural Manner with Emphasis on Consistency

Because suspiciousness and hostility are often associated with fear, it is best to approach the resident in as natural a manner as possible. If staff display their own fear and uncertainty, either by withdrawing support or through an overly solicitous, unnaturally cheerful approach, the resident will likely feel even more mistrustful and isolated. By maintaining a calm, consistent approach during frequent but relatively brief contacts, staff may be able to create an atmosphere where trust can begin to develop. When disruptions in the regular schedule are inevitable, the suspicious resident will benefit from an explanation that is not overly lengthy or apologetic. Contracting with a suspicious resident around specific issues is a useful technique, but before taking this approach, staff must be certain that they will be able to hold up their end of the bargain.

Developing a Profile of Behavior

As caregivers learn to recognize the signs that a particular resident is feeling threatened, they can gauge how much contact the resident can tolerate and when it becomes necessary to withdraw. Documenting the antecedents to episodes of agitation and suspiciousness and the outcomes of various interventions leads to the development of a behavior management approach that can be used even by staff less familiar with the resident (see Chapter 13, Behavioral Management Strategies).

Maintaining a Safe Distance

If someone gets onto an almost empty bus and sits down right next to you, it is quite natural to feel uncomfortable. Many suspicious individuals need to surround themselves with even more space than most of us do to maintain a sense of comfort. Intrusions into this personal space can result in agitation and even violence. Whenever the potential for violence exists, it is unsafe for the caregiver to come between the suspicious resident and the door, as this causes the resident to feel trapped. Ideally both staff and resident should have free access to an exit.

The use of touch can be a powerful and often very positive intervention when it is applied judiciously. Suspicious people sometimes experience touch as an attack, however, and respond accordingly. Extra caution should be exercised around the use of touch in this population.

When examining the resident or providing physical care, a brief explanation preceding each action provides reassurance. At times, some suspicious residents will refuse all care. This can result in potentially life-threatening situations and force caregivers to make difficult clinical decisions. Ethical and legal considerations, the resident's competence to make informed choices, the opinions of relatives and guardians, and the need to transfer to an acute care facility are factors that need to be addressed as part of the decision-making process.

Verbal Strategies

Any communication that takes place in the presence of suspicious residents not involving them as participants can add fuel to the fires of mistrust. Whispering and gesturing between staff should be avoided. When addressing the resident directly, every effort should be made to communicate in a clear, unambiguous manner. Consistent use of the pronouns "I" and "you" as opposed to "we" helps maintain a clear boundary between the speaker and the suspicious person.

Discussing Suspicions

When residents discuss their suspicious and delusional beliefs, it can be difficult to maintain an attitude of sympathetic listening. Arguing with suspicious individuals about their beliefs is not only futile, but often increases their feelings of isolation and inadequacy, while jeopardizing any basis for a positive alliance. Yet neither is it helpful to take sides with residents against the world by supporting their delusional perspective. To do so will undermine residents' already tenuous hold on reality and further strengthen their beliefs. Sometimes it is possible to listen without making more than a few neutral comments and then to redirect the conversation to another topic. When residents demand a response from staff about their suspicions, distraction is not always possible or appropriate. At such times, an honest, nonevasive response is best. For example, one might say, "You have described the way you see the situation and I understand things are very difficult for you at the moment. I don't share your view, but maybe you and I can still work on these problems together."

Giving Feedback to the Resident

When suspicious residents have behaved in a hostile or violent manner, it is often appropriate to inform them that their behavior affects others. Feedback is best given in the context of a quiet conversation, after the behavior has stopped. The time lag serves two functions. It allows the caregiver to reach a clinical decision regarding the extent to which the resident is able to take responsibility for the behavior, while the risk that the feedback will become punitive is reduced.

Focusing on Strengths

Residents may continue to function well in areas not involved in their suspicious beliefs. Whenever possible, areas of strength should be encouraged. This distracts residents from their preoccupation and provides an opportunity for building self-esteem and interacting with others in a more positive manner.

Supporting Those Around the Resident

Since being attacked leaves people feeling angry, frightened, and vulnerable, those who come into contact with the suspicious resident will need support. Staff should be encouraged to share their experiences with each other informally or in sessions scheduled for this purpose. This can happen only if caregivers feel confident that they are being supported at all levels within the institution, even when the resident's accusations involve politically sensitive issues.

Family members and other residents also need an opportunity to voice their fears. They may benefit from education designed to help them understand and respond to the suspicious person (see Family Information Sheet).

Biological Strategies

Identifying and Treating Underlying Disorders

The medical and/or psychiatric disorders identified in association with the suspiciousness should be treated where possible. Certain conditions such as delirium or mood disorder may be fully reversible and their treatment will result in the resolution of suspiciousness. Unfortunately, in other situations, little can be done to reverse or even halt the progression of the underlying disease. It is still possible, however, to provide relief from anxiety and discomfort and thereby achieve a significant amelioration of the suspiciousness.

Identifying and Reducing Sensory Impairment

Identification and treatment of visual and hearing impairments can reduce the risk that the suspicious resident will misinterpret sensory cues.

Using Medications to Manage Suspiciousness

The use of medication is an option in managing suspiciousness. The potential benefits of using medication must always be weighed against the risks of producing side effects and toxicity, especially when the medication is being used for symptom control rather than as a definitive treatment for the underlying condition. Moreover, not all forms of suspiciousness respond to medication. Once a medication has been started, its effects should be monitored and the ongoing need for its use reassessed at regular intervals (see also Chapter 11, Principles of Geriatric Psychopharmacology).

Antipsychotic medications can be very effective when psychotic symptoms are present. Not only do they reduce agitation, but they also have a specific antipsychotic effect. This is true whether the psychosis originates from a medical condition, as in delirium, or from a psychiatric disorder. Generally, the reduction in agitation is seen well before the persecutory delusions disappear. In some cases the delusions never go away but they do become less troublesome to the resident. The presence of delusions does not automatically indicate a need for treatment. Long-standing delusions and those that do not result in distress are often best left alone.

In the absence of psychosis, antipsychotics are rarely indicated in the treatment of suspiciousness. When anxiety is prominent, suspicious residents sometimes respond favorably to a brief course of an intermediate-acting benzodiazepine. In other cases, however, the anxiolytic and sedative effects of these medications undermine the resident's subjective sense of being able to guard against danger and may actually increase the level of agitation. Thus, before initiating benzodiazepines, the physician must decide how important it is to a particular resident to be able to remain alert and vigilant.

Suspicious people often agree to take medication if it is presented as something that might help reduce their agitation and suffering. The medication should be administered in such a way that the resident can see and count the pills. The resident should also be informed about changes in dosages, times and the form in which the medication is dispensed. Sometimes residents will only agree to take medication from certain trusted staff or family members. When residents refuse medication, the same considerations must be applied as when other aspects of care are refused.

Case Illustration: Tolerating Risks

Miss G., an 85-year-old single woman, was admitted to a nursing home when she was evicted from her apartment for failing to pay the rent. The apartment was badly neglected and filled with hoarded objects and old newspapers. A distant cousin described Miss G. as a lifelong loner who had become increasingly eccentric and reclusive since retiring 20 years earlier.
On admission, Miss G. was found to be unkempt and malnourished. She refused to participate in any aspect of the assessment and accused staff of meddling in her affairs. She insisted that she was vacationing in a hotel and would soon return home. Offers of assistance with personal care were politely but firmly refused. She walked unsteadily, refusing to use aids, and did not participate in social activities. When challenged, Miss G. became extremely angry, lashing out at staff verbally and physically.

Comment

Miss G. has a long-standing pattern of suspicious behavior. In addition, she may have acute nutritional, medical, and/or psychiatric disorders, but without a full assessment, any hypothesis remains tentative. She is clearly least distressed when left to her own devices and is having difficulty adapting to her new environment. Her pride and suspiciousness interfere with her judgment, and her competence to make informed decisions is in doubt. The potential that she will harm others, especially if they cross her, is significant.

Are there ways of facilitating Miss G.'s adjustment?
Allowing Miss G. as much independence as possible while attempting to maximize her safety is all that can be done. In order to preserve her dignity, Miss G.'s insistence that she is "on vacation" should not be challenged. Encouraging her to join group activities would likely be very threatening to her and contrary to her lifelong pattern of keeping people at a distance.

Miss G. may gradually develop some degree of trust that those around her will not violate her privacy and dignity, and then begin to accept occasional assistance with certain aspects of personal care. If possible, the cousin could be involved in this process. It is unlikely that Miss G. will ever engage fully with those around her or accept care easily.

Does it make sense to contract with Miss G.?
Yes. Allowing Miss G. to participate in decisions around bathing and other aspects of personal care will increase her sense of control and enlist her as an ally rather than an adversary. For example, it may be possible to arrange a regular bathing time by allowing Miss G. to choose her preferred time from a number of options, and then placing copies of the agreed upon schedule in her room and at the nursing station.

How do staff decide when to intervene?
This is an extremely difficult decision to make at both the ethical and clinical levels. Although Miss G. is clearly at risk, this risk was likely much greater when she was still alone in her apartment. Caregivers may have to learn to tolerate their own anxiety as Miss G. teeters down the hall, simply because there is no safer alternative. Careful documentation of the situation and discussion with the cousin are recommended.
Should Miss G. develop a medical emergency or suffer a fracture, interventions will be necessary. She may be more willing to accept care for a clearly identifiable and symptomatic illness but if not, temporary restraint may be necessary. Her relative should be kept informed as the situation unfolds.

Is there a role for medication in this case?
Even if she agreed to take them, antipsychotic medications will most likely have no effect on Miss G.'s chronic suspiciousness and may result in troublesome side effects.

Case Illustration: A Case of Missing Underwear

Mr. N. is a moderately demented 77-year-old widower who has lived in the institution for some years. Although forgetful, he is generally cheerful and appears to enjoy social activities. His vision is failing. Mr. N. frequently misplaces personal belongings. Whenever this happens, he becomes very distressed and agitated. Lately, he has started to accuse others of stealing the objects. At first, the accusations were not directed at specific people, but this morning he threatened to hit his room-mate for stealing his underwear. Responding to this situation, the staff located the garment under his bed.

Comment

Mr. N.'s failing vision and memory have left him floundering and unable to hold onto either his thoughts or his belongings. Accusing others of stealing protects him from an awareness of this painful reality.

What can be done to deal with the consequences of the morning's events?
If Mr. N.'s memory remains sufficiently intact that he is able to recall the morning's events, he could be confronted gently with the seriousness of the threat and its effects on his room-mate. Mr. N. should be

encouraged to report any missing articles to staff. This message will have to be reinforced over the coming days. The key to Mr. N.'s cupboard could be put on a cord so that he can wear it around his neck at all times. Staff should check whether the lighting in Mr. N.'s room is adequate, and perhaps encourage a trusted family member to come in and help him sort through his belongings.
At the same time, Mr. N.'s room-mate should be reassured that steps are being taken to prevent further incidents and informed that if Mr. N. does threaten him again, he should get out of the way immediately and report to staff.

What can be done when Mr. N. comes to the desk two days later shouting that his room-mate has stolen his glasses?
Rather than confronting Mr. N. with the likelihood that he has misplaced the glasses, the caregiver should calmly offer assistance in retrieving them. If they cannot be found, Mr. N. could be reassured that everything will be done to locate them. This may be sufficient to reduce Mr. N.'s agitation. It may then be possible to distract him by changing the topic or involving him in an activity. If Mr. N. continues to rail against his room-mate, it will be necessary to remind him that threats and violence are unacceptable. If he is unable to calm down, Mr. N. may have to be moved to another room temporarily.

What can be done if the relationship between Mr. N. and his room-mate continues to deteriorate?
If violence is an ongoing risk or has actually occurred, a permanent separation may have to be arranged. Although Mr. N. may begin to accuse his new room-mate of stealing, this is by no means the inevitable outcome of such a move. Moreover, as Mr. N.'s dementia progresses, he will likely become less aware of and distressed by his losses.

Case Illustration: A Little Contact Goes a Long Way

Mrs. W., an 89-year-old widow, has lived in the institution for 10 years. She has Parkinson's disease for which she takes several medications. For the last 6 years, she has been convinced that a group of unknown assailants comes into her room every night, ties her to her bed and begins to inject noxious chemicals into her body. She points to her varicose veins as "proof" that this is taking place.
The onset of the delusions coincided with the death of her sister and the initiation of medication for Parkinson's disease. Her delusions and the distress associated with them become much more pronounced when there is a crisis in her life. There has been a dramatic rise in symptoms recently. Staff have finally been able to link these symptoms to the upcoming departure of a caregiver who was in the habit of occasionally spending a few minutes with Mrs. W., listening to her talk about the horrible nights.

Comment

Mrs. W.'s delusions are elaborate, stable, and well circumscribed. The medication used to treat Parkinson's disease can cause psychotic symptoms as a side effect and may be an etiologic factor. Psychosocial variables clearly affect the intensity of the delusions and the level of Mrs. W.'s distress.

What can be done to alleviate Mrs. W.'s distress?
The departing caregiver has been providing Mrs. W. with psychotherapy, albeit informally. It would be

helpful if this person could meet with Mrs. W. a few more times in order to say good-bye. The recognition by the staff of the importance of this loss for Mrs. W. will allow the latter to begin the process of mourning that may eventually enable her to talk about her sister.
Since Mrs. W. has derived so much benefit from this contact, it would be useful to reinstate some form of ongoing psychotherapy. Whoever provides Mrs. W. with this contact should have a capacity to listen and be able to make a commitment to see her on a consistent basis.

Would antipsychotics be useful?
The delusions from which Mrs. W. suffers might respond to antipsychotic medication, but these medications would also have the effect of worsening the Parkinson's disease. Before considering an antipsychotic, the antiparkinsonian medication should be reassessed and reduced if possible. If Mrs. W. responds to psychotherapy with a significant decrease in her distress, it may not be necessary to use medications to treat the delusions.
Atypical antipsychotics such as olanzapine are less likely to exacerbate the Parkinson's disease. Even so, the use of antipsychotics should be limited as much as possible, unless the consequences of the psychosis become more serious and disabling than those of the Parkinson's disease.

Might Mrs. W. be suffering from a depression?
A careful injury into this question might reveal the presence of a depression. A trial of an antidepressant might be considered as an adjunct to the psychotherapy. Mrs. W. would have to be monitored closely to ensure that the medication does not worsen her psychosis.

Case Illustration: Dangerous Loyalties

Mr. and Mrs. A. moved into the institution when Mrs. A. became too demented to manage her household any longer. They share a room. Mrs. A. is diabetic, while Mr. A. is in excellent health apart from mild cognitive impairment.
Several months after admission, Mr. A., who spends all his time with his wife, begins to accuse male staff of raping her. He has barricaded himself into the room with Mrs. A. and refuses staff any access to either of them. Although he allows meals to be left at the door, Mr. A. would not let staff in to give Mrs. A. the oral hypoglycemic medication that controls her diabetes.

Comment

Mr. A. has decompensated under the stresses of his wife's ongoing decline, the move to the institution and his own failing cognitive capacity. His behavior is placing both himself and especially his wife at risk. The potential that he might attack anyone who tries to intervene is considerable.

What can be done to break the deadlock?
Female staff can try to engage Mr. A. in a conversation, find out what he fears might be the consequence of letting someone in, and reassure him if possible. Mr. A. might respond to the suggestion that he will be better able to look after his wife if he gets some rest and that there are others willing to share with him the task of watching over her and ensuring her safety. Another approach would be to discuss Mrs.

A.'s need for medication, enlisting Mr. A.'s help by asking him to be present when the medication is being given.
If these strategies do not work, and the risk to Mrs. A. is considered high enough, staff may have to force their way into the room and be prepared to restrain Mr. A. if necessary. It is possible that Mr. A. has been so frightened by the situation, that he may begin to calm down as soon as he senses that others are taking control. If not, sedation with an antipsychotic is an option, although if Mr. A. refused medication, legal and ethical considerations may necessitate a temporary transfer to an acute care facility.

Can anything be done to prevent further crises?
After the crisis, it may help to tell Mr. A. gently that he placed his wife at risk, even though he was clearly trying to protect her. If Mr. A. can be convinced to share the task of looking after his wife, he could begin to participate in activities that might distract him and provide him with the opportunity to establish some positive contacts. Eventually he could be encouraged to express his confusion and grief.
If Mr. A. does not respond to this approach, he may have to be moved to a separate room to ensure his wife's safety. His access to his wife's room would have to be carefully planned, negotiated, and monitored. As the conditions of both Mr. and Mrs. A. deteriorate, new difficulties will arise.

Is there an ongoing role of medication?
It is possible that Mr. A. might respond to a small regular dose of an antipsychotic medication until the effects of this crisis have abated, at which point the need for the medication would have to be reassessed. He might be more amenable to taking something if it is explained to him that the medication will help calm him thereby giving him more strength to help his wife and cope with his difficult situation.

References

1. Forsell, Y., Henderson, A.S. (1998). Epidemiology of paranoid symptoms in an elderly population. British Journal of Psychiatry, 172:429–432.
2. Howard, R., Rabins, P.V., Seeman, M.V., Jeste, D.V. and the International Late-Onset Schizophrenia Group. (2000). Late-onset schizophrenia and very-late onset schizophrenia like psychosis. American Journal of Psychiatry, 157:172–178.

Suggested Readings

1. Burnside, I.M. (1981). Paranoid behavior in the elderly. In I.M. Burnside (Ed.), Nursing and the aged (pp. 157–165). New York: McGraw Hill.
   Humanistic overview of responding to and managing suspicious residents.
2. Grossberg, G.T., Manepalli, J. (1995). The older patient with psychotic symptoms. Psychiatric Services, 46:55–59.
   Provides a good overview of psychosis in the elderly.
3. Verwoerdt, A. (1987). Psychodynamics of paranoid phenomena in the aged. In J. Sadavoy, M. Leszcz (Eds.), Treating the elderly with psychotherapy (pp. 67–93). Madison: International Universities Press, Inc.
   An interesting look at paranoid phenomena from a psychodynamic perspective, that can increase the ability to understand this population.

Suspiciousness – Family Information Sheet*

What Is Suspiciousness and What Causes it? A certain amount of suspiciousness about other people and their motives is essential to well-being. Nobody wants to be duped or robbed, or to have their secrets betrayed because they trusted unwisely or too much. Suspiciousness becomes problematic only if it reaches levels that interfere with day to day functioning. Suspiciousness is a symptom, not an illness. It can be caused by many different things. Some people are suspicious all their lives. Either it is part of their character or the symptom of a chronic psychiatric illness. Other people become suspicious as they age, perhaps as a side effect of medication or temporarily, as part of a medical illness. People with cognitive impairment, especially if they also have visual or hearing impairment may start accusing others of stealing the things they misplace, or of plotting against them.

What Do I Need to Know? Since suspiciousness occurs in so many different conditions, it is important for you to ask staff to explain their understanding of what underlies your relative's symptoms. Because suspicious people often need to keep others at a distance, staff have to develop a unique care plan that delivers important aspects of care without creating undue agitation. Depending on the cause of the suspiciousness, medication may be very helpful and can markedly reduce the suspiciousness. In other conditions medication will have no benefit. It will help your relative and the team if you are familiar with the care plan and the rationale for it.

Why Do Suspicious People Sometimes Become Angry or Violent? When we feel threatened or attacked we defend ourselves. Suspicious people may experience our care as an attack and will respond accordingly. If they perceive us as dangerous, it is quite natural for them to refuse the medications we offer and even to attack us when we approach. Deeply suspicious people will not be helped by being told their suspicions are unfounded. They may feel you are trying to trick them and become agitated. They will certainly feel more alone with their worries.

What Do I Say when my Relative Wants to Discuss the Suspicions? Try to just listen and then distract your relative with a different topic or perhaps an activity. Do not agree with the suspicions if you think they are unfounded. A false alliance that is not based in reality can only make things worse. If your relative insists on a response from you, you could say something like, "You have described the way you see the situation and I understand things are very difficult for you at the moment. I don't share your view, but maybe you and I can still work on these problems together."

How Else Can I Help? Staff are sorting out what condition is at the root of your relative's suspiciousness. Their interventions may include a careful review of the history and the medication, and if indicated and tolerated a physical examination and laboratory tests. You can help the staff by providing them with information about what your relative was like before admission, and whether there have been any changes in medication that you are aware of. Even over-the-counter medications and alcohol may be relevant.

* From *Practical Psychiatry in the Long-Term Care Home: A Handbook for Staff* (D.K. Conn et al., Eds.). ISBN 978-0-88937-341-9. © 2007 Hogrefe & Huber Publishers.

8 The Resident with Personality Disorder

Anne Robinson and Barbara Schogt

Key points

- Personality disorders are pervasive, life-long patterns of perceiving, relating to, and thinking about others that cause significant functional impairment and/or subjective distress.
- Personality disorders can coexist with and complicate the diagnosis and management of other psychiatric disorders.
- The development of personality disorders has been linked to deficits in the childhood environment. Constitutional factors may also play a role.
- Because of the rigid way in which people with personality disorders cope with living, they are very vulnerable to breaking down under stress. To adapt to the losses, role changes, and dependency that come with aging is particularly difficult for this population.
- The demands of institutional living cause ingrained behavior patterns to surface and because these residents are unaware of their contribution to their problems, they will blame caregivers for all that goes wrong.
- If the powerful impact of these behavior patterns on staff is not understood, it can interfere with clinical judgment, team functioning and the resident's care.
- Setting realistic treatment goals involves accepting the resident's limitations and working within these limitations to promote the optimal coexistence of the resident with others in the institution. Improving communication at various levels, applying behavior management strategies and occasionally using psychoactive medications and/or formal psychotherapy are important aspects of a comprehensive approach to management.

Just as we recognize a face without consciously analyzing its features, we experience a person's character as unique without enumerating its traits. So intrinsic is the concept of personality to our appraisal of others that we rarely pause to wonder what personality is. To continue with the analogy, expressions alter the appearance of a person's face while the underlying facial structure remains constant and always recognizable. In the same way, personality or character is a stable structure upon which different moods are superimposed. As described in the Diagnostic and Statistical Manual of Mental Disorders (DSM-IV-TR), "personality traits are enduring patterns of perceiving, relating to, and thinking about the environment and oneself that are exhibited in a wide range of important social and personal contexts" [1].

Our character, comprised of numerous personality traits, determines how we interact with others and how we adapt to changing circumstances. Aspects of our character may facilitate or complicate our interactions, enrich or impoverish our journey through life. When personality traits are so inflexible and maladaptive that they cause significant functional impairment or subjective distress, they constitute a personality disorder. The manifestations of personality disorders are often recognizable by adolescence, and continue throughout adult life into old age. This chapter will focus on the problems that arise when elderly individuals with personality disorders enter long-term care settings.

Identifying a Personality Disorder

Personality determines both our capacity to adapt and our unique ways of doing so. This is equally true whether things are going well for us or whether we are suffering from a physical or mental illness. Whatever is going on in the foreground will be colored by the backdrop of character. If this backdrop is ignored, it becomes difficult to understand, for example, why one person's recovery from an uncomplicated hip fracture is so much stormier than that of another. The treatment team that fails to identify the presence of a personality disorder cannot modify its management plan to try to prevent or mitigate such storms.

People with depression often report to us that they feel terrible. The symptoms of schizophrenia are usually quite obvious to observers. But people are generally no more aware of their own personality than of the way they walk. Even for the observer, personality disorders are easy to miss. In the DSM-IV-TR, personality disorders are classified separately from other mental disorders to ensure that they will not be overlooked. Psychiatrists first identify the disorder(s) in the foreground, such as depression, schizophrenia or delirium, and classify these disorders on Axis I. The psychiatrist then comments separately on the presence or absence of a personality disorder which is classified on Axis II. This separation from other diagnoses emphasizes that personality disorders can coexist with any other mental disorder. It also encourages clinicians to remember the importance of character as it contributes to and interacts with Axis I diagnoses.

That being said, it can be very difficult to diagnose a personality disorder during an acute episode of another mental disorder. Too much turmoil in the foreground can distract from and obscure the background. Many features characteristic of personality disorders may also be seen in people ill with an acute episode of, for example, mania or schizophrenia. The diagnosis of personality disorder should be made only when the characteristic features are stable "over time and across different situations" [1]. Staff in long-term care settings working with residents over extended periods are in a unique position to comment on personality.

People with personality disorders have difficulty with interpersonal relationships. They interact with the people around them in ways that create tension. They may be experienced by others as needy or unpleasant, seductive, threatening, or intrusive. It is unsettling for us to experience others in such negative terms, especially if we are care-givers engaged with them on a daily basis in intense and very personal interactions. These residents threaten our image of ourselves as capable, caring professionals. To preserve our cherished self-image we may end up avoiding the offending residents, blaming them and punishing them. We may also react with guilt, punishing ourselves in various ways for having feelings we consider unacceptable.

When a personality disorder is correctly identified, the tensions between the resident and others are now placed in a context where they can be understood. Staff are both challenged and encouraged by this diagnosis to try to understand the resident and to explore their own previously disavowed feelings and reactions. However painful, this exploration eventually reduces tension. It also leads to the development of a management plan that acknowledges the resident's unique set of needs and balances them with what staff can realistically provide.

Classifying Personality Disorders

If no two people have the same character, how can we develop a classification of personality disorders? We do know that certain personality traits are likely to occur together. A rigidly controlling person is more likely to be a perfectionist and a stickler for details than is an intensely dramatic and emotional individual. In the DSM-IV-TR, traits commonly encountered together are grouped to define the different personality disorders. Each personality diagnosis or grouping of traits is associated with a particular style of behavior, functional impairment, and kind of distress. To facilitate diagnosis, the personality disorders have been grouped into three clusters. There can be considerable overlap between different personality disorders, especially within one of the clusters and individuals can be diagnosed as having more than one personality disorder. Other individuals have clinically significant personality traits without meeting the diagnostic criteria for a full-blown disorder. A brief description of the different personality disorders is given in **Table 1**. Full diagnostic criteria for each of these disorders are listed in the DSM-IV-TR [1].

Table 1 Personality Disorders

Cluster A: Often Appear Odd or Eccentric to Others

Paranoid Personality Disorder
These individuals have a pervasive tendency to interpret the actions of others as deliberately demeaning or threatening. They do not trust other people and are reluctant to confide in them. They are easily slighted and bear grudges.

Schizoid Personality Disorder
These individuals have a pervasive pattern of indifference to social relationships and a restricted range of emotional experience and expression. They have no close friends, are cold and aloof, do not appear to have strong emotions and almost always choose solitary activities.

Schizotypal Personality Disorder
These individuals are acutely uncomfortable in close relationships. They have peculiar ideas, beliefs, and experiences such as clairvoyance, telepathy, and sixth-sense experiences. They may display eccentric behavior, speech, or appearance.

Cluster B: Behavior is Often Dramatic, Emotional, and Erratic

Antisocial Personality Disorder
Criteria for this disorder are more stringent that for other personality disorders. Individuals show evidence of a conduct disorder in childhood as indicated by a history of such things as truancy, running away, fighting, cruelty to animals, lying, stealing, etc. As adults they fail to conform to social norms, fail to honor obligations, are reckless, violate the rights of others, and lack remorse. They are unable to sustain consistent work behavior or function as a responsible parent.

Borderline Personality Disorder
These individuals show a pervasive pattern of instability of mood, interpersonal relationships, and self-image. Their relationships are intense and alternate between extremes of overidealization and devaluation. They are impulsive and prone to inappropriate, intense displays of anger. Suicidal threats, gestures, and self-mutilating behavior may occur.

Histrionic Personality Disorder
These individuals have a pervasive pattern of excessive emotionality and attention-seeking. They demand constant reassurance, approval, or praise. They may be inappropriately sexually seductive and exaggerated in their expression of emotion, while at the same time being self-centered and shallow.

Narcissistic Personality Disorder
These individuals show a pervasive pattern of grandiosity (in fantasy or behavior), lack of empathy, and hypersensitivity to the evaluation by others. They react to criticism with feelings of rage, shame, or humiliation (even if not expressed). They exploit others to achieve their own ends, believe themselves to be unique, special and entitled, and are preoccupied with feelings of envy.

Cluster C: Often Appear Anxious and Fearful

Avoidant Personality Disorder
These people show a pervasive pattern of social discomfort, fear of negative evaluation, and timidity. They are easily hurt by criticism and have no close friends. They avoid involvement with others unless they are certain of being liked and fear being anxious or embarrassed in front of people.

Dependent Personality Disorder
These individuals have a pervasive pattern of dependent and submissive behavior. They are unable to make everyday decisions or initiate activities on their own. They allow others to make their important decisions and agree with people even when they believe them to be wrong, because they fear being rejected or abandoned. They go to great lengths to avoid being alone.

Obsessive-Compulsive Personality Disorder
These individuals show a pervasive pattern of perfectionism and inflexibility. Their perfectionism interferes with task completion and they are overly preoccupied with details, rules, and schedules. They are excessively devoted to work, indecisive, overly conscientious, and restricted in the expression of affect. They want others to submit to exactly their way of doing things and may be unable to delegate.

Adapted from DSM-IV-TR, American Psychiatric Association, 2000.

The Development of a Personality Disorder

The question of how personality disorders arise has yet to be resolved. A growing body of theory and clinical data suggests, however, that early childhood deprivation, abuse, and neglect are important etiological factors. Why are infancy and early childhood so significant for future development? Very young human beings are neurologically immature and utterly dependent on those around them for survival. Their understanding of themselves and of others is just beginning to form. They are easily overwhelmed not only by the things that happen to them but also by the unmodulated intensity of what they feel.

Through countless interactions with caregivers, patterns are laid down. For children whose needs are usually understood and who come to expect a response attuned to those needs, the world gradually becomes a more predictable place. They gain confidence in their ability to manage their urges and longings, as well as in their capacity to adapt to an increasing range of challenges in their interactions with the world around them.

What happens to the child who is neglected or abused, whose longing for affection is rebuffed or who meets with an overstimulating, sexualized response? How are children affected when they are valued not for themselves but for what they can do, or when their self-esteem is relentlessly undermined? The development of these children is both thwarted and distorted. As a result of repeated failures, their capacity to manage or even identify their needs and impulses is impaired as is their trust in the people around them. Unmet needs which cannot be voiced or understood become the enemy. To avoid being overwhelmed as adults, some cling frantically to other people, overwhelming them instead. Some sexualize every interaction to become Don Juans and femmes fatales. Others try to satisfy their hunger through addictions; or they may disavow their needs altogether by martyring themselves to others or withdrawing into the splendid isolation of pseudo-self-sufficiency. These largely unconscious coping strategies constitute some of the symptoms of personality disorders. Later in life, the often rigid defensive structure that has developed leaves the individual ill-equipped to engage in satisfying relationships with others and vulnerable to breakdown under stress. Early world views, once established, are hard to modify. Just as it is more difficult for adults than for children to learn a foreign language, a new emotional language is also not easily acquired later in life.

We cannot predict what kind of personality disorder will result from any particular set of difficult childhood circumstances. We cannot even predict with certainty that unhappy children will develop a personality disorder. But we can say that the likelihood is greater. There are many different reasons why the environments in which people grow up fail to meet the criteria necessary for healthy development. These reasons range from a physical and/or emotional illness in caregivers to socioeconomic upheaval and war.

Apart from environmental variables, there may be genetic and other constitutional factors that predispose to the development of a personality disorder. The possibility that abnormalities in brain biochemistry underlie some of the symptoms is leading to an increasing focus on pharmacological interventions [2]. The notion that problems arise when an infant's temperament and particular needs do not "fit" well with what its environment can provide has also been explored. It is not possible to say, however, that there are any inherent factors that predispose to the development of a personality disorder.

The Impact of Aging

Aging is associated with many changes, and change is particularly difficult for those with personality disorders. As people age, they generally incur an increasing number of losses. Death of loved ones, loss of important roles, physical deterioration, and, in the case of nursing home residents, institutionalization all threaten a person's sense of self. To mourn these major losses without succumbing to hopelessness and despair requires strengths many people with personality disorders do not possess. The individual's usual means of defending against loss may be curtailed by ill health and changes in mobility and financial status. The socialite can no longer ward off loneliness by entertaining extravagantly. Flights from reality involving drug abuse, sexual promiscuity, or traveling become less feasible. As the aging body becomes a focus of concern, emotional distress may be expressed increasingly in somatic terms. Age- and illness-related changes in brain biochemistry are sometimes an additional complication, affecting the expression of the personality disorder.

Elderly people all have to redefine their role in relation to others, a challenge that involves letting go of cherished aspects of the self: What it meant, for example, to have been a boss, a teacher, a valued employee, or manager of a large household. Many have to turn increasingly to others to survive. Individuals with personality disorders, having problems in their interpersonal relationships, often lack the kind of support network that would allow them to continue to function in the community. Even if such networks exist, these individuals may have difficulty acknowledging a need for help. To do so would recall the failures of the early environment. Individuals with paranoid or schizoid tendencies may become reclusive, reject all assistance, and end up living in appalling conditions that sometimes lead to enforced institutionalization. At the other extreme, those prone to helpless panic rapidly exhaust their community resources. For these reasons, individuals with personality disorders are often less able than others to continue living in the community in the face of disability. As a result, they may be overrepresented in the nursing home population.

The Impact of Institutionalization

Moving into a long-term care setting is an extremely stressful experience often provoking intense feelings of loneliness and abandonment. For people with personality disorders, the difficulties of this process are compounded by their vulnerabilities. Bombarded by the sights, sounds, and smells of aging and thus reminded of their own aging and mortality, they are at the same time put in a situation of enforced dependency and intense, frequent interpersonal contact that resembles family life.

Direct caregivers provide daily intimate physical care requiring intrusions into privacy reminiscent of the nurturing care provided by a mother. For some residents, such care can arouse unconscious rage, grief, and disappointment at never having received the nurturing they craved. For others, caring may evoke feelings of shame, humiliation, and mistrust or precipitate regression and helplessness. The emotional demands of institutionalization may cause vulnerable residents to intensify their reliance on characteristic behavior patterns that give rise to symptoms and interpersonal conflict with staff and other residents. Unaware of their own contribution to their problems, these residents will blame those on whom they are now most dependent – the care providers.

Diagnosing Personality Disorders in the Long-Term Care Setting

A new resident enters the institution. What factors might alert staff to the possible presence of a personality disorder? There may be clues in the history. Childhood experiences of abuse or severe disruption in the continuity of parenting are often associated with problematic personality development. A history of difficulties in interpersonal relationships or an absence of connections to others is often present. Work histories can also provide useful information. Sometimes it is possible to get a sense from relatives or others that the person is "odd" or "difficult." It must be kept in mind, however, that such opinions are formed on the basis of many factors. Not all those judged by conventional norms as eccentric suffer from personality disorders.

As staff become familiar with the resident, certain persistent behavior patterns become apparent. What initially presents as the resident's conflict with a particular room-mate emerges as a pattern of failing to get along with any room-mate. Suspiciousness, inability to adapt to routines, excessive demands, rages, and difficulty establishing social contacts may all be symptoms of a personality disorder.

A personality disorder can also become apparent through powerful ways in which the resident affects others. Experienced clinicians learn to monitor their own feelings and behavior toward the individuals they work with. Strong, surprising, or unusual reactions are important diagnostic clues. When staff feel helpless or demeaned, when nothing they do for a resident is ever enough, or they find themselves consistently doing things the resident can do independently, then the question of a personality disorder should be raised.

In the case of a resident with borderline personality, the diagnosis sometimes becomes apparent when the treatment team finds itself split into feuding camps over how best to manage the resident's apparently insatiable needs. Some staff are experienced by the resident as allies, others as the enemy. When this phenomenon, termed splitting, is not recognized, staff begin to act out the roles in which the resident has cast them. Not surprisingly, chaos can ensue as staff members find themselves pitted against each other. The resident's care is compromised as staff fight among themselves.

Residents with personality disorders have been described in the professional literature as "difficult," "manipulative," "hateful," and "destructive." The feelings that these disturbed but vulnerable people evoke in those who work with them can cause staff to lose sight of and even disbelieve the fact that their behaviors are not intentional. Although they may be defined as maladaptive by the institution's standards, the behaviors represent the resident's attempt to cope. Defenses like splitting are unconscious and beyond the individual's ability to control at will.

Once a personality disorder has been identified, its manifestations become easier to recognize. Although the risk exists that these diagnostic terms may be used in a pejorative fashion to vent frustration and anger, establishing a diagnosis should lead to greater understanding and the development of a sound approach to management.

Differential Diagnosis

Care must be taken to identify other psychiatric disorders whose symptoms may overlap with those of personality disorders. Depression, which unlike a personality disorder often resolves with antidepressants, also interferes with a resident's interpersonal relations and ability to adapt. Suspicious residents or those with odd behavior may have a psychotic disorder responsive to antipsychotic medication. The rigid behavior, attacks of rage, and other symptoms associated with dementia can make it difficult to differentiate from a personality disorder without a careful history and cognitive assessment. Any of these other psychiatric disorders may coexist with a personality disorder leading to particularly difficult diagnostic and management challenges.

Management

General Considerations

Any development of a comprehensive treatment approach must begin with an understanding of the resident's limitations. Life-long patterns of behavior are deeply ingrained and exceedingly difficult to modify. To expect a resident who has been a loner all his life to adapt to an active schedule of group activities is not realistic. Those who have always been perfectionistic and governed by strict rules will not be able to "relax" or "let got" when their personal routines come into conflict with those of the institution. Someone who was never able to be sensitive to the feelings of others will not suddenly learn tolerance of and consideration for fellow residents. Residents who come with a history of having been impossible for their families will likely be impossible for staff.

Unrealistic expectations can result in feelings of alienation and abandonment on the part of the resident, and feelings of anger, frustration, and helplessness on the part of the staff. By setting more workable goals, staff strive to minimize tension while finding ways for the resident to coexist optimally with others in the institution. Several important aspects of management will be described in the following sections.

Clarity, Consistency, and Communication

One aspect of developing a management approach involves identifying problem areas and developing strategies to deal with them as described in Chapter 13, Behavior Management Strategies. Clarity is essential when working with this population. Only if the treatment goals are clearly articulated and documented will staff have an opportunity to evaluate various approaches without losing their sense of direction.

Although staff must be flexible in acknowledging a resident's problems and defining their expectations, once a particular treatment direction has been chosen, consistency is important. For example, if a decision is made to respond to a particular resident's need for control by allowing her some choice around certain aspects of daily care, the areas of choice must be clearly specified and consistently communicated to the resident, lest a battle for control develop around other issues such as medications and smoking.

There must be extensive communication among staff in order for the management plan to be applied consistently. This involves charting plans, communicating approaches to consultants who are not familiar with the situation, and reporting between shifts. Particularly in cases where the potential for splitting is high, communication must extend to all those involved, including family and administrative staff. Special meetings may have to be scheduled. The resident, also informed about aspects of the plan, may become a willing ally if the plan is felt to be a means of achieving desirable common goals. Even when such an alliance is not possible, clear and consistent communication to the resident of staff intentions is essential.

Staff Support

Most of us need to have some sense that the work we do is valued by others. Being compassionate, caring, and helpful are all part of being a caregiver. The meaning and fulfillment we derive from our role depends to some extent on confirmation from those around us that we are doing a good job. Residents with personality disorders often fail to give us the appreciation we may expect, deserve, and need. Instead, they demean, accuse, demand, and seem oblivious to our efforts. Those providing direct physical care have to cope with these reactions on a daily basis. Nondirect caregivers may become the recipients of a litany of complaints about the direct caregivers. This can lead to divisiveness among staff as the team is split along professional lines. Typically, nursing staff are pitted against physicians, social workers, and administrative staff. Staff meetings, by providing an opportunity for interdisciplinary communication, can foster greater understanding of the resident's impact on care and care providers.

Understanding the Role of Psychoactive Medications

In the face of the stress of caring for these residents, it can be tempting to seek "magical" solutions for complex problems. Physicians may feel pressure to "do something" in response to a sense of helplessness, urgency, or angry frustration in themselves or staff. A prescription for a psychoactive medication, however appealing, rarely resolves the problems and may complicate the situation. Apart from producing side effects and possibly leading to addiction, the medication may become a powerful symbol to the resident. While the medication represents a sign of caring for some, others interpret it as evidence they are being controlled, silenced, or dismissed as "mental cases."

There are, nevertheless, situations where the use of medications can be helpful. Whenever another psychiatric disorder is superimposed on a personality disorder, the acute illness must be treated in the usual manner, even as staff keep in mind that taking medication is an aspect of relating to others and can become a focus of conflict. Less commonly, the symptoms of the personality disorder itself may be an indication for using medication. Extreme anxiety, agitation, or occasionally even psychotic symptoms can be precipitated by stressful events. A brief course of anxiolytic or antipsychotic medication can help to reduce these symptoms and restore a sense of control to the resident. The use of long-term pharmacotherapy to manage specific aspects of different personality disorders such as impulsivity and dysthymia remains under investigation [2].

The Use of Psychotherapy

Where resources permit, the use of formal psychotherapy can be considered. Experience and skill are necessary in deciding when psychotherapy may be helpful, and if so, what kind of psychotherapy is indicated. When used inappropriately, insight-oriented therapy can be experienced as very intrusive or exacerbates an already difficult situation by uncovering needs and longings that cannot be met. Evidence supports the use of approaches focused on symptom relief and improved adaptation using a variety of supportive, cognitive, behavioral, and interpersonal techniques with the judicious use of insight [2]. Expecting major shifts in life-long personality patterns through psychotherapy is usually not realistic. Yet even modest successes can make an enormous difference to the resident, family, and caregivers.

Case Illustration

Mrs. A., a gaunt 80-year-old resident with chronic obstructive pulmonary disease, led a chaotic life characterized by interpersonal difficulties and disappointment in those around her. She berates and demeans her two daughters for not visiting or caring enough. Although the younger daughter, confined to a wheelchair, visits when she can, Mrs. A. is unable to appreciate the effort. Her relationship with her elder daughter is characterized by demands that her daughter intervene and insist that the administrators of the institution accede to Mrs. A.'s every wish.

The daughters tell staff their mother left them with their grandmother, in order that she might travel the globe with her husband. The marriage was chaotic. When infidelity eventually led to separation, Mrs. A. threatened suicide and took an overdose of medication. Yet Mrs. A. idealizes the relationship describing it as "special, like no other marriage; he adored me." Unable to maintain a steady job because of her explosive reaction to any criticism, Mrs. A. was barely able to make a living after the separation. Although clever and articulate, she alienated those around her by demanding their undivided attention and blaming them when things went wrong. Angry and alone, demanding more than the family could provide, she was admitted into a long-term care facility.

Her pattern of relating is replicated with the staff. She hurls insults at them and comments in a demeaning and derogatory fashion on appearance, race, and ethnic background. No staff member escapes her anger. She often refuses to be bathed, forgetting that she had agreed to a particular schedule earlier. She accuses staff of preferring other residents over her. She makes demands incessantly and attempts to keep staff in her room with numerous requests for assistance. She charges staff with taking belongings she has misplaced, but will not allow them to tidy her room. She pits staff against one another, alternating praise with criticism. Staff are never sure where they stand with her, and no one wants to be assigned to provide her care.

Comment

Mrs. A.'s manner of relating to others, her affective instability and her history of self-harm are typical of borderline personality disorder. The diagnosis helps caregivers understand that her behavior is not new or purposefully directed at them, and that they did not provoke her responses because they are inept. At this point, staff need assistance in containing and responding to Mrs. A.'s behavior. The following can be considered:

1. Providing consistent caregivers as opposed to rotating assignments involving the whole team, will give Mrs. A. the opportunity to begin to develop a relationship with a few of the staff. Because Mrs. A. is so difficult to work with, thought and discussion must take place within the team before the new approach is implemented.

2. The plan of care should be structured so that all staff can agree upon it and will follow it in a consistent manner. Posting a copy of the care plan in Mrs. A.'s room and having a copy readily available in the nursing station will ensure that it will be used on a daily basis and provide staff with the structure they need when caring for Mrs. A. If it is presented to Mrs. A. in a constructive rather than a punitive manner, the care plan may be reassuring to her, and serve as a concrete sign that she is not being abandoned.
3. As part of the care plan, the verbal abuse may be targeted for behavior management using the techniques described in Chapter 13. Based on their assessment of the behavior, whenever Mrs. A. yells, screams, insults, and makes racial remarks towards staff, she is told that they will leave the room until she is in control, at which time they will return to continue her care.
4. To help reduce the tendency for splitting, whenever Mrs. A. attempts to talk about one staff member to another, she is gently told to redirect her remarks to the caregiver she is discussing. If she continues, the staff member leaves the room until she stops.
5. Administration should be informed of the plan of care and asked to support it by redirecting complaints back to the unit providing the care. Meetings between Mrs. A.'s family and administration should always include a representative from the team providing the care.
6. The daughters can be assisted in setting appropriate limits on their contact with Mrs. A. by involving them as part of the team effort to cope with Mrs. A.'s needs.

Case Illustration

Mrs. B, a beautiful 85-year-old woman, is described by her daughter as always needing to be the most important person in the family. She remembers how both she and her father struggled to prove to Mrs. B. how much they loved her. Later, Mrs. B. was unable to be genuinely interested in her grandchildren, seeing them as competition for her daughter's time and attention. Living in an long-term care facility where she is one of many residents is difficult for Mrs. B. She is easily offended and reacts to perceived insults vigorously by screaming or refusing to do what is asked of her. She demands instant gratification of her needs, constant flattery, and insists she is not "like those others with no brains," but "of a superior class." She places great emphasis on her beauty and has a portrait of herself on her bedroom wall to which she constantly refers. She refuses to look in the mirror. Mrs. B. has cognitive deficits. She is often unaware that her clothes are soiled and that she needs bathing. She sometimes resists care, insulting and hitting out at staff. At other times, she flatters staff and cooperates with them. Because Mrs. B. is so unpredictable and difficult to work with, staff have come to believe that she is a nasty self-centered old woman who makes their lives miserable on purpose.

Comment

Mrs. B.'s sensitivity to criticism, her need to be special, her sense of entitlement, and her disregard for others characterize her as having a narcissistic personality disorder. It is difficult for staff to understand that her behavior is not purposeful but a function of her dementing process superimposed on a personality that feels entitled to be treated as a special person. Management is based on the understanding that underlying her need to emphasize her superiority and beauty is a deep-seated fear of worthlessness.

1. Given Mrs. B.'s vulnerability in the face of multiple assaults on her fragile sense of self, staff can help her by supporting her defenses. This could involve encouraging her to talk about her past accomplishments or discussing her clothes, her picture, and other areas of interest that give her pleasure. Pushing Mrs. B. in the direction of facing truths about her aging and decline would overwhelm her already tenuous ability to hold onto a positive image of herself. What might be construed in a less vulnerable individual as coming to terms with painful realities, would in Mrs. B.'s case likely lead to despair, anger, and an exacerbation in interpersonal difficulties.
2. Understanding that Mrs. B.'s feelings about herself, and her ability to accept the care she needs, fluctuate with her self-esteem, will prepare staff for Mrs. B.'s unpredictability. In this case, the unpredictability is also a function of cognitive difficulties. In order to maintain consistency, the management plan should anticipate conflicts by spelling out, for example, how staff can respond in case Mrs. B. refuses a certain aspect of care. As in the previous case, certain behaviors may be targeted for modification.
3. As in Mrs. A.'s case, Mrs. B. will benefit from continuity and consistency in caregivers. Gradually she may begin to build relationships in which she can feel safe with a few of the staff. Through such relationships, staff may begin to understand Mrs. B. a little better. For example, Mrs. B.'s consistent battle over bathing might be reassessed when it becomes known that she never liked to be touched and that she never bathed except in absolute privacy. Using this knowledge, bubble bath and perfumed soap could be added to the bathing routine. Staff could make sure to turn their backs as much as safety will allow. Although with these changes Mrs. B.'s aggression may decrease, it would be unrealistic to expect it to go away.

Case Illustration

Mrs. C., an 82-year-old widowed woman, currently lives in the long-term facility that a decade earlier she had visited every day for 4 years until her husband died. Although at the time her children and others encouraged her to take time for herself she was unable to do so. She felt she would be criticized for being a bad wife and said that her husband cried whenever she raised the issue of not coming in the next day.

Mrs. C. was admitted to residential care after she broke her hip. Although competent, she gave her daughter financial power of attorney, feeling she did not want to make decisions about selling her home or managing her money. Since admission, Mrs. C. has been disappointed that staff encourage her to be independent in activities of daily living. She experiences this as staff "not caring" about her or "being lazy."

She has a long history of depression. She tells staff she had a very hard life and "never a happy day." Whenever she is alone she becomes "very nervous." She often mistakenly refers to he daughter as "my mother."

She has some problems with recent memory and worries about becoming like the others who have "lost their minds." She is aware of her need for others and says that, "being between people helps." She goes to craft class and recreation programs and likes to knit when alone.

No amount of family contact diminishes her wish to be with them or her feeling that she is neglected by them. This way of relating to others is replicated in her relationship with the staff. She is disappointed in the direct caregivers whom she perceives as not doing enough for her. Yet she does not tell them this directly, feeling that they will reject her if she does. Instead she becomes unhappy and irritable, expressing her distress in the form of physical symptoms.

Comment

Mrs. C. has a dependent personality disorder. Her behavior is characterized by dependency, submissiveness, and an inability to make important decisions on her own. Her attachments to others have a clinging, helpless quality. She is unable to tolerate being alone. Helping Mrs. C. involves the following:

1. An assessment of Mrs. C.'s needs would identify clearly those areas in which she needs assistance, while functions that she can carry out independently will become apparent. Care can then be planned to ensure that Mrs. C. receives help where she needs it. By coming to Mrs. C.'s assistance before she asks for help, staff can begin to build for Mrs. C. a sense that her needs are being taken seriously and attended to promptly.
2. Sharing the results of the needs assessment with Mrs. C. is an important aspect of this approach, because it establishes clearly those areas in which Mrs. C. will be expected to function independently. Whenever Mrs. C. requests help around one of these functions, staff can remind her gently of the assessment and assist her in finding ways to overcome the problem on her own.
3. Mrs. C.'s tendency to somatize (i.e., to express her distress in the form of physical symptoms) can present a significant management challenge. Even though staff recognize that when Mrs. C. says "I feel weak, my head is spinning and I can't breathe," she is unconsciously voicing her fear of being alone, staff cannot dismiss these symptoms without investigating them. In giving her the concern and caring she craves through the investigation, staff unfortunately reinforce Mrs. C.'s tendency to somatize. Particularly in the elderly such patterns can be difficult to avoid. Investigations can, however, be done in a judicious and conservative manner once staff become more familiar with Mrs. C.'s symptoms. Moreover, by linking crises such as her daughter's holidays with an escalation in Mrs. C.'s physical symptoms, staff can anticipate problems. It may be possible to modify the approach during difficult periods by, for example, spending a little extra time with Mrs. C. and acknowledge her feelings about her daughter.
4. Mrs. C.'s character structure and behavior may be difficult to differentiate from depression and may predispose her to developing clinical depression. A trial of antidepressant therapy may be considered, even in situations where depressive symptoms appear to be very long-standing.

References

1. American Psychiatric Association. (2000). Diagnostic and statistical manual of mental disorders (4th Ed. – Text Revision). Washington, DC: American Psychiatric Association.
2. De Leo, D., Scocco, P., Meneghel, G. (1999). Pharmacological and psychotherapeutic treatment of personality disorders in the elderly. International Psychogeriatrics, 11(2):191–206.

Suggested Readings

1. American Psychiatric Association. (2000). Diagnostic and statistical manual of mental disorders (4th Ed. – Text revision). Washington, DC: American Psychiatric Association.
   Provides comprehensive listing of the criteria by which personality disorders can be diagnosed.
2. Adshead, G. (1998). Psychiatric staff as attachment figures. Understanding management problems

in psychiatric services in the light of attachment theory. British Journal of Psychiatry, 172:64–69.
Explores the nature of attachments patients (residents) make to the staff working with them. Discusses staff response and implications for management.

3. Groves, J.E. (1978). Taking care of the hateful patient. New England Journal of Medicine, 298:883–887.
This classic paper provides an excellent and readable discussion of the problem of the individual with a personality disorder within the institutional setting, with special emphasis on patient–staff dynamics.
4. Sadavoy, J. (1987). Character disorders in the elderly: An overview. In J. Sadavoy, M. Leszcz (Eds.), Treating the elderly with psychotherapy (pp. 175–227). Madison: International Universities Press, Inc.
Provides a more in depth look at personality disorders in the elderly, highlighting the problems seen in borderline and narcissistic personality disorders.

9 Alcohol Use and Misuse

Ken Schwartz

Key Points

- Alcohol use by nursing home residents can have beneficial or detrimental effects.
- To maximize the benefits and to minimize the harm, nursing homes must implement alcohol policies that take into account their obligation to meet residents' social, emotional, and psychological needs while also ensuring the safety and well-being of their residents.

Historically, society has placed little emphasis on the aged and their mental health needs [1]. The importance of alcoholism as a mental health problem in the elderly is also not adequately recognized [2]. The misuse of alcohol remains a common but often overlooked, potentially preventable cause of morbidity and mortality among residents in nursing homes [3]. This is unfortunate because nursing homes are in the position to be an important component in the provision of mental health care to an increasingly frail and aging resident population with a multitude of medical, cognitive, social, and psychiatric problems, some of them alcohol related.

The use and misuse of alcohol among nursing home residents is probably underestimated. Figures from the United States have shown prevalence rates of alcohol misuse ranging from 2.8 to 15 percent. The highest rates of active alcoholism are in nursing homes with a population of male veterans, while lower figures exist in other long-term care facilities [4]. The estimated prevalence of problems in these facilities is significantly lower than that in the community, which is probably an artifact of study methodology and is associated with an underdiagnosis of problems [5]. The Diagnosis and Statistical Manual of Mental Disorders (DSM-IV-TR) has criteria for five categories of alcohol use disorders [6] (see **Table 1**). The categories include the need for academic, occupational, marital, legal, or social dysfunction to be present for a diagnosis to be made. Criteria that emphasize the need for occupational and social disability have little relevance in establishing a diagnosis of alcohol dependence for a retired nursing home resident with few social contacts [7].

Table 1 DSM-IV-TR Categories of Alcohol Use Disorders

Category	Definition
Dependence	At least three of the following: Tolerance; withdrawal symptoms; impaired control; preoccupation with acquisition and/or use; persistent desire or unsuccessful efforts to quit; sustains social, occupation, or recreational disability; or use continues despite adverse consequences
Abuse	At least one of the following: Fails to fulfill occupational or social obligations due to drinking; use occurs in physically hazardous situations or leads to recurrent legal problems; or use continues despite persistent social or interpersonal problems
Harmful use	Evidence that use is causing adverse consequences (physical or psychological harm)
Hazardous use	Quantity and/or pattern of use that places patients at risk for adverse consequences
Heavy drinking	Quantity of consumption that exceeds a defined threshold

Adapted from DSM-IV-TR, American Psychiatric Association, 2000.

Who Is at Risk?

Nursing homes can expect two groups of problem drinkers who may be differentiated by the onset of the disorder [8]. The life-long alcoholic, typically male, experiences a chronic and debilitating natural course with significant biopsychosocial problems. The late-onset drinkers more commonly experience stressors such as caregiver burden, loss of spouse, health problems, or depression prior to the onset of their drinking problems. They are less likely to have a family history of alcoholism or personal psychopathology.

Elderly alcoholics rarely identify themselves as addicts, instead focusing on physical or psychiatric symptoms [9]. These individuals inevitably are in denial about having an addiction or even a problem. Their drinking may occur with or without the knowledge of nursing home staff and administration, within or outside the facility.

The Recognition and Identification of Alcohol Problems in the Nursing Home

The recognition of elderly problem drinkers is a challenge for various reasons (see **Table 2**) [10, 11]. Many older alcoholics do not conform to the stereotype of late-stage alcoholics who are male and disheveled [12]. Instead they have a better socioeconomic background and work history, and a previously active social life.

Table 2 Challenges to the Recognition of the Nursing Home Resident with Alcohol Problems

- Many different types of alcohol-related presentations in the elderly
- Collusion of families
- Therapeutic nihilism
- Lack of assessment questionnaires
- Poor documentation of previous alcohol-related problems
- Limited education of nursing home staff
- Inadequacy of teaching on alcohol addictions in medical school and psychiatric curricula
- Infrequent requesting or unavailability of psychiatric consultation

Case Illustration

Mrs. C. was happily married for 55 years until her husband suddenly passed away three years previously. She said, "I miss him terribly. He was my life." Her loneliness was compounded by her only child being busy with his own family. As well, her arthritis limited her ability to leave the house. Initially Mrs. C. began using alcohol to help her sleep. Her son, now concerned about this new alcohol problem and his mother's increasing medical problems, arranged for her to move into a nursing home.

Comment

Mrs. C. is an example of a late-onset problem alcohol user. There is no previous personal or family history of alcohol misuse. When approached by her son and health care providers, she readily acknowledged both drinking too much and the need for help. Mrs. C. is fortunate that her son recognized the problem, because with social isolation problematic drinking may go undetected.

Case Illustration

Mr. B., a man with a history of interpersonal conflicts moved into the nursing home with various medical problems. His history included alcohol-related hospitalizations and an alcohol-related mild dementia. Mr. B. was once a high functioning executive who enjoyed managing others. In the nursing home, he struggled with staff who he believed were not respecting and listening to him. His drinking increased as he grew more frustrated. Following another alcohol-related hospital admission, he was seen in psychiatric consultation. He clearly stated, "I am an adult, I should be allowed to drink. I need some pleasure in what you call my home." Mr. B.'s drinking continued and his medical health worsened.

Comment

Mr. B. was unable to acknowledge the role he played in alienating others. Although able to previously work effectively, his drinking contributed to a divorce and a strained relationship with his adult children.

He tried to curtail his drinking upon entry into the nursing home, but struggled with the loss of control and independence associated with illness, aging, and institutional living. He insisted that his return to drinking, while exacerbating his medical and interpersonal problems, provided him with some solace.

Case Illustration

Mrs. A. was admitted to the nursing home with a left hemiparesis following a stroke. Although cognitively intact, she denied previous problems with alcohol that were documented on her chart. She participated in activities, but complained bitterly when her needs were not met. Subsequently, she would get drunk causing problems for both other residents and staff. The nursing home staff did not know where she was getting her alcohol. It was assumed she was getting it either from other residents whom she would pay to bring back alcohol, from family members, or from a private company that provided home delivery of alcohol.

Social work and psychiatric interventions were both unsuccessful. Mrs. A. made it clear that she did not want to stop drinking. Instead she focused solely on the pleasures associated with alcohol. She did not connect her complaints and alcohol use to a possible underlying depression. Her choice was a transfer to another facility.

Comment

Mrs. A. is typical in her complaining about other matters while denying, rationalizing, or minimizing alcohol misuse. The nature of denial in addictions makes it almost impossible to accurately evaluate some patients. The presence of depressive symptoms is difficult to assess in Mrs. A. If indicated, the use of antidepressant medication would have to be monitored carefully because of the risk of adverse interactions between alcohol and other medications. Health care providers must keep in mind that elderly adults are significantly more likely to have a dual psychiatric diagnosis compared with younger adults [13].

Therapeutic Use of Alcohol in Nursing Homes

It is expected that in the future there will be an increase in the number of older adults with well-established drinking patterns who move into nursing homes. While alcohol use carries the potential of being beneficial, its detrimental impact on social and physical functioning must be kept in mind. For example, while alcohol can be used to increase interpersonal relations, it can also be misused to self-medicate for pain control or as an ineffective antidote to depression and loneliness [14]. Misuse can result in addiction. The therapeutic use of alcohol in nursing homes remains controversial because these facilities have a dual mandate to provide a home-like environment while also promoting a safe environment for all of its residents [3]. Unfortunately, many facilities have been careless in allowing even residents with alcohol problems to participate and drink during happy hours [5].

Screening

Physicians must ask residents questions about the frequency and quantity of alcohol consumption while maintaining a level of skepticism and corroborating what they are told with others who know the resident well [8]. In other words, self-reported consumption is not sensitive in detecting alcoholism [15].

The use of formal screening tests pertaining to the effect of alcohol on the individual's life, health, and behavior increases the detection of alcoholism and perform well among older adults and nursing home residents [16]. Both the CAGE and MAST-G screening questionnaires have a high sensitivity and specificity with respect to a nursing home population [4]. For practical purposes, the CAGE screening instrument is especially brief, user friendly, and consists of only four questions (see **Table 3**) [17].

Table 3 CAGE Questionnaire

1.	Have you ever felt that you should **cut** down on your drinking?	C
2.	Have people **annoyed** you by criticizing your drinking?	A
3.	Have you ever felt bad or **guilty** about your drinking?	G
4.	Have you ever had a drink first thing in the morning to steady your nerves or to get rid of a hangover ("eye opener")?	E

Any one "yes" answer increases identification of potential problems and should lead to suitable prevention or treatment interventions. Others recommend more serious clinical intervention only if two or more "yes" answers occurred because a score of 2 is considered to be evidence of alcoholism [18].

If the CAGE is positive then it may be useful to use the Michigan Alcoholism Screening Test – Geriatric Version (MAST-G). The MAST-G is a 24 item yes or no scale used to diagnose alcohol problems in older adults [19] (see **Table 4**). A score of 5 or more "yes" answers indicates an alcohol problem.

Treatment of the Alcoholic Nursing Home Resident

Most nursing home residents with a history of alcoholism are admitted from another health care facility, so severe alcohol withdrawal occurs less commonly in the nursing home than in the acute care hospital [20]. Minor withdrawal symptoms may be treated symptomatically in the nursing home [3]. It is recommended that any newly admitted resident with a history of active alcohol dependence within the previous two years be treated with vitamins and appropriate nutritional supplements [5]. Continued alcohol use is problematic as it could result in unwanted interactions with medications, compound mental health problems such as depression or cognitive impairment, or create behavioral problems [21].

The family should be involved in obtaining a clinical history and at the same time be

Table 4 Michigan Alcoholism Screening Test – Geriatric Version

	Yes (1)	No (0)
1. After drinking, have you ever noticed an increase in your heart rate or beating in your chest?	___	___
2. When talking with others, do you ever underestimate how much you actually drink?	___	___
3. Does alcohol make you sleepy, so that you often fall asleep in your chair?	___	___
4. After a few drinks, have you sometimes not eaten or been able to skip a meal because you didn't feel hungry?	___	___
5. Does having a few drinks help decrease your shakiness or tremors?	___	___
6. Does alcohol sometimes make it hard for you to remember parts of the day or night?	___	___
7. Do you have rules for yourself that you won't drink before a certain time of the day or night?	___	___
8. Have you lost interest in hobbies or activities you used to enjoy?	___	___
9. When you wake up in the morning, do you ever have trouble remembering part of the night before?	___	___
10. Does having a drink help you sleep?	___	___
11. Do you hide your alcohol bottles from family members?	___	___
12. After a social gathering, have you ever felt embarrassed because you drank too much?	___	___
13. Have you ever been concerned that drinking might be harmful to your health?	___	___
14. Do you like to end an evening with a nightcap?	___	___
15. Did you find your drinking increased after someone close to you died?	___	___
16. In general, would you prefer to have a few drinks at home rather than go out to social events?	___	___
17. Are you drinking more now than in the past?	___	___
18. Do you usually take a drink to relax or calm your nerves?	___	___
19. Do you drink to take your mind off your problems?	___	___
20. Have you ever increased your drinking after experiencing a loss in life?	___	___
21. Do you sometimes drive when you have had too much to drink?	___	___
22. Has a doctor or nurse ever said they were worried or concerned about your drinking?	___	___
23. Have you ever made rules to manage your drinking?	___	___
24. When you feel lonely, does having a drink help?	___	___

Reproduced with permission from Blow, F. (1991). Michigan Alcoholism Screening Test – Geriatric Version (MAST-G). Ann Arbor, MI: University of Michigan, Alcohol Research Center.

informed of the diagnosis and the dangers of continued alcohol use. Nonetheless, some families choose to continue supplying their loved one with drinks, not wanting to deprive them of what they believe is one of their last pleasures in life.

Treatment of alcohol abuse is considered complete for residents with significant cognitive impairment when the resident is medically stable and not drinking. If there is coexisting depression, agitation, or psychosis, suitable medications can be administered once it is shown that these psychiatric problems are not present just because of the use or abuse of alcohol [5].

The more cognitively intact residents should be offered a full range of individualized treatment options even though treatment of the elderly alcoholic remains a challenge. The traditional approach to treatment continues to emphasize confrontation of the denial which is thought to be a universal attribute of alcoholics [22]. The resident is unlikely to be able to attend Alcoholics Anonymous meetings in a nursing home and attendance at community meetings is often impractical because of transportation problems or physical and mental health impairments. Besides appropriate treatment of any comorbid disorder, it is therefore suggested that individual psychotherapy based on the 12-step model of Alcoholics Anonymous [23] be used to break down the resident's denial, minimization, defocusing, rationalization, and the family's enabling behaviors [5]. Family members can be referred for psychological assistance to deal with the anger, guilt, or other feelings related to past or continuing use of alcohol by their family member. A referral to Alanon may also be appropriate.

A more controversial approach to hazardous or harmful alcohol use is setting a treatment goal of decreased drinking versus complete abstinence. The choice of approaches is based on the severity of the problem and the likelihood of achieving success with either goal [7]. This alternate approach emphasizes the existence of a continuum of alcohol use and uses brief techniques of motivational interviewing. These techniques are based on the concepts of patient autonomy, ambivalence, and intrinsic motivation [24]. The resident and therapist work together to achieve a mutual goal. The therapist's aim is to explore the individual's ambivalent feelings about drinking without imposing any judgment or assumptions about it being a "problem." It is the drinker who identifies the problem areas or reasons for concern and change.

General components of successful brief interventions are described using the acronym FRAMES (see **Table 5**) [25]. Although not tested in the nursing home population, brief interventions resulting in decreased alcohol use and decreased use of health resources have been shown to occur in several different primary care settings [24].

The actual stages of behavioral change have been described (see **Table 6**) [26]. The therapist's task is to help the patient set achievable goals and move to the next stage of change.

Table 5 FRAMES – Components of Successful Brief Intervention

F	Provide feedback on drinking behavior
R	Reinforce patient's responsibility for changing behavior
A	State your advice about changing behavior
M	Discuss a menu of options to change behavior
E	Express empathy for patient
S	Support patient's self-efficacy

Table 6 Options for Change According to Stage of Change

Stage of Change	Options
Precontemplation	– List pros and cons of drinking and not drinking – Keep diary of alcohol use – Agree to think about drinking behavior
Contemplation	– Options listed in precontemplation – Consider trial of abstinence for 2–4 weeks – Read pamphlets – Attend educational program on effects of alcohol or drug use
Determination	– Discuss available treatment options – Review family and social supports for change – Set goals for level of use or abstinence
Action	– Implement behavioral change
Relapse	– Understand relapse as a learning experience – Reassess goals – Return to action plan – Consider more intensive treatment

Similarly, another therapeutic approach stresses a need for caregivers to follow nine guidelines to gradually help the alcoholic in denial bring into consciousness the painful aspects of reality related to their drinking (see **Table 7**) [12].

Table 7 Guidelines for Working Through Denial

- Remember what realities and associated feelings are being denied, repressed, and fought against on an unconscious level
- View resolution of denial as a lengthy process rather than an event to be undertaken and concluded in one or two sessions
- In early discussions about the severity of drinking, use nonstigmatized, noncharged language
- Provide factual information about the differences between use, abuse, and addiction
- Illustrate the progress of symptoms of alcoholism with incidents from the drinker's own life
- Express concern for the patient's physical and emotional safety
- Avoid guilt-inducing statements aimed at motivating the patient
- Encourage patients to engage in an abstinence or reduced drinking experiment to gather data about the extent of the problem
- Integrate work on drinking issues with other issues and concerns to the patient

For some problem drinkers, a change in environment as afforded by the social milieu of a nursing home can be helpful in meeting their needs for acknowledgment and respect. Being cared for can contribute to increased self-esteem and lessen the need for alcohol.

This approach is effective without the use of disulfiram (Antabuse) which is not recommended for older adults because of the fear that associated medical problems might make the use of the drug too dangerous [27].

It is important to keep in mind a wide range of treatment options because nursing home residents with a multitude of medical and cognitive problems vary in their ability to benefit from the more traditional treatment interventions. Fortunately, some residents will achieve abstinence with minimal intervention, while unfortunately others continue to drink despite much time and help from nursing home staff.

Nursing Home Policies

It is generally accepted that nursing homes should have written policies governing alcohol use in their facilities. Meetings with the resident council of elected resident representatives help address autonomy concerns [3]. Collaboration with all involved health care providers is also recommended for policy development and implementation. Physician participation will ensure that they do not feel rules are being imposed upon them. Nursing staff and healthcare workers are encouraged to describe their existing problems and frustrations in dealing with residents who are problem drinkers.

Certain questions should be considered in developing a policy for alcohol use in the nursing home (see **Table 8**) [3].

Table 8 Questions to Consider in Developing an Alcohol Policy

- What are the characteristics of the nursing home?
- Are alcohol problems prevalent among the residents?
- How will alcohol be provided to residents?
- Will the facility furnish alcoholic beverages, or simply allow residents to keep their own supply for private use?
- Will physician's orders be required?
- How will adverse events such as resident intoxication or behavioral problems be handled?
- If alcohol consumption is not allowed, how will this rule be enforced?

A recent study examined the alcohol policies and practices of 111 immediate care facilities and homes for elderly people in the northeastern part of the United States [14]. The authors concluded that despite the problems reported at these facilities, screening and treatment of alcohol problems and training of staff were not adequate [14].

Example of a Nursing Home Alcohol Policy

A nursing home in Toronto, Canada, finally acknowledged that some residents' problems had become too great to ignore and deny. They drafted the following policy:

> "There will be no alcohol without a physician's order. The limit is two drinks per day. This does not include alcohol offered during recreational programs. The resident's alcohol will be labeled and kept locked at the nursing station. The alcohol will be dispensed by registered staff" [11].

The nursing administrator opted to choose for two drinks per day in the home's policy because the literature on optimal alcohol consumption is unclear as to the actual difference between one and two drinks per day with respect to the emotional and physical health of nursing home residents.

The policy now recommends the use of the CAGE screening instrument and in some cases, the MAST-G questionnaire. A closer look at the biopsychosocial needs of the residents identified as drinkers has placed this home in a better position to curtail alcohol misuse. At admission, the policy is clearly stated to all individuals and their families. Any difficulties in complying with the rules, whether by residents or their families, are addressed. If problems continue, measures are taken such as curtailing visits of any family member who might bring back the resident in an intoxicated state or sneak bottles into the nursing home. In more serious cases, residents may be assisted in looking for a home more able to deal with, or tolerant of, their drinking problems. For example, a home having a locked unit permitting closer monitoring of the resident might be more appropriate. Finally, the home has implemented an ongoing educational process to better train the staff to deal with alcohol-related problems. Contracts with hospitals wishing to admit problem drinkers into this nursing home are also now in place so that if problems arise, the hospitals must agree to readmit the resident.

Ethical and Legal Matters

What if drinking meets a number of the resident's emotional and psychological needs? What if drinking is regarded as "the last pleasure" of the resident's life [14]? Guided by legal and ethical concerns, nursing homes require rules and regulations in order to ensure the safety and well-being of all residents. Should these rules be extended to include the use of alcohol, which for many is a social beverage? Those who view drinking as a social issue and not a medical one will question a physician's right to write an order to determine who can drink how much, and who cannot drink. On the other hand, for those who view alcohol as a psychoactive drug of abuse, drinking becomes a medical issue. The establishment of drinking rules is a challenge because nursing homes house both social and problem drinkers.

A nursing home is expected to attempt to treat a resident's health care needs, including alcohol dependency. However, if residents are still competent to determine their own interests, the principal of autonomy must supersede the nursing home's determination of what is best for those residents, because decisions regarding care should be guided by the resident's need, not the homes' interest [28].

Nursing homes should be guided by the doctrine of "least restrictive alternative" which directs the decision maker to make decisions that are least restrictive of an individual's freedom and most appropriate in the situation [28]. Alternatively, a give-and-take discussion between resident and health care providers that more or less "splits the difference" between the two conflicting positions could be considered [28]. Such an approach might work better with alcohol users who are in denial and who become oppositional when confronted with nursing home concerns or policies. In this way, they feel at least their point of view is being heard.

Varying opinions exist about what a model alcohol policy should be. The different cultural and religious practices of residents and staff may influence compliance with any policy that is implemented. For example, those who come from a background where much drinking is accepted or considered normal will object to what seems to them a ridiculously low limit of two drinks per day. Conversely, others who come from a background where drinking is frowned upon would prefer a lower limit. It would be unethical for staff members who hold such beliefs to ask someone to give up alcohol. On the other hand, would it be unethical if the medical staff or administration encourages someone whose behavior goes against the social mores of the facility to give up alcohol for the good of the larger community? Similarly, would it be unethical for a nursing home to ask or demand compliance with this alcohol policy from a private company that provides home delivery of alcohol orders? What if the resident is competent to place and sign for receipt of that alcohol order? Or, when a competent resident continues to drink against physician's advice, what kind of medical or psychiatric care is a staff obligated to provide?

Legal obligations of a nursing home recognize that nursing homes have a duty to exercise reasonable care and that what is reasonable varies with residents' abilities to look after their own safety [28]. In other words, there is room for the nursing home to use discretion and implement individualized care. Occasionally, legal "waivers of liability" are used so that in optimizing the resident's quality of life, the home is also protecting itself from being sued if problems occur. Nursing homes must ultimately remember that a combination of good programming and polices, an attentive, respectful staff, and an administration that is genuinely interested in hearing from residents all contribute to residents' feeling they are more in a home and less in an institution [11].

References

1. Kim, E., Rovner, B. (1996). The nursing home as a psychiatric hospital. In: W.E. Reichman, P.R. Katz (Eds.), Psychiatric Care in the Nursing Home (pp. 3–9). New York: Oxford University Press.
2. Hirata, E.S., Almeida, O.P., Funari, R.R., Klein, E.L. (2001). Validity of the Michigan Alcoholism Screening Test (MAST) for the detection of alcohol-related problems among male geriatric outpatients. American Journal of Geriatric Psychiatry, 9(1):30–34.
3. Joseph, C.L., Horvath, T. (1998). Alcohol and drug misuse in the nursing home. Journal of Mental Health and Aging, 4(2):251–269.

4. Joseph, C.L., Ganzini, L., Atkinson, R.M. (1995). Screening for alcohol use disorders in the nursing home. Journal of the American Geriatrics Society, 43:368–373.
5. Solomon, K., Shackson, J.B. (1996). Substance abuse disorders. In: W.E. Reichman, P.R. Katz (Eds.), Psychiatric Care in the Nursing Home (pp. 165–187). New York: Oxford University Press.
6. American Psychiatric Association. (2000). Diagnostic and statistical manual of mental disorders (4th Ed. – Text Revision). Washington, DC: American Psychiatric Association.
7. Reid, M.C., Anderson, P.A. (1997). Alcohol and other substance abuse. Medical Clinics of North America, 81(4):999–1016.
8. Liberto, J.G., Oslin, D.W. (1997). Early versus late onset of alcoholism in the elderly. In A.M. Gurnack (Ed.), Older adults' misuse of alcohol, medicines, and other drugs: Research and practice issues (pp. 94–112). New York: Springer Publishing.
9. Solomon, K., Manepalli, J., Ireland, G.A., Mahon, G.M. (1993). Alcoholism and prescription drug abuse in the elderly. St. Louis University Grand Rounds. Journal of the American Geriatrics Society, 41:57–69.
10. Christie, D. (1997). Alcohol abuse in the elderly: Making a difference. Canadian Journal of Canadian Medical Education, 9:101–114.
11. Schwartz, K.M., Lasky, N. (2002). The development and implementation of an alcohol policy in a nursing home: Overcoming denial. Journal of Geriatric Psychiatry, 35(2):151–167.
12. Amodeo, M. (1990). Treating the late-life alcoholic: Guidelines for working through denial integrating individual, family, and group approaches. Journal of Geriatric Psychiatry, 23(2):91–105.
13. Solomon, K., Stark, S. (1993). Comparison of older and younger alcoholics and prescription drug abusers: History and clinical presentation. Clinical Gerontologist, 12(3):41–56.
14. Klein, W.C., Jess, C. (2002). One last pleasure? Alcohol use among elderly people in nursing home. Health and Social Work, 27(3):193–203.
15. Midanek, L. (1982). The validity of self-reported alcohol consumption and alcohol problems: A literature review. British Journal of Addiction, 77:357–382.
16. Buchsbaum, R.G., Buchanan, R.G., Walsh, J., Cantor, R.M., Schnoll, S.M. (1992). Screening for drinking disorders in the elderly using the CAGE questionnaire. Journal of the American Geriatrics Society, 40:662–665.
17. Ewing, J.A. (1984). Detecting alcoholism. The CAGE questionnaire. Journal of American Medical Association, 252:1905–1907.
18. Mayfield, D.G., McLeod, G., Hall, P. (1974). The CAGE questionnaire: Validation of a new alcoholism screening instrument. American Journal of Psychiatry, 131:1121–1123.
19. Blow, F. (1991). Michigan Alcoholism Screening Test – Geriatric Version (MAST-G). Ann Arbor, MI: University of Michigan, Alcohol Research Center.
20. Rubenstein, L.Z., Ouslander, J.G., Wieland, D. (1988). Dynamics and clinical implications of the nursing home – Hospital Interface. Clinics of Geriatric Medicine, 4:471–491.
21. Atkinson, R.W. (1991). Alcohol and drug abuse in the elderly. In: R. Jacoby, C. Uppenheimer (Eds.), Psychiatry in the elderly (pp. 819–851). Oxford: Oxford University Press.
22. Fox, R. (1973). Treatment of the problem drinker by the private practitioner. In: P.G. Bourne, R. Fox (Eds.), Alcoholism: Progress in Research and Treatment (pp. 227–243). New York: Academic Press.
23. Alcoholics Anonymous. (1976). Alcoholics Anonymous, 3rd Ed. New York: Alcoholics Anonymous World Service.
24. Barnes, N.H., Samet, J.H. (1997). Brief interventions with substance-abusing patients. In: J.H. Cullen (Ed.), The medical clinics of North America (pp. 867–879). Philadelphia: W.B. Saunders.
25. Miller, W.R., Rollnick, S. (1991). Motivational interviewing preparing people to change addictive behavior. New York: Guildford Press.
26. Prochaska, J.O., Diclemente, C.C. (1983). Stages and processes of self-change of smoking: Toward an integrative model of change. Journal of Consulting Psychology, 51:390–395.

27. Sckuckit, M.A. (1990). Introduction: Assessment and treatment strategies with the late-life alcoholic. Journal of Geriatric Psychiatry, 23(2):83–89.
28. Priester, R. (1990). Leaving homes: Residents on their own recognizance. In R.A. Kane, A.L. Caplan (Eds.), Everyday ethics: Resolving dilemmas in nursing home life (pp. 155–164). New York: Springer Publishing Company.

Suggested Readings

1. Gurnack, A.M. (1997). Older adults' misuse of alcohol medicines, and other drugs. New York: Springer Publishing Company.

10 Sexuality and Sexual Behavior

Ken Schwartz, David Myran, and Marcia Sokolowski

Key Points

- Myths exist that elderly nursing home residents are "asexual."
- When these myths are challenged, nursing homes can design policies that facilitate the rights of residents to sexual expression while safeguarding vulnerable residents from exploitation or abuse.
- While rapid interventions are often demanded to manage sexual disinhibition, it is necessary to proceed systematically with a good understanding of the behavior before attempting appropriate behavioral or medication interventions.

Residents of nursing homes have physical, social, cognitive, emotional, and sexual needs that facilities attempt to address. However, sexual needs are not adequately being met leading to the neglect of an important aspect of emotional health and self esteem [1]. A review of the literature on the quality of life in older adults shows few studies regarding sexuality, and even fewer studies examining the sexual needs of nursing home residents [1]. Intimacy, sexuality, and sexual behaviors consequently remain some of the most sensitive and controversial health care issues in nursing homes [2]. When individuals enter nursing homes, their sexuality may become more public and staff and families both struggle with accepting that residents have the right to seek out and engage in sexual expression [3]. No mention is made of any right to privacy and sexual expression for individual residents in the Bill of Rights for residents of long-term care facilities in Ontario, Canada [4]. Regardless, it is suggested that sexuality is an integral part of human life throughout all stages of the life span [5]. The expression of sexuality in cognitively impaired residents, however, may result in behaviors that are difficult to manage.

Barriers to Sexual Expression for Cognitively Intact Residents in Nursing Homes

If it is true that an important component of a good quality of life for some nursing home residents includes having meaningful relationships and engaging in sexual activities, then it is important to recognize barriers to sexual expression. Physical changes associated with normal aging, medical illness, medication, anxiety, depression, and ageism all contribute to decreasing sexual interest and functioning among residents [6]. Conditions within the nursing home environment such as limited privacy, conflict with the personal values of staff and administration, and concerns about the consent of cognitively impaired residents

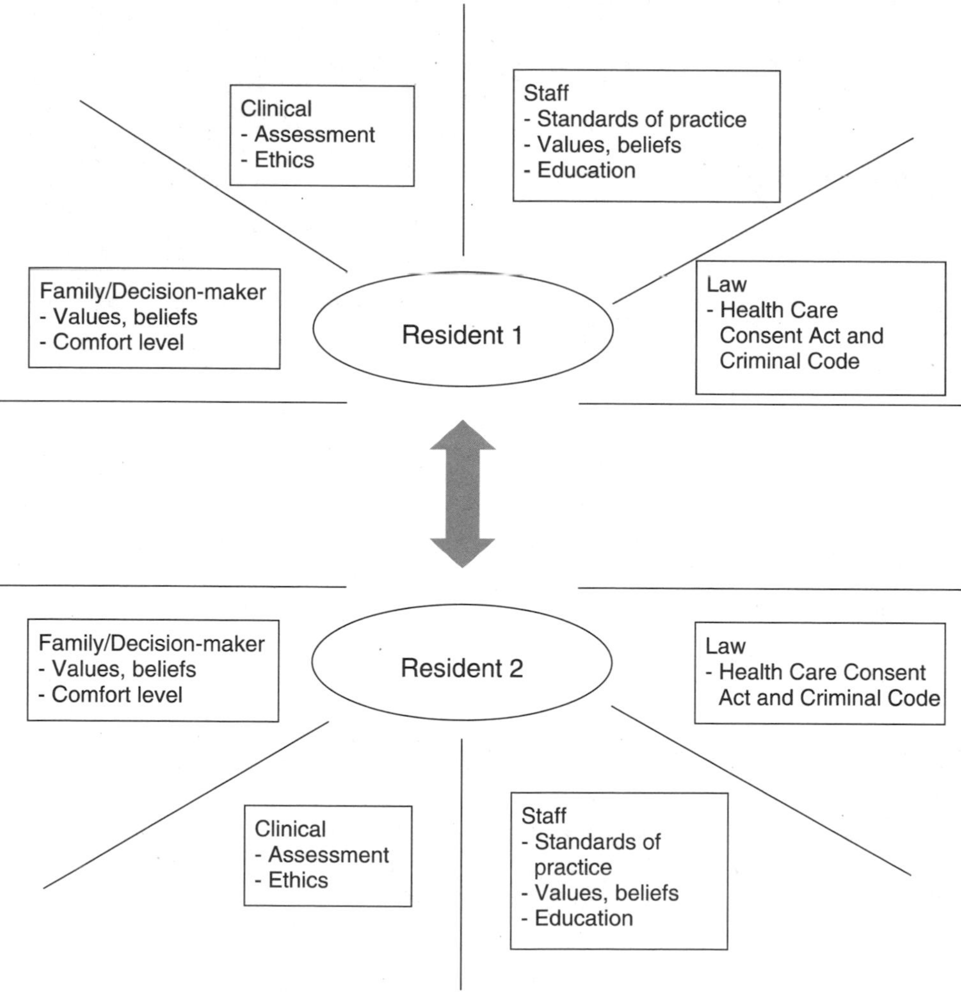

Figure 1 Issues Related to Sexuality in Long-Term Care

further restrain the sexuality of residents [7]. Institutions may respond to constraints placed by family members who believe seniors no longer have sexual interests. Or perhaps family members believe that their parents must remain forever faithful to their deceased spouses. It is the responsibility of nursing homes to address the various institutional, staff, resident, family, clinical, ethical, and legal issues (see **Figure 1**) [2].

Ethical Issues of Resident Rights Versus Concerns Over Resident Exploitation and Abuse

Often of great concern is the issue of competence and the resident's ability to consent to sexual activity with another person. The principle of protection is often cited when there is question about the resident's awareness of who the sexual partner is, and whether or not the resident's desire to have such a relationship is based upon a delusional belief (for example, a resident might be under the delusion, even occasionally, that her partner is her husband).

While these concerns would exist in the situation where both residents are cognitively impaired, the challenges are often exacerbated if there is a real or perceived difference between the two individuals' cognitive abilities, and there is a heightened risk of one resident exploiting the other (not to infer however that the potential of exploitation only occurs when there is a cognitive differential; one may be more emotionally vulnerable than another and thus at greater risk of harm, though we seem to focus more on the need to protect the "incompetent" person.

Case Illustration

Mrs. A., frail and tired from her caregiver role to her cognitively impaired husband, entered the nursing home shortly after her husband. The couple resided on separate floors because a room they could share was unavailable. Mrs. A., healthier and more mobile, spent most of the day visiting her husband but returned at night to sleep in a room she shared with another woman. Mrs. A. missed the "private time in and out of bed" that she once enjoyed with her husband. She believed she still would have this in a single room.

Comment

The issue of room allocation is vital because the nursing home room is the only personal place a resident or couple enjoys [8]. Physical intimacy goes hand in hand with emotional intimacy and commitment to lifelong caring for many married couples [9]. However, when a spouse is affected by cognitive impairment and loss of capacity for emotional intimacy, various responses in the healthier partner regarding sexuality may be seen. It is agreed when possible, that couples wishing to stay together be allowed to share private rooms [1]. The autonomy of all residents can still be respected by the communitarian allocation of rooms [9]. This entails the overriding of other residents' preferences be reserved only for situations of dire scarcity, such as couples being allowed to share a room [10]. Unfortunately, such rooms still lack space for a larger bed and a lock on the door. Privacy could be provided by putting up signs that say "do not disturb" [1], but these signs often attract attention or are not respected. Staff should therefore be reminded to first knock and wait for permission to enter the room in cases when safety is not an issue. Another option is having a "private room" at another location in the nursing home where couples could choose to "book time" for private meetings with their spouses or other partners [10].

Case Illustration

Mr. C., a 75-year-old widower of three years displays few residual symptoms of a minor stroke and is minimally cognitively and physically impaired. Mrs. D., a 73-year-old widow of five years and resident for one year, enjoys good physical health but has moderate Alzheimer's disease.

Mr. C., although tearful when asked about his late wife, did not speak of loneliness or looking for a partner. Upon meeting Mrs. D., he developed an obvious liking for her and began escorting Mrs. D. to activities. They soon held hands and he openly complemented her. She was quieter but enjoyed his attention. After a few months, they became engaged and wished to share a room.

In separate interviews, Mrs. D. stated "being engaged means we care for each other. I know I have Alzheimer's, but it's not that bad because I'm living with it." Mr. C. stated "I have worries about her health, but I can cope with it. She has Alzheimer's and forgets. She will forget more some day, but it won't stop me from loving her. She remembers she's engaged and we both want to share a room, with one bed if possible. We want to always be together. We kiss now, maybe one day we'll do more but I wouldn't touch her if she wouldn't want me to. I would respect her feelings."

Comment

Residents with dementia who wish for a romantic sexual relationship present a unique challenge to caregivers and institutions in terms of obligations for the resident's quality of life, safety, and well-being [11]. Staff initially found it "cute" that the couple spent time together holding hands. They only expressed concern when the couple announced their engagement and wish to share a room. They were particularly concerned about Mrs. D.'s capacity to give consent and shared these concerns with the families. Mr. C.'s daughters were supportive, while Mrs. D.'s son wished for the couple "to go slower" and not live together or get married.

Without the co-operation of staff and Mrs. D.'s son, the couple is no closer to sharing a room or getting married. Staff is concerned about the cognitive decline of Mrs. D. and wonder about transferring her to another floor one day. If so, they know they would be disregarding the couple's wish "to always be together." However, they worry that the level of care the couple might require means that one would be out of place if they remained on the same floor.

Case Illustration

Mrs. L., a 74-year-old woman with a six-year history of Alzheimer's disease has resided in a nursing home for four years since her husband died suddenly. She adjusted well to the nursing home, but her ability to consistently identify family members was waning and occasionally she was found roaming the hallways searching for her room.

Six months ago Mrs. L. met Mr. O., aged 78, a married man who had a wife hospitalized with severe dementia. He moved into the nursing home because he became lonely after her hospitalization and was requiring nursing support for heart problems. Cognitively he remained quite intact. Initially he seemed depressed and experienced difficulties initiating new friendships. His two sons visited weekly and were relieved to learn that recently their father's general mood was better. He had developed a budding friendship with Mrs. L., who increasingly sought him out. He seemed to respond positively to her warm and outgoing nature. Recently they took to walking the hallways together, arm in arm.

Last week the couple was discovered by a nurse in his room, lying on his bed. Partially disrobed, they were engaged in sexual exploration. The nurse immediately yelled for them to stop their activity, ordered them to dress, and promptly removed Mrs. L. from Mr. O.'s room, telling them both to behave themselves and ordering them to "never do that again!" Both were visibly shaken.

Comment

The nurse reported their behavior in a team meeting and expectedly there was a range of emotions and responses. Several staff felt very uncomfortable discussing the topic of sexuality, while others normalized the notion of residents desiring sexual activity and emphasized that their needs be respected by allowing for privacy rooms. In retrospect, the nurse reconsidered her angry spontaneous reaction and wondered whether her own personal values were being inappropriately placed upon the couple. Some staff suggested that guidelines be established. If so, there was unanimous agreement amongst all team members that certain cautions ought to be recognized, so that while residents would have their rights to consensual sexual activity respected, when appropriate, due vigilance would be applied to trying to balance these rights with the right to protection, as needed.

Mrs. L. and Mr. O.'s adult children were met with separately. Her two daughters were outraged to learn that their mother had engaged in sexual activity. They both believed the myth that seniors were "asexual," and determined that the fact that Mr. O. was still "okay in his mind" and that their mother was "clearly not" constituted evidence of his exploitation.

Mr. O.'s sons reacted differently. Both were delighted that their father's depression had lifted, and attributed this to his new romance. They argued against any claim of exploitation, believing that their father would never do such a thing, and that in fact they imagined that she must have been the initiator, as their dad was quite passive. One son however felt that their father's romance was disloyal to their mother, who, although cognitively impaired, was "very much our father's wife." He was ambivalent about what role, if any, the staff should play in either encouraging or discouraging their relationship, and ultimately felt it was his father's private business. The other son basically felt that their parents' marriage was "over and dead" since their mother was "no longer the same person who married our dad," in fact "incapable of being a wife" and thus their was no real relationship for their father to be disloyal to.

The Development and Implementation of a Policy on the Management of Normal and Inappropriate Sexual Behavior in the Nursing Home Setting

The wishes and values of staff, residents, and families often conflict when cognitively impaired residents express sexual wishes and needs. It is important that nursing homes develop a resident-oriented policy that balances the rights of residents with the missions and goals of their institutions so that vulnerable residents will be protected from unwanted sexual advances [6].

Initial Steps

Facilities can follow several steps in setting up policy guidelines. Initially, a team ideally comprised of a nurse, physician, social worker, administrator, family member, health care aide, and if possible, an ethicist meet and agree to read and discuss pertinent articles related to the topic, including sexual policies from other facilities [2]. This process encourages the identification of personal biases and openness. Often of great concern are the issues of competence and consent. Sexuality, intimacy, and sexual behaviors to be considered as normal or requiring assessment also need to be defined [2]. While it initially appears straightforward, it is difficult to formulate a clear definition of inappropriate sexual behavior which operationally has been defined as that which is judged inappropriate for the environment in which it occurs often as a function of the values, religious beliefs, and training of the staff. There is little agreement in the literature as to what constitutes sexually inappropriate behavior which makes it difficult to estimate the prevalence of the problem. Johnson [12] estimates that upwards of 7% of cognitive impaired elderly exhibit sexually disinhibited behaviors and that geriatric offenders account for 1.7% of all reported sex crimes. In contrast, others find that only 1.8% of residents in nursing homes exhibit inappropriate sexual behavior [13].

When a Potential Problem Occurs

When a sexual behavior of concern occurs, whether in an individual or in a couple, a three part process is suggested: A team meeting, a family meeting if necessary, and an ongoing assessment of the effectiveness of the initial plan to address any changes in the individual or the situation [6].

In the team meeting, the behavior is thoroughly documented and discussed as to what occurs, when, why, and who was involved (see **Table 1**) [14].

The assessment of the risks and benefits of the behavior must be weighed in view of other competing principles and values, including the right to privacy, the right to experience a loving relationship with another, the right to make one's own decisions even if others consider them to be "bad" ones. One must be careful not to project one's own religious, cultural, gendered, or personal beliefs onto another.

Table 1 Areas to Assess in Evaluating a Sexual Behavior Problem

- Describe and document the behavior accurately
  - What occurs, when, where, and how often?
  - Who (residents, staff, family, visitors) are the involved parties?
  - Who else (residents, staff, family) is indirectly affected?
  - What responses have staff observed in the participants?
- Consider the reactions of others (family, staff, visitors, other residents)
  - What are the reasons for their reaction ? Inconvenience, moral objections etc.
- Identify why the behavior is occurring
  - Who is initiating the behavior(s)?
  - What needs are being met?
  - What is the sexual history of participants? Is this behavior consistent with the way participants acted prior to the onset of dementia?
- Evaluate competency and consent
  - Are all participants willing? Is consensual behavior being demonstrated?
  - What is the competency status of participants? Is there legal incompetency and guardianship? What are the participants' abilities to express desires and wishes and/or issues, ability to make choices?
- Evaluate risks and benefits
  - What are the potential risks of allowing the behavior to continue?
  - What are the potential benefits for the participants if the behavior is allowed to continue?
  - Is anyone being exploited?
- Report team's assessment back to resident and their family

Types of Sexual Behaviors

There are four categories of sexual expression that all need to be assessed so it can be determined if interventions are necessary [15].

- *Level 1:* Intimacy, courtship behaviors: consensual kissing, hugging, fondling, and cuddling
- *Level 2:* Verbal sex talk: nonaggressive flirting or use of suggestive language
- *Level 3:* Physical sexual behaviors directed toward self or toward coresidents who are in agreement or masturbating or exposing oneself during personal care tasks
- *Level 4:* Unwanted overt sexual behaviors directed toward others

Interventions

The first three categories of sexually inappropriate behavior seldom require intervention that involves the use of medications, and can frequently be handled with behavioral interventions.

Physically sexual intimate behaviors involving two residents imply a moderate level of risk and staff must monitor for any signs of intimacy overtures that are unwelcome [15]. It is suggested that the following questions be asked to identify under what conditions and circumstances a relationship between coresidents be allowed and/or encouraged to continue [16].

1. Resident's awareness of the relationship
   (a) Is the resident aware of who is initiating sexual contact?
   (b) Does the resident believe that the other person is a spouse and thus acquiesce out of a delusional belief, or are they cognizant of the other's identity and intent?
   (c) Can the resident state what level of sexual intimacy they would be comfortable with?
2. Resident's ability to avoid exploitation
   (a) Is the behavior consistent with formerly held beliefs/values?
   (b) Does the resident have the capacity to say no to any uninvited sexual contact?
3. Resident's awareness of potential risks
   (a) Does the resident realize that this relationship may be time limited (placement on unit is temporary)?
   (b) Can the resident describe how they will react when the relationship ends?

Whether competency is an issue or not, there is a tendency to compare the current behavior and values of the resident with those that he/she previously held and displayed. If discordant, there is a general tendency to interpret the difference as evidence that the resident is not "acting as him- or herself" and would be appalled to learn about his/her aberrant behavior. However, it can be argued that the changed beliefs and/or values that residents might be experiencing in the present ought to be respected, with a view to acknowledging that we do shift our beliefs and values, and that it would be unfair to assume that the beliefs and values held later on in life, even while "incompetent" should be accorded with any less moral status than earlier held beliefs.

Regardless, if both residents appreciate the situation and are both consenting, they have the right to privacy and liberty in pursuing their activities as long as the rights of others are not compromised [6]. An assessment tool to help staff in long-term care facilities decide if two residents are capable of making decisions to engage in a sexual relationship has been described [17]. If the team, however, deems either resident as vulnerable to exploitation, the relationship is immediately ended and the resident's family or substitution decision maker are involved [6].

When family is met with, their values, beliefs, and level of comfort is determined in order to identify the need for support and education [15]. However, caution also needs to be heeded when speaking to families because, although it is essential that staff apprise relatives of their family member's sexual activities with other residents, issues of protection, respect for privacy, and integrity of the resident must be balanced out. While it could be considered ethically wanting for staff to not alert unsuspecting adult children regarding expressions of care between their parents and other residents, it could be considered a privacy boundary violation to tell anything, never mind to "tell all," to family members without appropriate recognition of the resident couple's intimacy needs, especially if there is consent between residents.

For self-stimulation, behavior which is inappropriately frequent and/or is performed in public, interventions need to be employed which respect the dignity and autonomy of the involved residents while acknowledging the needs of others using the area, who find the situation awkward and embarrassing [6]. In such cases, staff needs to point out to the involved parties that the behavior is not appropriate for common areas and should encourage them to go to a private space such as their own room, or their own bed with the curtain drawn if they share a room. Also, if the resident or residents are able to understand, it is appropriate to discuss the reasons for the interventions [6]. Staff are also encouraged to ensure that the meaning behind the behavior is acknowledged and unmet needs are addressed [6]. Education is important to increase staff awareness of sexuality and intimacy so they can better understand and respond to sexual behaviors and/or advances [3].

Sexually Aggressive Behaviors

Nonconsensual, overt physical behaviors involving touching another resident in a way that is unwelcoming and upsetting are high risk behaviors that staff must immediately respond to by immediately ending the exploitive relationship [15].

While sexual aggression by residents in a long-term care environment is relatively rare, a crisis atmosphere is often generated when residents exhibit this degree of sexually inappropriate behavior. In many cases there is a request made to psychiatry that the person, usually a male with dementia, be treated with hormonal medications in order to control the behavior. Given this sense of urgency, it is easy to rush into an intervention without doing a thorough history and assessment. However, it is always important, as already discussed, to establish a clear description of what was observed, by whom, and the circumstances, including antecedents and consequences of the behavior. It is also crucial to obtain a comprehensive psycho-social history that includes a past sexual behavior that is obtained either from the resident or a relative. In anticipation of problems, the sexual policy for a dementia unit includes taking a sexual history for new admissions as this helps to articulate and sensitively respond to later problems [14]. It is also important, if available, to examine previous records for any indication of a history of difficulty. Finally, psychological, biological, and social factors that could be contributing to the behavior need to be looked for.

Causes of Inappropriate Sexual Behavior

Inappropriate sexual behavior can have a number of causes. It is important to check if the individual has had a past history of sexual aggression and treatment. Violent, habitual sexual offenders may require management in secure settings. There are a number of possible causes of inappropriate sexual behavior in geriatric residents [18]. Causes include medications, in particular dopaminergic agents for the treatment of Parkinson's diseases. In the case of new onset sexually disinhibited behavior, the possibility of a manic disorder, delirium, surreptitious use of alcohol, benzodiazepines, or other substances should all be considered. Residents suffering from a delirium can exhibit disinhibited behavior with sexualized content. Assessing and treating the underlying delirium is crucial both to manage the behavior and because of the high morbidity and mortality associated with delirium.

Misidentification, a common syndrome associated with dementia, can result in residents approaching others in a sexualized fashion, believing that the object of their attention is their spouse. Disinhibition associated with a dementia is yet another cause.

As well, it is important to assess that what is perceived as inappropriate sexual behavior is not due to physical discomfort in the genital region on the part of the resident or related to poor self care. For example, residents may frequently touch themselves in the genital region because of discomfort or irritation leading to the perception that they are stimulating themselves. Addressing the cause of the discomfort leads to the stopping of the behavior. Occasionally, some residents dress inappropriately and walk into public areas with genitalia exposed as a result of difficulty with appropriately adjusting clothing after toileting [19].

Behavioral and Medication Interventions

Intervention in managing inappropriate sexual behavior should first employ behavioral strategies. The first behavioral intervention often consists of redirection. It can be helpful to redirect the behavior, verbally or physically, by moving the resident to another room, and informing them of the behavior that was perceived as inappropriate. It can also be helpful to isolate the resident from others who are likely to be targeted by the resident. It may be necessary for care to be provided by a staff of a different sex than the one targeted. Clothing that opens in the back can be especially helpful for male residents who expose genitalia or masturbate publicly. A general helpful strategy is to ignore unwanted behaviors and encourage appropriate behavior through rewards and attention. When behavioral strategies have been implemented and have failed, it is appropriate to consider pharmacological intervention.

A variety of classes of medications have been utilized to treat hypersexuality in nursing home settings after nonpharmacological means of treatment have been attempted. A review of treatment of sexual disinhibition in geriatric patients suggests treatment first with serotonin reuptake inhibitors before using hormonal treatment, taking advantage of the well know adverse effects on sexual desire and function that can arise in as many as one third of patients taking SSRIs [20]. It is suggested that SSRIs be initiated at ¼ to ½ the normal starting dose, and that the patient be stabilized on the lowest possible dose. If the treatment with SSRIs fails, then the patient can be treated with hormonal medications. An estrogen patch is recommended if the patient is likely not to comply with oral medications. It is recommended that the patch be placed on the back, where the patient is not able to remove it easily. The usual patch strength utilized varies from 0.05 to 0.10 mg. If the patient is willing to take oral medications, then 0.625 mg of estrogen daily is the suggested dose. Side-effects include an increased risk of deep vein thrombosis, nausea, fluid retention, vomiting, and gynecomastia. The use of anti androgen medication is recommended if more rapid onset of treatment is required [20]. DepoProvera (medroxyprogesterone acetate) has been used in doses of 200–300 mg/week intramuscular (IM). It is a potent progestogen that decreases testosterone levels by inhibiting pituitary luteinizing hormone (LH) and follicle-stimulating hormone (FSH) resulting in decreased testosterone production in the testes. Side-effects include sleepiness, mild diabetes, increased appetite, weight gain, hair loss, and mild depression. Lupron (leuprolide) is a luteinizing hormone-releasing hormone (LHRH) agonist that can be given as an intramuscular injection at the dose of

11.25 mg every three months. It decreases testosterone production by suppression of LH and FSH secretion. There is a risk of osteoporosis on this medication. The antiandrogen Androcur (cyproterone acetate) at doses of 10–300 mg/day blocks testosterone at the receptor level and has been used in the management of sexual acting out in males. One review of several cases suggests that much lower doses of 10–100 mg daily can be effective with minimal side effects [21]. It is necessary to monitor liver function on this medication. Other side effects can include fatigue, weight gain, transient depression, and gynecomastia.

Case reports of treatment with psychotropics suggest benefits with mood stabilizers (valproate and carbamazepine), antidepressants (paroxetine, fluoxetine, and clomipramine) and atypical antipsychotics (quetiapine and olanzapine). In many cases the resident is not capable of making his/her own medical decision. It is necessary to have a substitute decision maker who is informed of the risks of the medication treatments. Hormonal treatments essentially work by causing chemical castration and recommendation for their use is based solely on case reports or uncontrolled case studies.

To demonstrate how and when to use medication and behavioral interventions, two examples will now be provided. The first example illustrates a case where the resident exhibited clear cut sexual aggression and where medication was necessary. The second case, by contrast, dealt with a resident where education and redirection were possible because of the resident's partial insight, and medication was unnecessary.

Case Illustration

Mr. Z., an 83-year-old single male was recently admitted to a long-term care facility with Alzheimer's disease. An urgent consultation was requested because he was sexually touching staff and female residents. In addition he was frequently masturbating in public areas and was suspected of having sex with a very impaired coresident. When confronted, he denied everything. Staff reacted with both anger and fear and provided him with less personal care.

Information was obtained from his sister living in California, as the resident was a poor historian with gradual cognitive decline over the past four years. There had never been a history of sexual assault on his part, although his sister admitted she did not know very much about the nature of his relationships with women. He was a nondrinker and was on thyroid medication.

Comment

Upon assessment Mr. Z. was found not to have any delusions or delirium and clinically there was no suspicion of covert alcohol use or depression. He was found to be cognitively impaired with an MMSE [22] of 15 and did not appear to have any insight into the concerns about his behaviors. After careful evaluation of the antecedents and consequences of his sexual disinhibition, it appeared he engaged in sexual acting out only when females of any age interacted with him. When a female was within range he would touch them on the breast or buttock regions. This was especially true when females were in close proximity and providing personal care. When his sexual verbalizations were ignored they seemed to subside but if Mr. Z. was scolded they seemed to escalate.

Increased understanding of Mr. Z.'s behavior following the assessment resulted in more staff willingness to attempt a variety of behavioral interventions. However, attempts to reorient him as to the inappropriateness of his behavior were not successful. Mr. Z. was assigned a same sex personal care provider. Whenever he engaged in any sexual banter the verbalizations were ignored, but when he engaged in what was considered more appropriate behavior staff would interact with him. These interventions resulted in a decrease in the sexual behavior.

Despite the behavioral interventions, Mr. Z. remained periodically agitated and aggressive, especially when redirection from the room of female residents was attempted by his caregiver. He was given a trial of olanzapine for agitation, with the hope that there would be a reduction in his sexual acting out, but he developed extrapyramidal side effects.

There was discussion with his sister regarding hormonal treatment. She was not willing to provide consent as she was concerned about possible side effects. Instead Mr. Z. received a trial of the SSRI paroxetine 30 mg. There was considerable improvement with significant decrease of sexual behaviors.

Case Illustration

Mr. X., a 78-year-old widowed male with a history of Alzheimer's disease was admitted to a nursing home one year ago as he had been unable to live on his own. An urgent consultation was requested when he was observed by staff to be kissing and fondling a woman in a public area.

Comment

The resident's daughter was contacted and she was present for the interview with Mr. X. who was very fit for his age. A comprehensive psycho-social history was obtained from both the daughter and resident. Information from the daughter indicated that her father had always been very flirtatious with women, but had been very caring with his wife who had died several years earlier. There had been a change in his personality since the onset of his dementia. She felt that he would never previously have been as openly affectionate in a public area. Mr. X. indicated that he felt flattered by the attention of several women who would approach him, but he understood that the open affection was offending some people, in particular staff and visiting family members.

The first intervention consisted of providing feedback to staff regarding the results of the assessment. This resulted in a decreased sense of urgency and an increased willingness to attempt a variety of behavioral interventions. Based on the historical information and the resident's current level of awareness, the first intervention that was attempted involved discussing the situation with the resident. Mr. X. indicated that he had enjoyed the attention from the women, but agreed to try and stay out of the common areas. His inappropriate behavior resolved itself based on this meeting.

References

1. Spector, I.P., Rosen, R.C., Leiblum, S.R. (1996). Sexuality. In W.E. Reichman, P.R. Katz (Eds.), Psychiatric care in the nursing home (pp. 133–150). New York: Oxford University Press.
2. Continuing Gerontological Education Cooperative. (2002). Intimacy, sexuality and sexual behavior in dementia: How to develop practice guidelines and policy for long-term care facilities. Hamilton, ON: McMaster University Press. HQ 30–157. Available at www.fhs.mcmaster.ca/mcah/cgec/toolkit.pdf.
3. Molloy, W., Reich, M., Jacobson, J., Rock, S., Renaud, S., Milburn, G., Sheehan, C. (1999). Intimacy and sexuality in long-term care facilities. Windsor Essex Geriatric Assessment/Consultation Program.
4. Advocacy Centre for the Elderly (ACE) and Community Legal Education Ontario (CLEO). (2001). Every resident: Bill of rights for people who live in Ontario long-term care facilities. Available at www.cleo.on.ca/english/pub/onpub/PDF/seniors/everyres.pdf.
5. Butler, R.N., Lewis, M.I., Hoffman, E., Whitehead, E.D. (1994). Love and sex after 60: How to evaluate and treat the sexually active woman. Geriatrics, 49(11):33–42.
6. Doyle, D., Bisson, D., James, N., Lynch, H., Martin, C. (1999). Human sexuality in long-term care. The Canadian Nurse, January:26–29.
7. Richardson, J.P. (1995). Sexuality in the nursing home patient. American Family Physician, 51(1):121–124.
8. Tong, R. (1990). Till death us do part: Married life in nursing homes. In R.A. Kane, A.L. Caplan (Eds.), Everyday ethics: Resolving dilemmas in nursing home life (pp. 100–108). New York: Springer Publishing Company.
9. Montenko, A.K., (1989). The frustrations, gratifications, and well-being of dementia caregivers. Gerontologist, 29:166–172.
10. Miles, S.H., Sachs, G.A. (1990). Intimate strangers: Roommates in nursing homes. In R.A. Kane, A.L. Caplan (Eds.), Everyday ethics: Resolving dilemmas in nursing home life (pp. 90–99). New York: Springer Publishing Company.
11. Berger, J.T. (2000), Sexuality and intimacy in the nursing home: A romantic couple of mixed cognitive capacities. The Journal of Clinical Ethics, 11(4):305–317.
12. Johnson M. (1995). Clinical issues in the treatment of geriatric sex offenders. In B. Schwartz, H. Celini (Eds.), The sex offender: Correction treatment and legal practice. Civic Research Institute Inc. Kingston, NJ: Civic Research Institute, Inc.
13. Aliagkrishnan, K., Lim, D., Brahim, A., Wong, A., Wood, A., Senthilselvan, A., Chimich, W., Kagan, L. (2005). Sexually inappropriate behavior in demented elderly people. Postgraduate Medical Journal, 81(957):463–466.
14. Sloane, P. (1993). Sexual behavior in residents with dementia. Contemporary Long Term Care, 16(10):66, 69, 108.
15. Shalom Village Nursing Home. (2001). Intimacy and sexuality practice guidelines (revision). Hamilton, Ontario: Shalom Village Nursing Home.
16. Lichtenberg, P.A., Strzpek, D.M. (1990). Assessment of institutionalized patients' competency to participate in intimate relationships. Gerontology, 30:117–120.
17. Lichtenberg, P.A. (1997), Clinical perspectives on sexual issues in nursing homes. Topics in Geriatric Rehabilitation, 12(4):1–10.
18. Kamel, K., Hajjar R.R. (2004). Sexuality in the nursing home, Part 2: Managing abnormal behavior ethical and legal issues. Journal of American Medical Director Association, 5:S49–52.
19. Stern, B. (2003). Caring for your loved one: An education guide for caregivers of persons with dementia. Toronto: Baycrest Centre for Geriatric Care.
20. Lothstein, L.M., Fogg-Waberski J., Reynolds, P. (1997). Risk management and treatment of sexual disinhibition in geriatric patients. Connecticut Medicine, 61:609–618.

21. Hausserman, P., Goeker, D., Beir, K., Schroeder, S. (2003). Low-dose cyproterone acetate treatment of sexual acting out in men with dementia. International Psychogeriatrics, 15(2):181–186.
22. Folstein, M.F., Folstein, S.W., McHugh, P.R. (1975). "Mini-Mental State." A practical method for grading the cognitive state of patients for the clinician. Journal of Psychiatric Research, 12:189–198.

Suggested Readings

1. Gordon, M., Sokolowski, M. (2004). Sexuality in long-term care: Ethics and action. Annals of Long-Term Care, 12(9):45–48.
   This article addresses a number of ethical issues specific to the context of two residents experiencing different degrees of dementia wishing to engage in a romantic, and possibly sexual, relationship.
2. Ehrenfeld, M., Bronner, G., Tabak, N., Alpert, R., Bergman, R. (1999). Sexuality among institutionalized elderly patients with dementia. Nursing Ethics, 6(2):144–149.
   This article examines the subject of sexuality among elderly patients with dementia, focusing on two main aspects: The sexual behavior of institutionalized elderly people with dementia; and the reactions of other patients, staff and family members to this behavior.

11 Principles of Geriatric Psychopharmacology

Nathan Herrmann

Key Points

- Psychotropic medications are considered to be only one part of a multi-faceted treatment program, and should only be initiated after a careful review of risks and benefits.
- Specific target symptoms should be chosen for monitoring, and reassessment of efficacy should occur regularly.
- Because the elderly are extremely sensitive to the side effects of psychotropic medications, staff should be vigilant for these adverse drug reactions.

Introduction

The introduction of psychoactive medications in the 1950s and 1960s revolutionalized the treatment of psychiatric illness. With the help of antidepressants and antipsychotic drugs the chronic in-patient population of mental hospitals declined dramatically. Consequently, the percentage of residents with psychiatric disturbances in nursing homes, rest homes, and homes for the aged increased markedly. Because of the scarcity of resources in many of these facilities, pharmacological management of emotional and behavioral disturbances is often the only form of therapy these residents receive. Despite the potential benefits for some residents, there is data to suggest, that psychoactive drugs are at times misused, occasionally abused, and often administered by individuals with limited knowledge of their indications and side effects [1].

When indicated, the use of psychoactive medications for treatment of depression, anxiety, or control of behavioral symptoms, should be viewed as only one component of a treatment plan made up of multiple modalities. Often, as in the case of residents with dementia, these medications should not be considered the treatment of first choice. The institutionalized elderly are a population at high risk for side effects, particularly in the presence of physical illness and multiple medical drug use. Safe and effective use of psychotropics requires careful observations and regular periodic reappraisal of effectiveness.

Principles of Pharmacotherapy in the Elderly

Table 1 Factors Affecting Drug Metabolism in the Elderly

- Decreased lean body mass
- Increased body fat
- Decreased serum albumin
- Changes in absorption
- Changes in liver function
- Decreased kidney function
- Changes in drug receptor sensitivity
- Changes in amount of neurotransmitters

The elderly experience many physiological changes that can alter the way drugs are metabolized. Some of the factors that effect drug handling in the elderly are listed in **Table 1**. As a result of these changes, many psychotropic medications will have prolonged effects, and tend to accumulate more in the elderly than in younger individuals. The elderly are very susceptible to side effects; even so-called "therapeutic" doses of common psychotropic medications may lead to complications such as delirium or hypotension. All these factors highlight the need for careful administration of psychotropics with close monitoring [2].

Prior to initiating pharmacotherapy, the clinician should establish the relative indications and contraindications of drug use in each resident. Indications should include a specific diagnosis as well as a number of target symptoms that can be used to monitor the efficacy of treatment. Target symptoms should be easily measurable and could include weight changes, hours of sleep, number of aggressive outbursts, frequency of shouting, participation in social activities, etc. Nursing staff and other members of the treatment team should work with the treating physician to establish appropriate target symptoms, and then record changes in their frequency and severity in the chart. Relative contraindications to specific medications depend on individual characteristics that may place the resident at greater risk (e.g., those residents with preexisting cardiovascular or renal disease, or those residents on numerous medications maybe more susceptible to serious side effects).

If the potential benefits outweigh the risks, the clinician must then choose an appropriate medication. There are many psychotropic medications that are better tolerated than the older traditional medications such as amitriptyline, chlorpromazine, haloperidol, and diazepam. For the elderly the drugs of choice should (1) have fewer active metabolites, (2) accumulate in the body to a lesser extent, (3) have shorter action, and (4) be less prone to causing side effects such as hypotension, falls, and confusion. The drug should be started at very low dosages and increased slowly while monitoring for side effects. The effective dosage of many psychotropic medications is usually lower than in younger populations, and the medications can often be given in single daily dosages.

Psychotropic medication use should be reviewed on a regular basis. Because many conditions such as depression, or agitation associated with dementia are episodic, long-term treatment with these medications, which are prone to causing side effects, is not necessarily indicated. Attempts to reduce and even discontinue the drugs should be a regular part of the resident's management. The use of quarterly pharmacy rounds or drug reviews is highly recommended for this purpose.

Treatment of Depression

Depression is a common form of psychiatric illness in nursing home residents that can have serious consequences if it is untreated (see Chapter 5). Appropriate pharmacological management of depression is often extremely effective at ameliorating depressive signs and symptoms [3]. Although there are numerous medications available to treat major depression, the drugs used most commonly are the selective serotonin reuptake inhibitors (SSRIs), which have largely supplanted the tricyclic antidepressants (TCAs). TCAs such as amitriptyline (Elavil) and imipramine (Tofranil) were first introduced more than four decades ago, and while many new medications, such as the SSRIs, have been marketed no single drug has been shown to have consistently better efficacy than these original two agents. In view of this fact, how is a medication chosen for a specific resident?

- *Personal History:* If a resident has experienced a depression in the past which was successfully treated with a specific drug, that same medication should be considered the treatment of first choice. Occasionally, clinicians will carefully review a family history to determine if other family members have been successfully treated with certain types of antidepressants, and choose the same one for the resident.
- *Side-Effect Profile:* The elderly are extremely sensitive to the side effects of antidepressants (see **Table 2**); those medications with the fewest bothersome side effects will therefore be better tolerated. Occasionally, the presence of side effects can be a positive indication for choosing a particular agent (e.g., the depressed resident with severe insomnia may benefit from a drug that causes more sedation).
- *Concomitant Medications:* The presence of other medications for the treatment of chronic medical conditions increases the risk of drug interactions. Some of the SSRIs for example, like fluoxetine and paroxetine, are more likely to be involved in such reactions than citalopram or sertraline. Working closely with the facility pharmacist can help alert clinicians to potential drug interactions and suggest the safest choice of drug for the individual resident.

Table 2 Antidepressant Side Effects

Tricyclics	anticholinergic effects, sedation, orthostatic hypotension, cardiac arrhythmias
SSRIs	nausea, vomiting, loose stools, weight loss, insomnia, hyponatremia, sexual dysfunction
Venlafaxine	nausea, hypertension, tremor, sweating
Mirtazapine	excessive sedation, weight gain
Bupropion	insomnia, agitation, nausea
MAOIs	orthostatic hypotension, dizziness, insomnia

All antidepressants require several weeks until they are completely effective. Sleep and appetite may improve within the first two weeks of treatment, but it may take up to 6–8 weeks until there is complete objective and subjective improvement. It is therefore important to allow this amount of time to pass before switching to another medication.

Selective Serotonin Reuptake Inhibitors (SSRIs)

SSRIs are among the most commonly prescribed antidepressants today, largely based upon their perceived safety and ease of administration. The SSRIs citalopram (Celexa), fluoxetine (Prozac), fluvoxamine (Luvox), paroxetine (Paxil), sertraline (Zoloft), escitalopram (Lexapro/Cipramil) specifically block the reuptake of the neurotransmitter serotonin. These medications are usually well tolerated in the elderly with the most common side effects being gastrointestinal (nausea, vomiting, loose stools), insomnia, and sexual dysfunction. Less common but potentially serious effects include hyponatremia, gait unsteadiness, and weight loss (the latter most frequently noted with fluoxetine). The ease of use of the SSRIs relates to their relatively flat dose-response; the starting dose is often the effective dose, with little need for dose titration. Based on studies of drug metabolism the doses of paroxetine and citalopram should be significantly lower in the elderly while doses of sertraline, fluvoxamine, and fluoxetine may be similar to younger populations. Starting all SSRIs at lower doses would be prudent in the very old, frail, or medically ill.

Another major advantage of the SSRIs is their marked safety in overdose. The SSRIs have several important drug interactions that must be avoided, however. For example, if SSRIs are prescribed concomitantly, or in close proximity to a monoamine oxidase inhibitor antidepressant, a potentially fatal interaction can ensue. This interaction, called the "serotonin syndrome," is characterized by anxiety, restlessness, confusion, incoordination, and insomnia. The SSRIs also variably effect the hepatic cytochrome P450 system which is responsible for metabolizing many drugs, leading to the potential for drug interactions with a variety of frequently coadministered psychoactive medications (e.g., alprazolam, haloperidol, risperidone) and drugs for medical conditions (e.g., metoprolol, quinidine, warfarin). Because the risks of such interactions vary with each SSRI and each concomitant medication, it is highly recommended that clinicians carefully review the pharmacopoeia and/or consult with a pharmacist prior to starting an SSRI.

Tricyclic Antidepressants (TCAs)

Prior to the introduction of the SSRIs, the TCAs were the most frequently prescribed antidepressants. While most reviews of the controlled trials of antidepressants in the elderly have failed to show any differences in the efficacy between SSRIs and TCAs, age- and disease-specific characteristics may limit the use of TCAs in the elderly. The most common troublesome side effects of the TCAs are sedation, orthostatic hypotension, and anticholinergic effects.

Orthostatic hypotension is a drop in blood pressure that occurs when a resident rises from a chair or gets out of bed. It is easily measured by taking the resident's blood pressure while lying or sitting, asking the resident to stand, and after waiting one minute, measuring the pressure again. A drop of systolic pressure greater than 10 mmHg associated with complaints of dizziness or light-headedness is indicative of this side-effect. Residents with this problem should be warned to get out of bed slowly, rising to a sitting position, prior to standing up. The dizziness caused by orthostatic hypotension can be a serious problem in the elderly leading to falls and possible fractures. Management usually involves reducing or discontinuing the medication. Because orthostatic hypotension is a common potentially serious problem, all residents on antidepressants and antipsychotic medication should have regular monitoring of their blood pressures while lying and standing.

Table 3 Anticholinergic Side Effects

- Dry mouth
- Blurred vision
- Constipation
- Tachycardia
- Urinary retention
- Sweating
- Exacerbation of narrow angle glaucoma
- Anticholinergic delirium (delirium, disorientation, confusion, cognitive impairment)

Anticholinergic side effects are a common problem caused by many antidepressants and antipsychotics (**Table 3**). The most frequent complaints include dry mouth, blurred vision, and constipation. Although these problems are not serious, they can be very bothersome; constipation can be extremely distressing to the elderly who often focus on bowel function. The elderly are also more susceptible to the more serious anticholinergic side effects: confusion and delirium (see Chapter 4).

Amitriptyline (Elavil) and imipramine (Tofranil) appear to cause side effects more frequently and clinically they are not well tolerated in the elderly. Unless there is a clear history of previous response to these medications, they should not be considered agents of first choice. Nortriptyline (Aventyl, Pamelor) conversely, has a relatively low frequency of side effects and tends to be well tolerated. Nortriptyline can be initiated at a dose of 10 mg h.s. and increased slowly to a dose of 50–100 mg h.s. The blood level of this medication can be checked, as several studies have shown that serum levels 50–150 ng/ml (150–500 nmol/L) are associated with therapeutic efficacy, while levels above or below this "therapeutic window" may be ineffective.

While use of the TCAs has been waning since the introduction of the SSRIs, they may still be used occasionally for the treatment of conditions other than depression including chronic pain syndromes and urinary incontinence.

Other Antidepressants

There are many other antidepressants with different chemical structures and hypothesized actions. Several so-called "second generation" antidepressants were marketed prior to the introduction of the SSRIs and include maprotiline (Ludiomil) and trazodone (Deseryl). Trazodone is no longer used frequently as an antidepressant because of its sedating effects, orthostatic hypotension, and short action which necessitates multiple daily dosing. Trazodone is still frequently prescribed, however, for the treatment of agitation in dementia or as a sedative for patients with insomnia. Newer, nonSSRI antidepressants include bupropion, venlafaxine, and mirtazapine. Bupropion (Wellbutrin) is well tolerated in the elderly. It is nonsedating and can cause insomnia, headache, and seizures if the dosage is raised too quickly or when administered at dosages above 450 mg/day. Venlafaxine (Effexor) blocks both serotonin and noradrenaline reuptake. It is well tolerated with the most common side effects being nausea, somnolence, insomnia, dry mouth, dizziness, and anxiety. Occasionally, at higher dosages, it can also cause sustained increases in blood pressure that may necessitate discontinuation especially in patients with preexisting or poorly controlled hypertension. Mirtazapine (Remeron) is a noradrenaline and specific serotonin antidepressant. In a large recent trial it was shown to be safe and effective in the elderly. Its side effects include sedation and weight gain. It is well tolerated in doses of 15–30 mg per day, with the unusual effect of lower doses occasionally causing more sedation than higher doses.

Another class of medication which has been used to treat depression in the elderly is the monoamine oxidase inhibitors (MAOIs). These medications are only being prescribed infrequently and usually by consulting psychiatrists. The MAOIs phenelzine (Nardil) and tranylcypromine (Parnate) are well tolerated and extremely useful for residents whose depression has not responded to other agents. The MAOIs have fewer anticholinergic and cardiac side effects, but can cause significant orthostatic hypotension and insomnia. All residents treated with MAOIs should, therefore, have their blood pressure measured sitting and standing. The major concern with MAOIs, however, is the potential to cause a hypertensive crisis when taken with foods that contain the compound tyramine. Residents taking MAOIs therefore must adhere to certain dietary and medication restrictions (**Table 4**). Any resident on an MAOI who complains of an acute severe headache (usually at the back of the head), stiff neck, nausea, or vomiting must have their blood pressure checked. If this is significantly elevated the physician should be notified immediately or the resident should be transferred to an emergency department for treatment and monitoring. A revers-

Table 4 MAOI Dietary Restrictions

Foods to avoid:

– Aged or matured cheeses (e.g., Cheddar, Blue, Swiss, etc.)

– Aged or fermented meats and fish (e.g., pepperoni, corned beef, pickled herring, etc.)

– Meat and yeast extracts (e.g., Bovril, Marmite, Oxo, etc.)

– Broad bean pods

Medications to avoid:

– Cold medications

– Decongestants (including nasal sprays)

– Asthma medications

– Narcotic analgesics (especially meperidine [Demerol])

– Appetite suppressants and stimulants

N.B. Many other foods and drugs have been implicated in causing MAOI adverse reactions. For a list of these foods and drugs please refer to Suggested Reading 1 at the end of the chapter.

ible, selective MAOI moclobemide (Manerix) (not available in USA), has much less potential for drug interactions and does not require the dietary restrictions of the other MAOIs. It is extremely well tolerated in the elderly and may cause insomnia, nausea, headache, and dry mouth but little orthostatic hypotension, unlike the other MAOIs. Similarly, another MAOI, selegiline, has recently been approved in the USA as a patch formulation that will also not require dietary restrictions. While its safety and efficacy in elderly depressives remains to be determined, it may have significant advantages in some long-term care patients who cannot swallow because of neurological problems, or refuse to eat because of depression.

The psychostimulants methlyphenidate (Ritalin) and dextroamphetamine (Dexedrine) are occasionally used as antidepressants in the elderly. Some studies have shown them to be particularly effective in patients who are elderly, medically-ill, withdrawn, and apathetic. These medications are well tolerated and cause few side effects when used at low doses. Some residents may experience insomnia or agitation, and occasionally delirium may be precipitated. The patient should also be monitored for tachycardia and hypertension. They are given orally, usually in two daily doses (the last dose given no later than the early afternoon to avoid insomnia). In contrast to the previous classes of antidepressants described, if no therapeutic effect is noticed within the two weeks, these medications should be discontinued.

Mood Stabilizers and the Treatment of Mania and Bipolar Affective Disorder

While there are no controlled studies of the treatment of elderly patients with bipolar affective disorder or mania, treatment with a mood stabilizer (e.g., lithium, valproic acid, carbamazepine) is recommended both acutely and for long-term prophylaxis. Acutely, adjunctive medication such as benzodiazepines and antipsychotics may be necessary to manage agitation, psychosis, and insomnia [4].

Lithium carbonate is used to treat acute mania, as prophylaxis against manic and depressive episodes, and can be added to an established course of antidepressants to improve efficacy. The administration and monitoring of lithium requires special consideration in the elderly. With aging, renal functioning becomes progressively compromised; the dose of lithium, which is excreted solely by the kidneys will need to be markedly reduced. The elderly are also more sensitive to lithium's side effects and therefore should be maintained at lower serum levels than younger populations. All patients on lithium therapy must have periodic measurements of blood levels of lithium, best examined 12 hours after the last dose. The vast majority of elderly require 150–600 mg o.d. to attain 12-hour serum levels of 0.5–0.8 mmol/l (mEq/L) (a level considered safe/effective in this population).

Lithium can cause numerous side effects the most common being nausea, a fine tremor of the hands, urinary frequency, and thirst (see **Table 5**). Signs of lithium toxicity include coarse tremor, slurred speech, ataxia, confusion, and drowsiness. Lithium toxicity should be considered a medical emergency necessitating holding of the drug and immediate measuring of the serum level. Although toxicity develops in adults at levels between 1.5 and 2 mmol/l, the elderly may experience these same effects at levels as low as 1.0 mmol/l.

Table 5 Side Effects of Lithium

Gastrointestinal	Central Nervous System
Nausea	Fatigue
Abdominal pain	Restlessness
Diarrhea	Stupor or coma
Vomiting	Confusion
Constipation	Dizziness
Metallic taste	Blurred vision
	Slurred speech
Neuromuscular	**Endocrine**
Muscular weakness	Hypothyroidism
Tremor	
Abnormal involuntary movements	
Renal	**Other**
Reduced concentrating ability	ECG changes
Polyurea (urinary frequency)	Skin rashes
Polydipsia (thirst)	Exacerbation of psoriasis
	Weight gain
	Baldness

Changes in lithium levels and toxicity can be caused by many factors including dehydration, vomiting, and diarrhoea. Drugs that interact with lithium and can potentially lead to toxicity include diuretics (e.g., hydrochlorothiazide, furosemide), angiotensin-converting enzyme inhibitors (e.g., ramapril) and some nonsteroidal anti-inflammatory drugs.

Besides regular monitoring of serum lithium levels, all residents taking lithium should have yearly checks of serum creatinine and urine osmolality for lithium induced renal impairment, and thyroid function tests for lithium induced hypothyroidism.

While treatment with lithium carbonate is potentially problematic in the elderly, there has been little study of the other frequently used mood stabilizers carbamazepine and valproic acid. Carbamazepine (Tegretol) can cause confusion, ataxia, hepatotoxicity, and leukopenia as well as the potential for multiple drug interactions. Serum levels above 38 mmol/L (9 mg/L) are associated with increased risk of side effects in the elderly. Because of those concerns, valproic acid (Depakene, Depakote, Epival) has received more attention recently. It is generally recommended to use the divalproex sodium preparation starting at 250 mg twice daily with titration up to a usual dose of 500–2000 mg/day given in two or three doses. Serum levels between 200–700 mmol/L (35–100 ng/ml) are thought to be effective and well tolerated. Side effects include sedation, unsteadiness, tremor, nausea, and thrombocytopenia.

More recently, the atypical antipsychotics such as risperidone, olanzapine, and quetiapine (see below for more details) have been demonstrated to be effective mood stabilizers in younger manic patients. While they are being used increasingly frequent in elderly bipolar patients, there is little available data on their efficacy and long-term safety in this population.

Treatment of Psychosis, Agitation, and Aggression

Psychiatric symptoms such as delusions and hallucinations, can occur in a variety of illnesses including depression, mania, schizophrenia, paranoid disorders, delirium, and dementia. Antipsychotics (AP) are used to treat psychosis, as well as the agitation and aggression associated with dementia. The first AP introduced to North America in the early 1950s was chlorpromazine (Thorazine, Largactil). Since that time numerous APs were marketed and all shared equal efficacy though with slightly different side-effect profiles. In the past decade, however, a new class of APs has been introduced referred to as "atypical antipsychotics" which have potential advantages compared with the older "typical" APs. Advantages include fewer side effects and efficacy with respect to negative symptoms (e.g., blunted affect, emotional withdrawal, apathy, etc.) and treatment refractory patients [5].

There are many studies which have demonstrated the APs' effectiveness in reducing and eliminating hallucinations and delusions in schizophrenia and affective disorders, and many recent studies on their usefulness in treating agitation and other behavioral disturbances associated with dementia. Unfortunately, while many of these trials have documented efficacy, results from pooling the safety findings from the studies of patients with dementia suggest there is a small but significant increased risk of cerebrovascular adverse events and mortality associated with atypical APs. Despite this, atypical APs are currently the most commonly prescribed drugs for treating agitation, aggression, and psychosis in dementia patients in long-term care institutions. Because of these concerns, APs should only be prescribed when symptoms are serious and place the patient, other residents and/or staff at risk of harm. APs should only be considered as part of a management plan that includes environmental, behavioral, and other psychosocial treatments. Finally, while typical APs will be reviewed next, since they are still used frequently by some clinicians, it is this author's opinion that atypical APs should be used preferentially for elderly patients.

Typical Antipsychotics

Since all typical APs are equally effective, the choice of drug for an individual resident should be based on the medication's side-effect profile (see **Table 6**). The typical APs can be classified on the basis of their relative potency. In general the low potency typical APs (e.g., chlorpromazine) produce the most sedation, hypotension, and anticholinergic effects, while the high potency typical APs (e.g., haloperidol [Haldol] and trifluoperazine [Stelazine]) produce the greatest amounts of extrapyramidal symptoms. Regardless of choice,

Table 6 Antipsychotic Side Effects

Side-Effect	Comment
Anticholinergic effects	see Table 3
Extrapyramidal symptoms: – dystonias – parkinsonism – akathisia – tardive dyskinesia	more common with typical antipsychotics
Neuroleptic Malignant Syndrome	
– Elevated temperature, muscular rigidity, increased CPK, tachycardia, altered consciousness	more common with typical antipsychotics
Sedation	
Hypotension	
Weight gain	
Diabetes	
Hyperlipidemia	
Cerebrovascular adverse events/mortality	reported in dementia trials

these medications must be prescribed in very small doses as the elderly are exquisitely sensitive to side effects; even small doses (e.g., haloperidol 0.5–1.0 mg h.s.) may cause excessive daytime sedation, confusion, or severe parkinsonism with stiffness and rigidity.

Antipsychotic-induced extrapyramidal reactions include dystonias, parkinsonism, akathisia, and tardive dyskinesia. Dystonias, which occur relatively infrequently in the elderly, are dramatic, acute, sustained contractions of specific muscle groups. These distressing reactions occur within the first days of treatment and can involve the muscles of neck, mouth, and eyes. Antipsychotic-induced parkinsonism is extremely common in the elderly presenting with rigidity, slowed movements, tremor, shuffling gait, stooped posture, an inexpressive face, and drooling. Akathisia is motor restlessness in which the resident feels compelled to keep moving and pacing. Residents often complain about feeling anxious and being unable to sleep. In younger adults these symptoms are often treated with anticholinergic agents such as benztropine (Cogentin), diphenhydramine (Benadryl), and trihexyphenidyl (Artane). Because the elderly and patients with dementia are so prone to developing confusion and delirium with anticholinergic medications, the use of these agents is not recommended. When extrapyramidal symptoms are prominent, the dose of the typical AP should be reduced, or an atypical AP should be substituted.

The other serious extrapyramidal symptom is tardive dyskinesia. This syndrome appears gradually after prolonged use of typical APs (months to years) and can present with various abnormal, involuntary movements most often involving the tongue, mouth, and face (e.g., tongue-writhing, lip-smacking, facial grimacing). The risk factors for developing tardive dyskinesia include length of drug exposure, increased age of the patient, female gender, and the presence of dementia. In a significant percentage of patients this movement disorder may last for years or be permanent even after the discontinuation of medication. Because tardive dyskinesia can be permanent and because there are no really effective treatments available, prevention is essential. For the institutionalized elderly at high risk for tardive dyskinesia, prevention involves: (1) avoiding the use of typical APs if possible, (2) reducing and discontinuing the medication as soon as possible following amelioration of symptomatology, and (3) examining each resident receiving an AP regularly to determine if there is any evidence of abnormal involuntary movements.

Atypical Antipsychotics

The major advantage of the atypical APs compared to typical APs is their tendency to cause less EPS. As an example of the significant difference between typical and atypical APs in the elderly, one study compared the rates at which elderly patients developed TD with the typical AP haloperidol and the atypical AP risperidone (Risperdal). After nine months of treatment, 1/3 of patients treated with haloperidol compared with 3–4% of risperidone treated patients had developed TD [6]. Currently available atypical APs include clozapine (Clozaril), risperidone (Risperdal), olanzapine (Zyprexa), quetiapine (Seroquel), ziprasidone (Geodon – not available in Canada) and aripiprazole (Abilify – not available in Canada).

Clozapine was the first atypical AP to be developed and while it is still considered the "gold standard" with respect to efficacy and low rates of EPS, its use is limited in the elderly. Clozapine is very sedating, highly anticholinergic and requires frequent regular monitoring of complete blood counts because of its tendency to cause leukopenia and potentially life-threatening agranulocytosis. There is some suggestion that the risk of leukopenia is actually higher in the elderly compared with younger patients. Risperidone is relatively nonsedating and causes little EPS when used at low doses in the elderly. The efficacy of risperidone in treating agitation, aggression and psychosis in patients with dementia has been demonstrated in several large well-designed studies. At doses of approximately 1 mg/day risperidone was well tolerated and effective. Side-effects include somnolence and EPS, both of which are dose-dependent. Risperidone can also cause orthostatic hypotension. Olanzapine is slightly more sedating than risperidone and is also well tolerated in the elderly. Elderly patients with schizophrenia or mood disorders with psychosis can be treated with 5–15 mg/day while agitation, aggression and psychosis in dementia patients should be treated with 2.5–10 mg/day in most cases. Higher doses of olanzapine may be associated with increased EPS as well as confusion secondary to anticholinergic effects. Quetiapine should be started at very low dosages (e.g., 25 mg at bedtime) because of significant initial sedation (most patients quickly adjust to this effect). This low potency medication has a very wide dose range (25–300 mg/day) and while some elderly patients can be maintained on dosages around 100 mg/day, higher doses may be required for optimal efficacy. Quetiapine has remarkably little EPS over its whole dose-range, though sedation and orthostatic hypotension may be troublesome. There is no published data on the use of ziprasidone in the elderly, and only one published study of aripiprazole in dementia that demonstrated only questionable efficacy at average doses of 10 mg/day.

Some atypicals have been associated with significant weight gain, diabetes and hyperlipidemia, though these adverse events appear to be uncommon in the elderly. As noted previously however, drug regulatory authorities have recently issued warnings about the use of all atypical antipsychotics for the treatment of elderly dementia patients. Results from controlled trials suggest increased risks for cerebrovascular adverse events (e.g., stroke, transient ischemic attacks) and mortality. What is not yet clear is whether the typical antipsychotics lack these risks and in fact preliminary evidence suggests similar or greater risks compared with the atypicals [7]. It is clear, however, that the atypicals offer significant advantages for the elderly who are at a high risk for falls secondary to drug-induced EPS, and tardive dyskinesia. If residents have been treated successfully with typical APs for lengthy periods of time, and demonstrate no evidence of TD, there is not much reason to switch to an atypical. Treatment of new onset psychosis or severe agitation and aggression with dementia however, should begin with an atypical AP, and residents currently treated with typical APs who are still symptomatic or have demonstrated EPS should probably be switched to an atypical.

A significant number of patients with dementia, agitation and aggression may not respond or tolerate treatment with APs, and given the recent safety warnings, physicians and families may prefer to avoid these drugs. A variety of other psychotropic medications have been used for this purpose [8]. Treatment with the antidepressant trazodone in doses ranging from 25 mg at bedtime to 100 mg three times daily may be effective, though residents must be monitored for excessive sedation and orthostatic hypotension. The SSRIs can also be used, as some studies have suggested they decrease irritability, anxiety and agitation in some patients with dementia. Several studies have noted that carbamazepine, in doses of approximately 100 mg three times daily, is effective and well tolerated when treating elderly nursing home residents with dementia and agitation. Valproic acid has also been recommended for this indication, though several recent trials in dementia patients suggest it is not effective or well tolerated. A variety of other medications such as beta-blockers, lithium, buspirone, estrogen, and anti-androgens have all been used though appropriate trials to document their efficacy and tolerability are not available. Finally, the benzodiazepines are still frequently used for agitated patients with dementia despite limited evidence of efficacy and significant potential side effects (see below). Benzodiazepines can be useful for short-term use on an as needed basis, in emergency situations or for sedation when a resident must undergo a procedure (e.g., dental work, x-ray, etc.).

Treatment of Anxiety and Insomnia

The most commonly used agents to treat anxiety and insomnia are the benzodiazepines. Prior to the introduction of the benzodiazepines in the 1960s the drugs of choice for these problems were the barbiturates, known for their tendency to produce addiction, severe withdrawal reactions, and extreme lethality in overdose. Compared to the barbiturates, the benzodiazepines are more effective and far safer. Benzodiazepines are the most commonly prescribed psychotropic agents and there is good evidence that the elderly receive a disproportionately high percentage of these prescriptions, both in the community and in long-term care. The efficacy and safety of this group of medications therefore requires careful consideration.

The benzodiazepines can be grouped on the basis of their relative half-lives, a measure of how quickly the drugs are metabolized. In the elderly the rate of benzodiazepine metabolism is significantly slower than in younger populations; diazepam (Valium) which has a half-life of approximately 24 hours in a young adult may have a half-life of 90–120 hours in an 80 year old. The longer the half-life, the more likely a drug will accumulate in the body, potentially leading to increased risk of side effects. The drugs of choice for institutionalized elderly will therefore be the short or intermediate acting benzodiazepines such as lorazepam (Ativan) and oxazepam (Serax). Another group of drugs, with benzodiazepine-like actions has more recently been introduced. These include drugs like zopiclone (Immovane – not available in the U.S.), and zolpidem (Ambien – not available in Canada). While purported to have efficacy and safety advantages in the elderly over the standard benzodiazepines, this has not been clearly documented in clinical trials, and for the most part, their risks and benefits should be considered equivalent.

The major side effects of the benzodiazepines are excessive daytime sedation, confusion and disorientation, and withdrawal reactions. Excessive daytime sedation may account for the finding that these drugs have been associated with increased risks of falls and hip fractures in the institutionalized elderly. Withdrawal reactions usually occur after these medications have been prescribed for long periods, in high doses, and are then abruptly withdrawn. Signs and symptoms can include insomnia, anxiety, tremor, and tachycardia. In severe cases the resident may experience delirium, psychosis, or seizures. Treatment involves reinstituting the drug and then tapering it very slowly. A recent meta-analysis that reviewed the published studies of all the benzodiazepines and benzodiazepine-like drugs, conducted in elderly subjects, raised significant questions about their risk-benefit ratio, and suggested that there were relatively small benefits in relationship to rather significant potentially serious adverse events [9]. Their use in the elderly, and particularly the frail elderly in long-term care, should therefore be carefully considered.

Other medications which are used to treat anxiety and insomnia include trazodone, antihistamines, antipsychotics, and buspirone (Buspar). Trazodone, an antidepressant, can be effective in doses of 25–50 mg at bedtime for the treatment of patients with insomnia, or patients with dementia who become agitated prior to bedtime. The antihistamines such as hydroxyzine (Atarax) and diphenhydramine (Benadryl) are highly anticholinergic and should therefore not be considered agents of first choice in the elderly. Although antipsychotics can be helpful in treating severe anxiety and agitation, there are many risks associated with their use that have been described previously. Buspirone, a nonbenzodiazepine anxiolytic, is nonsedating and nonaddictive. It is extremely well tolerated in doses of 5–10 mg three times daily but onset of anti-anxiety effect is 2–4 weeks and it may not be very effective in patients who have previously been treated with benzodiazepines. While numerous medications have been described for the treatment of insomnia, pharmacotherapy should not be considered until other measures have been exhausted. Studies suggest that behavioral and environmental interventions, which improve sleep hygiene, are effective with long-lasting benefits and no potential side effects [10]. This is clearly the treatment of choice for insomnia in the elderly.

Treatment of Cognitive Impairment

The treatment of the cognitive deficits associated with Alzheimer's disease has become a reality only in the last few years. At the present time there are two classes of drugs marketed for this indication, the cholinesterase inhibitors (ChEI) and memantine (Ebixa/Namenda) [11]. The ChEIs such as tacrine (Cognex – not available in Canada), donepezil (Aricept), and rivastigmine (Exelon), and galantamine (Reminyl), potentially offer modest improvements in cognitive function, behavior and activities of daily living. These drugs have been tested mostly in patients with mild to moderate cognitive impairment (MMSE scores 10–26) raising the question about what role these drugs may play in nursing home patients, many of whom have moderate or severe dementia. In fact, some authorities have suggested that nursing home placement should be an indication for stopping these drugs. There have however, been a small number of recent studies that have examined the use of ChEIs in more severely impaired AD patients, including a recent nursing home study which demonstrated that donepezil was safe and effective, improving cognition and minimizing loss of activities of daily living.

All the cholinesterase inhibitors work by inhibiting an enzyme that breaks down acetylcholine, a neurotransmitter that is thought to play a key role in certain cognitive functions such as attention and memory. Increasing acetylcholine also leads to these drugs' characteristic side-effect profile which can include nausea, vomiting, loose stools, sweating, and muscle cramps. These medications must be used cautiously in patients with asthma, a history of GI bleeds, and certain cardiac arrhythmias.

Tacrine, the first available cholinesterase inhibitor marketed, causes significant gastrointestinal side effects and elevation of liver enzymes in many patients. As a result, it is used infrequently today. Donepezil, rivastigmine, and galantamine are much better tolerated. All the ChEIs are started at low doses (e.g., donepezil 5 mg) and increased slowly, no faster than every month. The typical therapeutic doses are donepezil 5–10 mg once daily, rivastigmine 3–6 mg twice daily, and galantamine 8–12 mg twice daily (or 16–24 mg once a day if the extended release formula is used). In order to accurately judge the effectiveness of these medications a variety of target symptoms should be considered including cognitive function (e.g., short-term memory, attention, concentration), behavior (e.g., apathy, agitation, hallucinations, delusions), and function (activities of daily living). Recent studies have suggested that these medications can effectively treat some behavioral disturbances such as hallucinations, and may be especially effective for patients with dementia with Lewy bodies (see Chapter 3). There is no persuasive evidence that one ChEI is more effective than another, though some patients may be able to tolerate and benefit from one drug but not another.

Memantine is an NMDA receptor antagonist and unlike the ChEIs whose therapeutic effects are mediated by acetylcholine, memantine has its effects on the neurotransmitter glutamate. The published studies of memantine have all included moderately to severe dementia patients and one was completed in a nursing home population. These studies demonstrate modest but significant benefits in cognition, function, and behavior, with an excellent safety profile. Agitation, in particular, appears to respond well to memantine. Memantine appears to work both by itself and in combination with the ChEIs. While the typical therapeutic dose of memantine is 10 mg twice daily, very old, frail, cachectic patients and those with compromised kidney function should be treated with lower doses.

HERMAN®

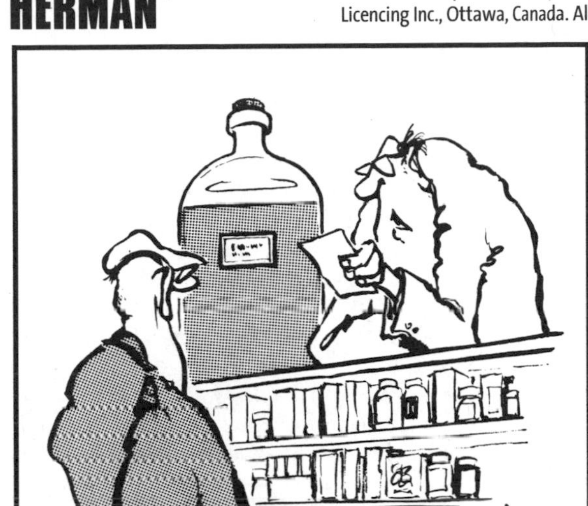

"That's what it says: 'one tablespoonful, 300 times a day'."

References

1. Avorn, J., Dreyer, P., Connelly, K., Soumeri, S.B. (1989). Use of psychoactive medications and the quality of care in rest homes. New England Journal of Medicine, 320:227–232.
This important study concludes that a large percentage of residents in these long-term care facilities are elderly and psychiatrically disturbed. It raises the important concern that such institutions frequently use psychoactive medications without adequate medical supervision, using poorly trained supervisory staff.
2. Zubenko, G.S., Sunderland, T. (2000). Geriatric psychopharmacology: Why does age matter? Harvard Review of Psychiatry, 7:311–333.
This comprehensive review of geriatric psychopharmacology includes details on age-related changes to drug metabolism, specific properties of commonly used psychotropics, and a helpful discussion on therapeutic compliance.
3. Alexopoulos, G.S., Katz, I.R., Reynolds, C.F., Carpenter, D., Docherty, J.P. (2001). Pharmacotherapy of depressive disorders in older patients. Postgraduate Medicine Special Report, (Special Issue):1–86.
This is a report form the Expert Consensus Guidelines which reviews the assessment and treatment of depression in the elderly and includes details about antidepressant therapy. Most useful is the Results and Commentary section of the Introduction, pages 10–16.
4. Sajatovic, M., Madhusoodanan, S., Coconcea, N. (2005). Managing bipolar disorder in the elderly: Defining the role of newer agents. Drugs and Aging, 22:39–54.
This article provides guidelines for the management of bipolar disorder in the elderly with a focus

on the use of lithium carbonate, valproic acid, carbamazepine, as well as newer mood stabilizers and the atypical antipsychotics.

5. Sweet, R.A., Pollock, B.G. (1998). New atypical antipsychotics: Experience and utility in the elderly. Drugs and Aging, 12(2):115–127.
   This comprehensive review covers the studies of atypical antipsychotic use in the elderly, including a focus on metabolism and drug interactions.
6. Jeste, D.V., Lacro, J.P., Bailey, A., Rockwell, E., Harris, M.J., Caligiuri, M.P. (1999). Lower incidence of tardive dyskinesia with risperidone compared with haloperidol in older patients. Journal of the American Geriatrics Society 47:716–719.
   This important study emphasizes the high rates at which elderly patients develop tardive dyskinesia when treated with typical APs, and the significant advantage that treatment with atypical APs provide with respect to this adverse event.
7. Herrmann, N., Lanctot, K.L. (2006). Atypical antipsychotics in the elderly: Malignant or maligned? Drug Safety, 29(10):833–843.
   This comprehensive review examines the safety of atypical antipsychotics in the elderly including mortality and cerebrovascular risks, comparing them with typical antipsychotics.
8. Herrmann, N. (2001). Recommendations for the management of behavioral and psychological symptoms of dementia. Canadian Journal of Neurological Sciences 28(Supplement 1):96–107.
   This article reviews the phenomenology, assessment, and management of behavioral disturbances in dementia including agitation and aggression.
9. Glass, J., Lanctôt, K.L., Herrmann, N, Sproule. B.A., Busto, U.E. (2005). Risk-benefit analysis of sedative-hypnotics in the elderly: A meta-analysis. British Medical Journal, 331:1169–1173.
   This study pooled results from all the published studies of benzodiazepines in the elderly, and raises concerns that their side effects may outweigh their potential benefits.
10. Morin, C.M., Colecchi, C., Stone, J., Sood, R., Brink, D. (1999). Behavioral and pharmacological therapies for late-life insomnia: A randomized controlled trial. Journal of the American Medical Association, 281:991–999.
    This study demonstrates that while treatment of insomnia is effective with both medications (benzodiazepines) and behavior therapy (including sleep hygiene) improvements are actually better sustained with the latter.
11. Cummings, J.L. (2004). Alzheimer's disease. New England Journal of Medicine, 351:56–67.
    This paper focuses on the pharmacological options for the treatment of Alzheimer's disease, but also nicely summarizes information on the diagnosis and pathophysiology of the disease.

Suggested Reading

1. Bezchlibnyk-Butler, K.Z., Jeffries, J.J. (Eds.). (2006). Clinical handbook of psychotropic drugs, 16th Edition. Toronto: Hogrefe & Huber Publishers.
   Although not specifically related to the elderly, this spiral-bound handbook reviews the major psychotropic drug classes with numerous handy charts and tables.
2. Sadavoy, J. (2004). Psychotropic drugs and the elderly: Fast facts. New York: Norton.
   A highly detailed reference manual which focuses specifically on geriatric psychiatric drugs.

Medications for Emotional and Behavioral Problems – Family Information Sheet*

- Emotional problems (e.g., depression, anxiety, suspiciousness, hallucinations) and behavioral problems (e.g., aggression, resistiveness to care) are common problems for residents in long-term care institutions.
- When these problems interfere with the resident's quality of life or when they represent danger to the resident, other residents, or staff, the team may recommend specific treatments.
- Such treatments will usually be recommended after the staff have considered the possible causes for the behavior which might include recent changes to the resident's physical health.
- Emotional and behavioral problems are best treated with a combination of approaches that may include changes to their rooms, their nursing care, their daily activities, and medications.
- Many people become extremely worried when medications for emotional and behavioral problems are recommended. They fear that their relative may become a "zombie," that the resident is somehow being punished, or they simply feel uncomfortable with their relative receiving a "psychiatric" medication.
- Medications for emotional and behavioral problems can be extremely helpful, can improve the lives of residents, and may help staff provide more effective care, without causing bothersome side effects. These medications should definitely not be considered "treatments of last choice."
- The physician will prescribe the lowest effective dose of the medication and with other team members will check to see if the medication is working and if there are any side effects.
- Depending on the medication, it might be worthwhile to try and discontinue it after a period of behavioral stability, e.g., 6 months.
- The physician and/or pharmacist will be able to tell you what the medication is supposed to do for your relative and what the most common side effects may be.
- You can help the team by reporting if you see any positive changes in your relative, or whether you notice any side effects. Your input is very important – after all, you know your relative best!

* From *Practical Psychiatry in the Long-Term Care Home: A Handbook for Staff* (D.K. Conn et al., Eds.). ISBN 978-0-88937-341-9.

Medications for Depression – Family Information Sheet*

- Medications for depression are called antidepressants.
- Antidepressants can be very useful for reducing sadness, tearfulness, anxiety, hopelessness, loss of pleasure and enjoyment and improving sleep, appetite, and energy.
- Antidepressants don't work immediately. Older people with depression treated with antidepressants may not improve significantly until they have been treated for 6 to 12 weeks.
- Different symptoms of depression respond differently to antidepressants. For example, sleep, appetite, and energy tend to improve in the first several weeks, while the feelings of sadness and hopelessness may require a month or more to improve. The depressed person is often the last one to recognize they feel better!
- All antidepressants have been shown to be equally effective. Unfortunately, only two-thirds of people treated, will respond to a given antidepressant. Your relative may, therefore, require more than one trial of an antidepressant.
- Antidepressants are not addictive or habit-forming. They are safe even after they have been used for many years.
- People treated with antidepressants may require the medications for months or even years to ensure depression does not return.
- The most commonly used antidepressants in long-term care belong to the "Prozac" type of drugs and include medications such as fluoxetine (Prozac), sertraline (Zoloft), fluvoxamine (Luvox), paroxetine (Paxil), citalopram (Celexa), and escitalopram (Cipralex, Lexapro). These drugs are also referred to as selective serotonin reuptake inhibitors (SSRIs).
- The SSRIs are effective antidepressants that generally cause few side effects for older people. The most common side effects might include upset stomach, nausea, and loose stools. Some people may also complain of headache or dizziness and they may be unsteady on their feet. Many of these side effects will go away with time or will improve if the dose is decreased.
- Other commonly used antidepressants include tricyclics [examples: nortriptyline (Aventyl, Pamelor), desipramine (Norpramine), imipramine (Tofranil), amitriptyline (Elavil)], trazodone (Desyrel), venlafaxine (Effexor), bupropion (Wellbutrin), mirtazapine (Remeron), and moclobemide (Manerix).
- Your relative's doctor can provide more information on any of these medications as well as explaining which symptoms you can help monitor for evidence of improvement. Another excellent source of information on these antidepressants is the facility's pharmacist.

* From *Practical Psychiatry in the Long-Term Care Home: A Handbook for Staff* (D.K. Conn et al., Eds.). ISBN 978-0-88937-341-9. © 2007 Hogrefe & Huber Publishers.

Medications for Anxiety and Sleep – Family Information Sheet*

- Commonly used medications for the treatment of anxiety and sleep difficulties belong to a group of drugs called "the benzodiazepines."
- These include drugs like lorazepam (Ativan), oxazepam (Serax), Temazepam (Restoril), clonazepam (Rivotril, Klonopin), and alprazolam (Xanax).
- Similar medications include zopiclone (Imovane), zolpidem (Ambien), eszopiclone (Lunesta), and zaleplon (Sonata, Starnoc).
- These drugs share many similar characteristics. They are very effective for reducing anxiety and helping people fall asleep. They work quickly and will often be effective after the first dose.
- Unfortunately these drugs have many potential side effects, especially in older people. These include daytime tiredness (or a "hangover" effect), unsteadiness which could lead to falls, and the possibility of causing a worsening of memory and concentration difficulties.
- These medications also have the potential to be habit-forming and they may cause withdrawal symptoms (such as increased anxiety or insomnia) if they are stopped abruptly.
- Because of these concerns, these drugs are often prescribed on an "as needed" basis instead of regular everyday use. They may also be prescribed regularly but for short periods of time (several days or weeks).
- Another commonly used medication is trazodone (Desyrel). This medication is actually an antidepressant that is effective for treating anxiety and insomnia in small doses. Possible side effects include daytime tiredness and low blood pressure which may lead to falls. It is generally considered safer than the benzodiazepines and is not habit-forming.
- Buspirone (Buspar) is another medication that is used for the treatment of anxiety. It has few side effects, but usually takes several weeks to work. It does not help with sleep problems.
- Sleep problems often respond to simple nondrug treatments such as avoiding caffeine, limiting drinking in the evening, avoiding daytime napping, and ensuring adequate exercise and stimulation during the day. It is always worthwhile to consider nondrug treatments for such difficulties before medications.

Medications for Aggression and Other Disturbing Behaviors – Family Information Sheet*

- Residents in long-term care, many with dementia, will at times have problems with aggression, restlessness, hallucinations (hearing or seeing imaginary things), and delusions (persistent false beliefs).
- The most commonly used medication for these problems are called "antipsychotics."
- Antipsychotics are divided into two groups called typical and atypical. Typical antipsychotics include drugs like haloperidol (Haldol), chlorpromazine (Largactil, Thorazine), and perphenazine (Trilafon). The atypical antipsychotics are newer drugs such as risperidone (Risperdal), olanzapine (Zyprexa), quetiapine (Seroquel), and aripiprazole (Abilify).
- While these medications can reduce the frequency and severity of aggressive behaviors and improve hallucinations and delusions, they have potential side effects.
- Besides effects such as sedation, they can also cause problems with movement. These include too little movement (stiffness, rigidity, and slowed movement) and too much movement (shaking and writhing). While some of these effects occur only while the patient is receiving medications, some may persist even after the medication is discontinued. The newer atypical antipsychotics are much less likely to cause the movement problems than older typical antipsychotics. There is some evidence that antipsychotics are associated with a small increased risk of strokes and mortality when used in patients with dementia.
- A variety of other medications may be used to treat aggression and disruptive behaviors including antidepressants such as trazodone (Desyrel), the "Prozac" type drugs, and anticonvulsants (e.g., carbamazepine (Tegretol), and valproic acid (Depakene, Depakote, Epival).
- All of these medications should be monitored closely for benefits and side effects and used in addition to other approaches such as changes to the environment, nursing care, and other activities.

* From *Practical Psychiatry in the Long-Term Care Home: A Handbook for Staff* (D.K. Conn et al., Eds.). ISBN 978-0-88937-341-9.

12 Optimizing the Use of Psychotropic Medications

David K. Conn

Key Points

- Residents in long-term care facilities represent a unique group for whom the prescribing of medications requires extra precautions.
- There is considerable evidence of inappropriate prescribing of medications, especially psychotropic medications, in nursing homes.
- Rates of use of psychotropic medications vary widely between comparable institutions and between countries.
- Approaches to maximize optimal prescribing include legislative approaches, such as OBRA 87 in the U.S., educational approaches and the use of drug audits.

Numerous studies have raised concerns about the quality of prescribing to elderly residents of long-term care facilities. Although criteria for "inappropriate prescribing" can be debated, there is general agreement that considerable improvement is required to ensure optimal prescribing. Several factors make the nursing home a unique setting for drug prescription. These include the extreme frailty of the patients, the complexity of the social institution, limited physician input, nonphysician's contribution to treatment decisions, the role of the pharmacist, limited staffing levels, and staff education.

Problems in Medication Use in the Elderly

The term "silent epidemic" has been used to describe the problems caused by adverse drug reactions. A 1998 report consisting of a meta-analysis of 39 prospective studies estimated the number of adverse drug reactions and deaths due to medications [1]. The study suggested that more than two million hospitalized patients had serious adverse drug reactions over a one-year period and that 106,000 died as a consequence. Even when the outcome is not fatal, medications can lead to disability, impaired function, confusion, and reduced independence in the elderly. The economic cost of these medication-related problems has been reported to total almost $85 billion annually in the United States.

Considerable concern has also been raised about prescribing for elderly patients living in the community. For example, a study by Tamblyn et al. [8] in Quebec of more than 60,000 elderly suggested that 52.6% experienced one or more events of high risk prescribing over a one-year period. High risk prescribing, defined on the basis of published data and expert review, was most prevalent for psychotropic drugs and "questionable prescribing" was more frequent than "rational prescribing" in this drug group. More than 30% of the total elderly population received benzodiazepines for more than 30 consecutive days and 12.9% received a long-acting benzodiazepine. Medications can cause motor vehicle accidents, home injuries, falls, and fractures. There is also evidence linking inappropriate prescribing to drug-related illness. Grymonpre et al. [9] reported that 19% of hospital admissions because of drug-related illness were attributed to inadequate or inappropriate drug therapy.

Eight general categories of medication-related problems have been described (see **Table 1**). Individuals over the age of 65 are particularly vulnerable to these problems because of age-related physiological changes, illness, and the large number of medications they take, both prescribed and over-the-counter. The elderly are especially vulnerable to the cognitive side effects of medications and at greatly increased risk of developing delirium.

Table 1 Categories of Medication-Related Problems

Untreated indication: Patient has medical problem that requires drug therapy but has not been prescribed medication for that indication
Improper drug selection: Patient has medical problem that requires drug therapy but is taking the wrong medication
Subtherapeutic dosage: Patient has medical problem that is being treated with inadequate dose of the correct medication
Failure to receive drugs: Patient has a medical problem that is the result of not receiving a drug that has been prescribed (e.g., for pharmaceutical, psychological, sociological, or economic reasons). This would include noncompliance.
Overdosage: Patient has medical problem that is being treated with too much of the correct drug
Adverse drug reaction: Patient has medical problem that is the result of an unintended and detrimental adverse drug effect
Drug interaction: Patient has medical problem that is the result of a drug-drug or drug-food interaction
Drug use without indication: Patient is taking a drug without a valid medical reason

Adapted from [20]

Addressing Problems in Medication Use

Increased education of healthcare professionals about medication effects in the elderly could begin to reduce the impact of the "silent epidemic" of adverse drug reactions. The Alliance for Aging Research notes that there are serious gaps in the current knowledge

Table 2 Questions for Evaluating Drug Use in a Nursing Home

- What is the target problem being treated?
- Is the drug necessary?
- Are nonpharmacologic therapies available?
- Is this the lowest practical dose?
- Could discontinuing therapy with a previously prescribed medication help to reduce symptoms?
- Does this drug have adverse effects that are more likely to occur in an older patient?
- Is this the most cost-effective choice?
- By what criteria, and at what time, will the effects of therapy be assessed?

Reproduced from Avorn, J., Gurwitz, J.H. (1995). Drug use in the nursing home. Annals of Internal Medicine, 123:195–204, with permission from the American College of Physicians.

base, which include: (1) insufficient research into the effects that age-related changes in body composition and functioning have on medication effects; (2) insufficient information about medication effects in elderly persons, especially the oldest age group, from premarketing clinical trials; and (3) lack of a system for collecting, processing, analyzing, and disseminating information about medication effects in the elderly population, especially after a medication is approved for marketing [2].

Avorn and Gurwitz [3] outlined some basic questions that should be asked prior to the prescription of any drug in the nursing home setting. These questions are listed in **Table 2**. Studies have shown that not infrequently there has been a failure to document reasons for prescribing medications in long-term settings. It is important to describe and document the target problem being treated, to consider alternatives to medications and to review potential adverse effects. It is especially important to determine by what criteria, and when, the effects of therapy will be reassessed. Rochon and Gurwitz [4] warn that a "prescribing cascade" can begin when an adverse drug reaction is misinterpreted as a new medical condition. Another drug is then prescribed, and the patient is placed at risk of developing additional adverse effects relating to this potentially unnecessary treatment (see **Figure 1**).

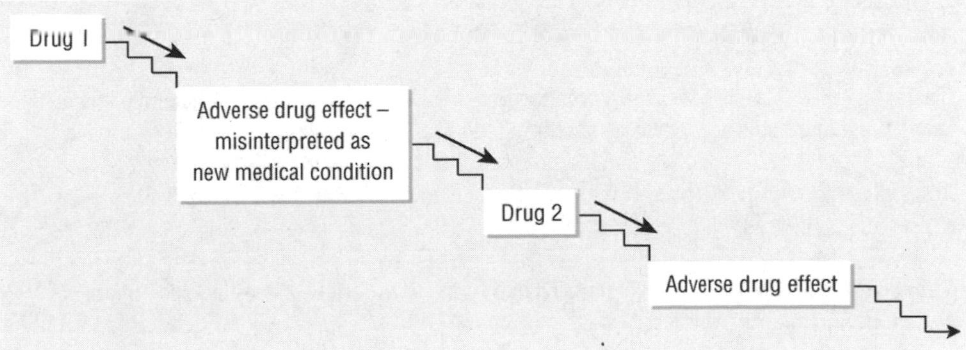

Figure 1 Prescribing Cascade (from [4]; British Medical Journal, 1997, 315:1096–1099, reproduced with permission from the BMJ Publishing Group)

Table 3 Drugs Potentially Inappropriate for Geriatric Use

Medication	Rationale	Medication	Rationale
Amitriptyline	A	Glutethimide*	B
Amobarbital*	B	Hyoscyamine	A
Belladonna alkaloids	A	Indomethacin	G
Butabarbital*	B	Isoxsuprine	F
Carisoprodol	C	Meperidine (oral)	G
Chlordiazepoxide*	D	Meprobamate*	B,G
Chlorpropamide	E	Metaxalone	C
Chlorzoxazone	C	Methocarbamol	C
Clidinium	A	Methyldopa	G
Cyclandelate	F	Orphenadrine	C
Cyclobenzaprine	C	Oxybutynin	A
Diazepam*	D	Pentazocine	G
Dicyclomine	A	Pentobarbital*	B,G
Dipyridamole	F	Propantheline	A
Disopyramide	A	Propoxyphene	G
Doxepin	A	Reserpine	G
Ergot mesyloids	F	Secobarbital*	B,G
Ethchlorvynol*	B	Trimethobenzamide	F
Flurazepam*	D		

Rationale Key:

A = Anticholinergic side effects
B = Addictive
C = Minimally effective and toxic
D = Increases risk of falls and fractures, short half-life benzodiazepines preferred
E = Excessive risk of hypoglycemia due to long half-life
F = Lack of evidence of effectiveness
G = Increased risk of toxicity; safer alternatives available

*Therapy should not be initiated with these agents in the elderly. When an elderly patient is already taking these medications, downward dose titration should be very gradual.

Drugs were included in this table on the basis of evidence provided by at least one of the following references [5, 21, 22, 23, 24, 25].

Adapted from [26]. Reprinted with permission of the American Society of Consultant Pharmacists, Alexandria, Virginia.

To prevent this cascade clinicians should always consider any new signs and symptoms as a possible consequence of current drug treatment.

Beers et al. [5] convened a panel of national experts in the United States in an attempt to reach a consensus on defining inappropriate medication use in the nursing home. While concurring on most questions, the panel failed to agree on several issues, including the use of antipsychotic medications for nonpsychotic patients. Using the agreed-upon criteria, they reported that more than 40% of residents in a group of California nursing homes had at least one inappropriate prescription. These criteria, developed by combining a literature review with the consensus of the expert panel, target 30 medications, excessive doses of medications or overly prolonged durations of therapy that potentially lead to unnecessary risks for nursing home residents. Beers and colleagues [6] then studied the characteristics and quality of prescribing by physicians practicing in nursing homes. They looked at the characteristics of physicians who prescribed most inappropriately and noted that they included older age, graduation from medical school before 1965, smaller nursing home practice and infrequent consultation with psychiatrists. A broad list of drugs which are considered to be *potentially* inappropriate for geriatric use is shown in **Table 3**.

The Beers criteria were recently updated [7]. From a psychotropic perspective medications added to the "to-be-avoided" list include: fluoxetine, buproprion in patients with seizure disorder, olanzapine in patients with obesity, conventional antipsychotics in patients with Parkinson's disease, some tricyclic antidepressants in patients with syncope or falls and stress incontinence, and benzodiazepines in patients with syncope or falls.

Use of Psychotropic Medications in Long-Term Care Homes

Most studies suggest that between 50% and 75% of nursing home residents have at least one prescription for a psychotropic medication. The patterns and rates of use of these medications vary widely from institution to institution and from country to country. Snowden [10] notes that factors which might explain these variations include differences in prevalence and severity of disorders, levels of physical disability, prescribing habits of physicians, involvement by pharmacists, number of untrained staff, size and design of institutions, funding and type of institutions, socioeconomic background of the residents, and policies regarding admissions. A comparison of rates of utilization of psychotropic medications in various countries is outlined in **Table 4** and it is evident that the rates vary widely in these studies. Concerns about the use of psychotropic medications have included the lack of a documented diagnosis, the high risk of complications, such as falls, fractures and movement disorders, that physician characteristics (rather than those of patients) predict drug dosage, and that mental health consultation is rarely available for nursing home residents. Particular concerns have been raised with regard to the use of antipsychotic (neuroleptic) drugs and benzodiazepines.

It should be noted, of course, that the management of behavior problems in nursing home residents, particularly those suffering from a dementing illness, is frequently described as the problem of *most* concern to nursing home staff. It should also be noted that until recently, well-designed studies of the use of psychotropic medications in nursing

Table 4 Rates of Utilization of Psychotropic Medications in Various Countries (% patients with prescription, scheduled or prn)

Authors, year of study publication	Type, number and location of institutions	Any psychotropic	Antipsychotics (neuroleptics)	Antidepressants	Benzodiazepines	Anxiolytics	Sedative/hypnotics
Nolan & O'Malley, 1989 [27]	11 Private Nursing Homes in Dublin, Ireland	65	27	13	42	–	–
Tyberg & Gulmann, 1992 [28]	32 Nursing Homes in Denmark	56	20	11	–	13	33
Snowdon et al., 1995 [29]	46 Nursing Homes in Sydney, Australia	65.9	36.6	15.6	–	14.3	39.2
Wancata et al., 1997 [30]	10 Nursing Homes in Vienna and Tyrol, Austria	72.1	32.1	21	–	26.3	22.1
Borson & Doane, 1997[a] (1992 data) [31]	39 Skilled Geriatric Care Facilities in Washington State	50	13.3	20.1	–	18.4	3.3
Tobias & Pulliam[b], 1997 [32]	878 nursing facilities in 40 States of USA (w/o specialized units)	–	14.2	26.3	–	10.9	2.7
Schmidt et al., 1998 [33]	15 Nursing Homes in Sweden after an educational intervention	77.1	32.6	25	–	43.8	32.2
Conn et al, 1999 [34]	10 Homes for the Aged and Nursing Homes in Ontario Canada	53.3	18.4	21.7	31.0	–	–

[a]These figures based on adding scheduled and prn data together; [b]Tobias and Pulliam reported percentage of residents with routine medication orders (shown here). Average prn orders per resident were also provided. Adapted from [34].

home patients have not been carried out. There is a need for future studies to consider the response of *specific* behaviors to different therapies, so that our interventions can be more directly targeted. The most commonly prescribed medications for behavior problems in this population traditionally have been neuroleptic (antipsychotic) drugs, even though the benefits of these medications are quite modest. A meta-analysis of controlled trials by Schneider and colleagues revealed that 58% of residents receiving antipsychotics showed some improvement compared to 40% of those receiving placebos [11]. Because of the often inadequate and unpredictable response to psychotropic medications, a growing list of different psychotropics are now given consideration for the treatment of these behavioral disorders (see Chapter 11). These include antidepressants and anticonvulsants, in addition to antipsychotics and benzodiazepines. For first line treatment, most consultants currently recommend either an atypical antipsychotic medication or an antidepressant such as trazodone or a serotonin reuptake inhibitor.

The American Society of Consultant Pharmacists (ASCP) have developed "Guidelines for the Use of Psychotherapeutic Medications in Older Adults" [12]. The eight guidelines are as follows:

1. Older adults should be screened for presence of affective, cognitive, and other psychiatric disorders.
2. Older adults who exhibit symptoms of psychiatric disorders should be thoroughly assessed by a qualified health care professional.
3. Behavioral symptoms in older adults should be objectively and quantitatively monitored by caregivers or facility staff and documented on an ongoing basis. When possible, psychiatric symptoms should also be monitored in this fashion.
4. If the behaviors do not present an immediate serious threat to the patient or others, the initial approach to management of behavioral symptoms in older adults should focus on environmental modifications, behavioral interventions, psychotherapy, or other nonpharmacologic interventions.
5. When medications are indicated, select an appropriate psychotherapeutic agent, considering effectiveness of the medication and risk of side effects.
6. Begin medication at the lowest appropriate dosage and increase the dose gradually.
7. Monitor the patient for therapeutic response from the medication and for adverse drug reactions.
8. The psychotherapeutic medication regimen should be routinely reevaluated for the need for continued use of medication, dosage adjustments, or a change in medication.

Legislation to Optimize Prescribing (OBRA-87)

Concerns about inappropriate and unnecessary prescribing of psychotropics as well as other concerns about psychiatric care of nursing home residents led to federal legislation in the United States entitled "The Omnibus Budget Reconciliation Act of 1987" (OBRA-87). The provisions of this legislation include strict guidelines for physicians with regard to the prescribing of psychotropic medications in nursing homes. Residents must not receive an "unnecessary drug," which is defined as any drug used (1) in excessive dosage;

Table 5 HCFA Interpretive Guideline: 483.25 (1) (2) (I) for U. S. Nursing Homes

Antipsychotic drugs should not be used unless the clinical record documents that the resident has one or more of the following specific conditions:

1. Schizophrenia
2. Schizo-affective disorder
3. Delusional disorder
4. Psychotic mood disorders (including mania and depression with psychotic features)
5. Acute psychotic episodes
6. Brief reactive psychosis
7. Schizophreniform disorder
8. Atypical psychosis
9. Tourette's disorder
10. Huntington's disease
11. Organic mental syndromes (including dementia) with associated psychotic and/or agitated features as defined by:
    (a) Specific behaviors as quantitatively (number of episodes) and objectively (e.g., biting, kicking, and scratching) documented by the facility which cause the resident to:
    – Present a danger to themselves,
    – Present a danger to others (including staff),
    – Actually interfere with staff's ability to provide care, or
    (b) *Continuous* crying out, screaming, yelling, or pacing if these specific behaviors cause an impairment in functional capacity and if they are quantitatively (e.g., periods of time) documented by the facility, or
    (c) Psychotic symptoms (hallucinations, paranoia, delusions) not exhibited as specific behaviors listed in (a) and (b) above, if these behaviors cause an *impairment in functional capacity.*
12. Short-term (7 days) symptomatic treatment of hiccups, nausea, vomiting, or pruritus.

(2) for excessive duration; (3) without adequate monitoring; (4) without adequate indication for its use; (5) in the presence of adverse consequences which indicate that it should be reduced or discontinued; or (6) any combination of the reasons above. The OBRA guidelines state explicitly that antipsychotic medications should only be prescribed for certain indications and should not be used for uncomplicated anxiety, wandering, insomnia, or agitation. The specific indications for the use of antipsychotics are listed in **Table 5**. Interestingly, a study of antipsychotic use in nursing homes in Scotland reported that in 88% of the residents receiving antipsychotics, the prescription would be classed as "inappropriate" according to OBRA guidelines [13]. The provisions of the OBRA legislation include screening of residents prior to entry into nursing homes and regular reviews by consulting pharmacists. The use of behavioral approaches and drug holidays are also required. Residents are comprehensively assessed by staff using the Resident Assessment Instrument (RAI) which includes the Minimum Data Set (MDS), Triggers and Resident Assessment Protocols (RAPS). The MDS contains more than 400 data elements which

include information regarding mood, cognition, communication, functional status, medications, and other treatments. Triggers are specific responses for MDS items that identify residents who may be at risk for specific problems and require further evaluation using RAPs, which are structured frameworks designed to form a basis for individualized care planning. There are 18 different RAPs (including cognitive loss, delirium, mood state, and behavior problem) that help staff to look for causal or confounding factors, some of which may be reversible.

The Health Care Financing Administration (HCFA) of the United States has recently revised its nursing home survey procedures and interpretive guidelines. Interpretive guidelines provide an outline regarding how to practically comply with the legislation. These procedures and guidelines provide federal surveyors with the tools required to implement HCFA's nursing home survey, certification and enforcement rules. As of July 1, 1999, quality indicators (QIs) based upon the MDS have been incorporated into the survey process. Five of these indicators relate specifically to medication use. These QIs include: (1) prevalence of symptoms of depression without antidepressant therapy; (2) prevalence of residents who take nine or more different medications; (3) prevalence of antipsychotic use, in the absence of psychotic or related conditions; (4) prevalence of antianxiety/hypnotic use; and (5) prevalence of hypnotic use more than two times in the previous week. The current list of antipsychotic drugs in the guidelines has been updated and new daily dosage levels for olanzapine (10 mg) and quetiapine (200 mg) have been added. The maximum recommended daily dosage for risperidone has been reduced from 4 mg to 2 mg. Drug therapy guidelines based upon the work of Beers have been added with regard to unnecessary drug use and for use in monthly drug regimen reviews.

A number of studies have assessed the impact of OBRA on rates of prescribing [14, 15]. These studies show a decrease of between 27% and 36% in the use of antipsychotic drugs. In general, this decrease has not been accompanied by an increase in the prescribing of other psychotropic drugs, although there has been an overall increase in the use of antidepressant medications during this period. One study in addition to showing a decrease in the use of antipsychotic medication found a strong association between increased staffing on night shifts and reductions in antipsychotic use. A recent study [16] suggests that during the initial period after OBRA the quality of care improved in more profitable nursing homes but had no effect more recently when the regulations were weakly enforced. The study also suggests that the legislation actually had a negative effect on the quality of care in less profitable homes.

Educational Approaches

Several studies have evaluated educational programs to try to improve prescribing in nursing homes. Avorn et al. provided an educational program for physicians and nurses in six nursing homes which were then compared with control homes [17]. The study monitored both drug prescriptions and clinical status. The educational program was successful in reducing the rates of "inappropriate" drug use as defined in the study. Ray et al. implemented an educational program in two rural community nursing homes that had high rates

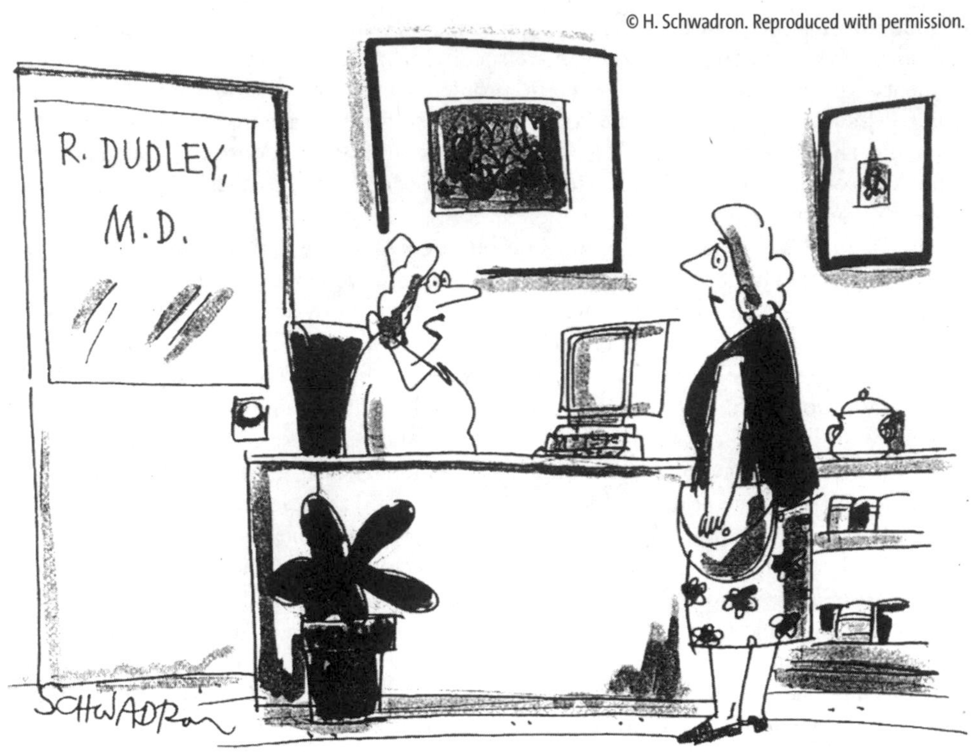

"Sorry, Dr. Dudley doesn't treat original diseases. He treats side effects from other doctors' treatments."

of antipsychotic use [18]. Days of antipsychotic use decreased by 72% in the homes receiving education vs. 13% in the control homes. The frequency of behavior problems did not increase in either group. In a Swedish study, Schmidt et al. used a similar approach and were also successful in reducing the rates of inappropriate psychotropic prescribing [19]. Avorn and colleagues described an approach called "academic detailing" in which the marketing techniques used by pharmaceutical company representatives are replicated in the teaching of nursing home staff. The approach appears to be successful because it takes into consideration the limited amount of time available for staff in nursing homes to participate in educational activities. In spite of these excellent examples, the amount of education available in most nursing homes around the world remains minimal. Hopefully, the problems of geography and limited availability of staff education might be overcome with the use of new technologies used for distance learning, e.g., the Internet or video conferencing.

Optimizing the Use of Psychotropic Medications in Your Institution

The following are suggestions regarding how to optimize psychotropic medication use:

1. Basic Questions
   Whenever starting a patient on a new medication, staff should ask themselves the questions listed in **Table 2**. It is particularly important to consider the target problem being treated. The final decision regarding the necessity of using a drug should always be based on a consideration of the potential benefits versus the risks.
2. Documenting Progress
   If practical, staff should try to document the progress of the resident using a standardized rating scale. Rating scales which can be easily and quickly filled out are most likely to be widely accepted and utilized. If this is not possible staff should try to document the specific changes that are observed, as accurately as possible.
3. Using Guidelines
   The use of clinical guidelines can be helpful and will encourage an evidence-based approach. Despite the somewhat overwhelming proliferation of published guidelines in recent years, the staff should reach a consensus on which guidelines are useful and make sense. Alternatively, a facility can develop its own set of guidelines based on the best available sources. Once approved, the use of guidelines should be monitored for levels of compliance. Guidelines are meant to assist in the decision making process. They are not meant to rigidly restrict clinical options.
4. Psychiatric Consultation
   In complex cases or those which are difficult to manage, it is advisable to obtain a consultation from a psychiatrist. Unfortunately, many institutions have limited ability to obtain such consultations. Sometimes administration must take steps to provide incentives which will encourage consultants to leave their office practices and venture into the long term care facility. Psychiatrists and pharmacists can provide helpful information for staff regarding optimal pharmacological approaches.
5. Education
   As described above, educational programs can help to reduce inappropriate prescribing. It is important to realize that all members of the team play a role in decisions regarding the use of medication. The opinions of family members are also critical. Therefore, educational programs should target all disciplines as well as relatives. Information sheets for family members regarding various classes of psychotropic medication are provided at the end of Chapter 11.
6. Drug Audits
   In countries lacking legislated surveys, staff may find it helpful to track the rates of use of psychotropic medications in their own facility. This can easily be carried out with the help of the pharmacist, the simplest method being a single-day survey. Data on the pattern of psychotropic drug utilization provides feedback to individual physicians, offers comparisons of prescribing rates between physicians, institutions or regions and can be used to monitor trends over time. Some institutions view this data as a method of quality assurance. It is particularly helpful to track the percentage of residents with prescriptions for particular classes of psychotropic medication (see **Table 4**).

Chart reviews can also be used to evaluate: the level of documentation with regard to diagnosis and reason for use of medication; target symptoms; frequency of follow-up and drug complications. The data can also serve as a means of monitoring inappropriate drug combinations and/or excessive dosages. Quality indicators can be developed as described above.

References

1. Lazarou, J., Pomeranz, B.H., Corey, P.N. (1998). Incidence of adverse drug reactions in hospitalized patients: A meta-analysis of prospective studies. Journal of the American Medical Association, 279:1200–1205.
2. Alliance for Aging Research. (1998). When medicine hurts instead of helps: Preventing medication problems in older persons. Washington, DC: Author.
3. Avorn, J., Gurwitz, J.H. (1995). Drug use in the nursing home. Annals of Internal Medicine, 123:195–204.
4. Rochon, P.A., Gurwitz, J.H. (1997). Optimizing drug treatment for elderly people: The prescribing cascade. British Medical Journal, 315:1096–1099.
5. Beers, M.H., Ouslander, J.G., Rollinger, I., Reuben, D.B., Brooks, J., Beck, J.C. (1991). Explicit criteria for determining inappropriate medication use in nursing home residents. Archives of Internal Medicine, 151:1825–1832.
6. Beers, M.H., Fingold, S.F., Ouslander, J.G., Reuben, D.B., Morgenstern, H., Beck, J.C. (1993). Characteristics and quality of prescribing by doctors practicing in nursing homes. Journal of the American Geriatrics Society, 41:802–807.
7. Fick, D.M., Cooper, J.W., Wade, W.E., Waller, J.L., MacLean, J.R., & Beers, M.H. (2003). Updating the Beers Criteria for potentially inappropriate medication use in older adults: Results of a U.S. consensus panel of experts. Archives of Internal Medicine, 163:2716–2724.
8. Tamblyn, R.M., McLeod, P.J., Abrahamowicz, M., Monette, J., Gayton, D.C., Berkson, L., et al. (1994). Questionable prescribing for elderly patients in Quebec. Canadian Medical Association Journal, 150:1801–1809.
9. Grymonpre, R.E., Mitenko, P.A., Sitar, P.A., Aoki, F.Y., Montgomery, P.R. (1988). Drug-associated hospital admissions in older medical patients. Journal of the American Geriatrics Society, 36:1092–1098.
10. Snowden, J. (1993). Mental health in nursing homes. Perspectives on the use of medication. Drugs and Aging, 3:122–130.
11. Schneider, L.S., Pollock, V.E., Lyness, S.A. (1990). A meta-analysis of controlled trials of neuroleptic treatment in dementia. Journal of the American Geriatrics Society, 38:553–563.
12. American Society of Consultant Psychiatrists. (1999). Guidelines for use of psychotherapeutic medications in older adults. Alexandria, VA.
13. McGrath, A.M., Jackson, G.A. (1996). Survey of neuroleptic prescribing in residents of nursing homes in Glasgow. British Medical Journal, 312:611–612.
14. Lantz, M., Giambanco, V., Buchalter, E.N. (1996). A ten-year review of the effect of OBRA-87 on psychotropic prescribing practices in academic nursing home. Psychiatric Services, 47:951–955.
15. Shorr, R.I., Gought, R.L., Ray, W.A. (1994). Changes in antipsychotic drug use in nursing home during implementation of the OBRA-87 regulation. Journal of the American Medical Association, 271:358–363.
16. Kumar, V., Norton, E.C., Encinosa, W.E. (2006). OBRA 1987 and the quality of nursing home care. International Journal of Health Care Finance and Economics, 6:49–81.

17. Avorn, J., Soumerai, S.B., Everett, D.E. (1992). A randomized trial of a program to reduce the use of psychotropic drugs in nursing homes. New England Journal of Medicine, 327:168–173.
18. Ray, W.A., Taylor, J.A., Meador, K.G., Lichtenstein, M.J., Griffin, M.R., et al. (1993). Reducing antipsychotic drug use in nursing homes: A controlled trial of provider education. Archives of Internal Medicine, 153:713–721.
19. Schmidt, I., Claesson, C.B., Westerholm, B., Nilsson, L.G, Svarstadt, B.L. (1998). The impact of regular multidisciplinary team interventions on psychotropic prescribing in Swedish nursing homes. Journal of the American Geriatrics Society, 46:77–82.
20. Hepler, C.D., Strand, L.M. (1990). Opportunities and responsibilities in pharmaceutical care. American Journal of Hospital Pharmacy, 47:533–543.
21. American Society of Consultant Pharmacists. (1995). Nursing Home Survey Procedures and Interpretive Guidelines. Alexandria, VA.
22. Beers, M.H. (1997). Explicit criteria for determining potentially inappropriate medication use by the elderly. Archives of Internal Medicine, 157:1531–1536.
23. McLeod, P.J., Huang, A.R., Tamblyn, R.M., Gayton, D.C. (1997). Defining inappropriate practices in prescribing for elderly people: National consensus panel. Canadian Medical Association Journal, 156:385–391.
24. Katz, I.R., Sands, L.P., Bilker, W., DiFilippo, S., Boyce, A., D'Angelo, K. (1998). Identification of medications that cause cognitive impairment in older people: The case of oxybutynin chloride. Journal of the American Geriatrics Society, 46:8–13.
25. Stuck, A.E., Beers, M.H., Steiner, A., Aronow, H.U., Rubenstein, L.Z., Beck, C.J. (1994). Inappropriate medication use in community-residing older persons. Archives of Internal Medicine, 154:2195–2200.
26. Buerger, D.K. (1998). Inappropriate Use Criteria: Covering all the bases. Consultant Pharmacist, 5:617–618.
27. Nolan, L., O'Malley, K. (1989). The need for a more rational approach to drug prescribing for elderly people in nursing homes. Age and Ageing, 18:52–56.
28. Tyjberg J., Gulmann, N.C. (1992). Use of psychopharmaceuticals in municipal nursing homes. A national survey. Ugeskr Laeger, 154:3126–3129.
29. Snowdon, J., Vaughan, R., Miller, R., Burgess, E.E., Tremlett, P. (1995). Psychotropic drug use in Sydney nursing homes. The Medical Journal of Australia, 163:70–72.
30. Wancata, J., Benda, N., Meise, U., Miller, C. (1997). Psychotropic drug intake in residents newly admitted to nursing homes. Pharmacology, 134:115–120.
31. Borson, S., Doane, K. (1997). The impact of OBRA-87 on psychotropic drug prescribing in skilled nursing facilities. Psychiatric Services, 48:1289–1296.
32. Tobias, D.E., Pulliam, C.C. (1997). General and psychotherapeutic medication use in 878 nursing facilities: A 1997 national survey. The Consultant Pharmacist, 12:1401–1408.
33. Schmidt, I., Claesson, C.B., Westerholm B., Nilsson, L.G., Svarstad, B.L. (1998). The impact of regular multidisciplinary team interventions on psychotropic prescribing in Swedish nursing homes. Journal of the American Geriatrics Society, 46:77–82.
34. Conn, D.K., Ferguson, I., Mandelman, K., Ward, C. (1999). Psychotropic drug utilization in long-term-care facilities for the elderly in Ontario, Canada. International Psychogeriatrics, 11:223–233.

Suggested Readings

1. Web site of the American Society of Consultant Pharmacists: http://www.ascp.com.
   An excellent resource. Filled with information and links regarding the use of medication in the elderly. Contains latest information on U.S. Government regulations regarding long-term care.
2. Avorn, J., Gurwitz, J.H. (1995). Drug use in the nursing home. Annals of Internal Medicine, 123:195–204.
   Useful article with practical advice on how to prescribe most appropriately in the long-term care setting.

13 Behavior Management Strategies

Dmytro Rewilak

Key Points

- Effective management of challenging behaviors in cognitively impaired residents requires attention to the following: (a) their cognitive deficits and the manner in which these compromise everyday functioning, (b) environmental factors that trigger and maintain challenging behavior, and (c) staff attitudes, perceptions, and expectations. Failure to attend to any one of the above can jeopardize the management program.
- Many challenging behaviors arise as a consequence of specific cognitive deficits and are not intentional. Labeling, however, affects how staff interact with residents and determines their emotional response to the challenging behaviors.
- Having cognitive deficits does not mean that residents have lost all capacity for change. While these deficits contribute significantly to the emergence of challenging behaviors, they are not the sole determinants. Important environmental events trigger and maintain all behavior. Changing these environmental events results in changes in behavior.
- When confronted with challenging behaviors, staff must adopt a scientific attitude. Challenging behaviors must be defined in specific and objective terms and be subjected to a functional, or ABC, analysis in order to determine the environmental variables that control them. Being scientific does not mean being uncaring or unsympathetic.
- An individualized management plan is developed which is based on the results of the ABC analysis and knowledge of cognitive deficits. Challenging behaviors require ongoing monitoring in order to determine the effectiveness of the program. Necessary adjustments are made as indicated.
- Staff perceptions of the challenging behaviors need to be examined, as these will affect their levels of stress. Challenging behaviors must be viewed as problems that require a solution. It is helpful to break down stressful interactions with a particular resident into a series of steps, for which coping self-statements are developed.

Introduction

A progressive deterioration of memory and other cognitive functions is a primary defining characteristic of dementia syndromes. This deterioration results in progressive inability to handle the demands of everyday life and contributes to the development of behavioral disturbances. The behavioral manifestations of dementia include psychiatric symptoms (e.g., delusions, hallucinations) and a broad range of agitated behaviors (e.g., wandering, kicking, screaming). Agitated behaviors are extremely difficult to manage. For this reason, we refer to them as challenging behaviors since, in every sense of the word, they challenge the knowledge, skills, creativity, and coping resources of caregivers. Challenging behaviors are a major risk factor for caregiver distress and nursing home placement, and they are extremely disruptive in an institutional setting.

Many challenging behaviors are magnified unnecessarily and result in what has been called "excess disability." Excess disability is defined as a degree of functional impairment in excess of that expected given the severity and duration of dementia. Contributing to excess disability are health, emotional, social, and environmental factors. The latter include not only the characteristics of the physical environment such as levels of noise, lighting, and temperature, but also the people with whom the individual interacts in that environment. In the nursing home setting, the resident's major interactions are typically with front-line nursing staff members who, in many cases, do not have an adequate spectrum of strategies for dealing with challenging behaviors.

Traditionally, challenging behaviors have been managed almost exclusively and preferentially through pharmacological means. Behavioral approaches, despite their extensive use and proven success with children and younger adults in a variety of clinical environments, have been under-utilized in geriatric and long-term settings. Given the frequently less than favorable risk-benefit ratio of most psychotropic drugs in older people, particularly those with dementia, the importance of behavioral approaches in helping an individual change socially significant behaviors cannot be overstated. Those individuals whose challenging behaviors have been successfully managed experience an improved quality of life. They have new opportunities to take part in social programming and functional tasks, they may experience less conflict with other nursing home residents, and they have improved interactions with both staff and family visitors. Successful management of challenging behaviors may also improve the safety of other residents and caregivers, thereby reducing the need for physical and pharmacological restraints. This chapter presents the behavioral approach to the management of challenging behaviors in cognitively impaired nursing home residents.

Overview

A comprehensive approach to the management of challenging behaviors in a resident with cognitive impairments should take into account: (a) the nature of the resident's cognitive deficits and their impact on everyday functioning, (b) the environmental variables that contribute to the expression and maintenance of the resident's challenging behaviors, and (c) staff's perceptions of these behaviors. This approach recognizes the complexity of human behavior, and takes into account important factors within individual residents, their caregivers, and their physical environments. Information about these factors is obtained through a cognitive assessment, a systematic behavioral assessment, and interviews with staff.

Cognitive Assessment

One of the most important determinants of challenging behaviors in cognitively impaired individuals in a nursing home setting is the integrity of their brain. Generally, the brain can be thought of as an organ that allows us to interact with and adapt to our environment. When it becomes dysfunctional, as in cases of Alzheimer's disease or stroke, this process of interaction and adaptation breaks down and results in challenging behaviors. Unfortunately, because the effects of individuals' cognitive deficits on their everyday functioning are often poorly understood, they tend to be misinterpreted. Terms, such as "senility," "dementia," and "organic" are too global and communicate little that can be of use in understanding specific behaviors. What once was called senility represents a multitude of different disease processes. Even in the case of Alzheimer's disease, there is evidence pointing to different subtypes. It is crucial, therefore, to describe the individual's impaired as well as spared cognitive functions, as these will have an important bearing on the success of any management strategies that are implemented.

A description of cognitive functions is achieved through a neuropsychological assessment. Two major patterns of neuropsychological impairment have been identified within the dementia illnesses and have been named according to what part of the brain is most involved. One pattern is called cortical, because it primarily involves the cortex (i.e., the surface areas of the brain that looks like the bark of a tree; *cortex* is Latin for the bark of a tree). Alzheimer's disease, which is the most well-known and most frequently occurring of all dementia illnesses, is a cortical dementia. The second pattern is called subcortical, because it primarily involves areas of the brain lying beneath the surface (*sub* in Latin means beneath). The dementia associated with Parkinson's disease is a subcortical dementia.

The importance of this distinction can be illustrated with reference to memory. Impaired memory is a symptom of all dementias. The nature of the impairment differs, however, depending on what brain areas are most affected. For example, the memory problems that are associated with Alzheimer's disease are different than those associated with Parkinson's disease. In Alzheimer's disease the person cannot form new memories, while in Parkinson's disease the person can form new memories but needs cues and prompts to retrieve them. A neuropsychological assessment helps to define the nature of the memory problem which has different implications for management.

The need to understand the underlying cognitive impairments is further illustrated with reference to fronto-temporal dementia, another cortical dementia. This type of dementia is characterized by the insidious onset and gradual progression of profound behavioral and personality changes in the absence of pronounced memory impairment in the first two years. This is different from Alzheimer's disease, in which a primary memory disturbance is typically the earliest sign indicating onset of the disease and in which prominent behavioral and personality changes may occur, but typically only much later in the disease process.

The behavioral and personality changes in fronto-temporal dementia are more likely than other symptoms of cognitive dysfunction to result in extreme levels of stress in care-providers, both professional and family, and lead to premature institutionalization. The behavioral and personality changes in this type of dementia are not uniform, but depend on what part of the frontal lobes is most affected.

There is a disinhibited type, in which the behavioral manifestations include impulsivity, emotional lability, and inappropriate laughing, crying, or sexuality. An attentional disturbance is also present, characterized by distractibility, or difficulty in selective attention. These behaviors contribute to poor social integration. Even though insight may be spared and individuals may be aware of their problem, they are unable to control their behavior. A second type is the apathetic type, in which the behavioral manifestations include indifference, psychomotor slowing, and impaired judgment and insight. Cognitive deficits include impairments in planning, goal-directed behavior, and keeping track of the temporal order of external and internal events. An attentional difficulty is present also in this subtype, but is one of difficulty sustaining attention. In the third type, difficulty in the initiation of motor and mental activity is the most prominent symptom. Difficulty programming motor acts is also characteristic.

Misinterpreting the underlying cause of the different behavioral disturbances associated with fronto-temporal dementia may lead to the wrong diagnosis and management. For example, a person with an apathetic type of this dementia could be diagnosed as suffering from depression.

The need to understand the contribution of cognitive deficits to challenging behaviors cannot be overstated. A full neuropsychological evaluation is time-consuming. In our setting, we have found that a comprehensive neuropsychological screening battery, which takes approximately one hour to administer, provides sufficient information that can be incorporated into a management plan. The battery assesses various aspects of the individual's orientation, attention, memory, language, constructional abilities, motor and sensory-perceptual functions, and abstract reasoning. If the services of a neuropsychologist are not readily available, valuable information about the individual's cognitive functioning can be obtained through a detailed mental status examination (MSE; see Chapter 2). The resident's medical record may also contain clues about the nature of the resident's cognitive impairments and should not be overlooked.

Behavioral Assessment

The behavioral assessment should be viewed as a companion to neuropsychological assessment. It is the best method of determining the practical functional consequences of the deficits identified by neuropsychological tests. For example, neuropsychological tests may identify the nature of a memory deficit or a deficit in self-monitoring, but they cannot really evaluate the disability – repeated requests for the same thing, getting lost in a particular environment, inappropriate social conduct – that results from them. To characterize the two types of assessment rather simply, the neuropsychological assessment is concerned with what impairments the person has, and the behavioral assessment is concerned with what the person does or does not do, in other words, the expression of the impairments in everyday behavior.

The behavioral assessment proceeds from the general to the specific. The starting point is the gathering of information from caregivers who are currently interacting with the individual exhibiting challenging behaviors. The caregivers' concerns and some of the context in which the challenging behaviors are occurring are clarified. It is not unusual to find that caregivers differ between themselves in their perception of how severe, stressful, or difficult to manage particular challenging behaviors are. Recognition of this provides an early hint to caregivers about how their approach to the provision of care may be contributing to the behaviors.

In addition to interviewing the caregivers, a thorough chart review also needs to be performed to glean as much information as possible about the individual's medical, social, and personal history. For example, the habits of a given individual (e.g., going to buy a newspaper at a particular time each day) may help to explain the temporal regularity of the individual's increased tendency to wander. It is particularly important to eliminate underlying physical factors, since many cognitively impaired individuals have at least one coexisting medical illness. The sudden emergence of a behavioral disturbance may be associated with such factors as urinary tract infections, exacerbations of pain, heart failure, constipation, and drug toxicity.

The next step in behavioral assessment is to perform a detailed and systematic analysis of a given challenging behavior and the events which both precede and follow it. What is meant by behavior? Behavior is anything a person does or says that can be observed, measured, and monitored. It does not occur in a vacuum, but has an impact on and is impacted on by the physical and social environment. The most important assumption of the behavioral approach is that behavior is lawful, in other words, its occurrence is systematically influenced by environmental events. Specifically, for every occurrence of a specific behavior there are events that trigger it and events that encourage its repetition. Triggering events are called **A**ntecedents, and events that maintain **B**ehavior are called **C**onsequences. In this approach, every behavior can be subjected to a functional, or an **ABC** analysis. An example is provided in **Table 1.**

The example in **Table 1** illustrates a number of important points. Recording the time of day a particular behavior occurs is important because it may reveal information about possible factors associated with the behavior. For example, the yelling may occur within a certain time following the ingestion of medication, food, or drink, or it may be more

Table 1 An ABC Analysis of Yelling Behavior

DATE	February 3, 1997
TIME	9:10 a.m.
ANTECEDENTS	Nurse enters room to provide a.m. care
BEHAVIOR	Resident yells: "What do you want, you (so and so) I don't belong here!"
CONSEQUENCES	Nurse responds: "What's the matter? You shouldn't use language like that. There, there now." Nurse strokes patient's arm.

frequent during shift changes. Regarding possible antecedents, the yelling may be associated with anyone entering the patient's room or just one particular individual. The yelling behavior has been described in specific and objective terms – it has been recorded verbatim. Finally, note the number of different responses on the part of the nurse to the yelling. It is important to remember that, whether the nurse appeals to the individual's reason, reprimands the individual, or attempts to reduce the individual's tension through touch, any response on the nurse's part is reinforcing, that is, it significantly raises the probability that the yelling behavior will be repeated.

While behavior is always observable, antecedents and consequences are not. For example, a particular thought (e.g., "he's going to attack me") can act as the trigger for evasive behavior, and the "high" that comes after smoking a cigarette can serve as a very powerful reinforcer of smoking. Through a behavioral assessment, an attempt is made to identify and measure the variables that control behavior. To illustrate, the antecedents that trigger the striking-out behavior of a cognitively impaired nursing home resident could include the nature of the resident's cognitive deficits, the time of day the behavior occurs, whether or not it is preceded by a stressful event, a particular location that is associated with the behavior, and the characteristics of the individual against whom the behavior occurs. Among the consequences that serve to maintain the behavior are the manner in which the behavior is handled, the amount of attention given to the behavior by staff, and staff's lack of attention to more appropriate behaviors. Only through a thorough and systematic analysis of a behavior is it possible to isolate the variables controlling it.

In carrying out an ABC, or functional, analysis of challenging behaviors, it is important to define them in specific and objective terms so that they can be measured. Terms such as "aggression," "dependence," and "agitation" are too vague and do not lend themselves to reliable measurement. They can be redefined, for example, as spitting or hitting (aggression), failure to self-feed (dependence), and pulling at hair (agitation).

Once the challenging behavior has been defined, a decision must be made about the best way to record the behavior. A number of different methods can be utilized. *Continuous* recording involves writing down everything a person says or does, a method which is not practical unless a highly specific analysis of a particular behavior is required. Recording the total length of time a behavior occurs is called *duration recording*. In *interval recording*, a period of time is broken down into blocks of five or 30 minutes, for example, and a record is made of whether or not the behavior occurred in that block of time. This type of recording does not measure whether a behavior occurred once or 50 times, it simply notes whether the behavior was present or absent during the stated interval. It usually is employed to assess behaviors occurring with a high frequency, such as constant yelling or screaming. *Momentary time sampling* involves checking for a behavior at the end of a predetermined block of time (e.g., at the end of every 10 minutes or every hour). The type of recording selected will depend on the behavior that needs to be assessed and managed.

Regardless of the recording method, the goal is to obtain baseline measurements of the challenging behavior. Monitoring of the behavior continues throughout the treatment period. This helps to determine the progress of treatment in an unbiased manner. If interventions are not monitored in this way, successful treatments may be overlooked and discontinued. In the case of yelling, staff might say that the individual is still yelling and conclude that the treatment has failed. If careful monitoring reveals that yelling is now occurring only 20 times per week rather than 55, however, staff would have direct proof that the frequency of yelling has been reduced substantially.

Staff Perceptions

When confronted with challenging behaviors in the cognitively impaired resident, it is crucial for the staff to examine their own perceptions, as these may be contributing to the problem. Under perceptions are included staff attitudes in general, staff interpretations of challenging behavior, and staff expectations of the cognitively impaired resident.

Attitudes are powerful determinants of behavior. For example, when an individual is introduced to somebody new she/he interacts briefly with that person, exchanges pleasantries, takes the person's phone number, and says goodbye, but not before having reached a conclusion about that person. The individual may label the person as a good or bad listener, as friendly or distant, as someone she/he could or could not trust. These conclusions, or labels, will determine whether the individual will call that person up on the phone and how she/he might feel (e.g., relaxed or tense) on meeting that person again.

One of the commonest forms of labeling relates to cognitive deficits. Many challenging behaviors are misconstrued as characterological when, in fact, they are the result of dysfunction in a particular cognitive domain. For example, consider the individual who has suffered a right hemisphere stroke and has difficulty attending to the left side of visual space. On his way to physiotherapy, he is wheeled along a corridor, attending only to the right side. On the return journey, what before was on the intact right side of space now is on the impaired left side. The individual begins to argue that this is not the way to his room, and staff tries to convince him to the contrary. The misinterpretations of his environment lead to increased agitation, and he becomes labeled as "confused," or even "aggressive" and "paranoid." These labels become a self-fulfilling prophecy. In the future, staff may become wary of him and stop interacting with him, because their expectations are now based on these labels. **Table 2** provides examples of common misinterpretations of challenging behaviors and suggestions for more appropriate and, consequently, more helpful in terms of management reinterpretations.

Table 2 Common Misinterpretations of Challenging Behaviors

Behavior	Misinterpretation	Reinterpretation
Asking repetitive questions	The person can control this but is doing it to annoy me	The person cannot keep track of things
Accusing caregiver of stealing	The person is paranoid and trying to embarrass me	This is the only way that the person can explain her/his memory failures
Hitting out	The person is trying to hurt me	Loss of control often results from brain damage

Adapted from Zarit, S.H., Orr, N.K., & Zarit, J.M. (1985). The hidden victims of Alzheimer's disease: Families under stress. New York: University Press

One of the functions of the cognitive assessment is to minimize the dangers of labelling, or rather mislabeling, by educating the staff about the nature of various cognitive deficits and their effects on psychosocial functioning. While it is recognized that the services of a psychologist are not routinely available to nursing homes, it remains crucial for staff to become more knowledgeable about cognitive impairments through different avenues, such as in-service education by invited professionals, attendance at workshops, or personal readings. A lack of understanding of cognitive deficits reduces the quality of life of residents and makes the job of providing care to them more difficult. Staff attitudes toward the behavioral management program are another important consideration. A common reservation raised by staff is, "How is it possible to change the behavior of residents with memory problems, when they will not remember either their behavior or the consequences following it?" Recent research suggests that individuals with severe memory disorders are capable of learning complex new skills even though they do not remember the training to learn them. The fact is that most people can learn new and unlearn old behaviors. Take the case of the so-called "screamer," constantly yelling out for cigarettes. Every nursing home probably has one such individual and the reader does not need to be reminded of the rebukes or commands to stop the yelling that follow this behavior. What happens when the individual is quiet? The first thought of staff is not to bother the individual, as this might trigger the screaming. The unfortunate result of these interactions or lack of interaction is that, through conditioning, the individual has learned that yelling is the only means of contact with the staff.

Another problem is the staff's reluctance to initiate behavioral management programs because of the additional work involved. For nursing home staff that often feels overworked and perhaps unsupported, systematically recording challenging behavior and providing consequences for them on a consistent basis requires considerable time and energy. Behavioral programs are most successful in settings where staff perceive the program as a treatment intervention that is essential for improving the quality of life of the cognitively impaired resident, just as important as insulin injections for a diabetic, for example. Their success can result in a sense of mastery and self-perceptions of increased capability and effectiveness. At a practical level, staff often perceive their workload to have decreased.

When staff attitudes are not dealt with, they detract from the potential effectiveness of any behavior management program. Left unattended, they can result in inconsistent recording of challenging behavior and inconsistent application of consequences, which may lead to exacerbations of the target behaviors. This could lead staff to conclude that the approach is ineffective and should be discontinued. The stress experienced by staff also has an important bearing on challenging behavior and the application of behavioral management programs. In order to reduce the level of stress in staff and enhance the effectiveness of a behavioral management program, it is helpful for staff to follow the stress inoculation paradigm [6]. In this paradigm, stressful situations are redefined as problems that require solutions. The solution is to break down a stressful event into a series of stages and use internal dialog, or self-talk, to cope with the stress.

The stages are: (a) preparing for the stressful event, (b) confronting and handling the stressful event, (c) coping with feelings of being overwhelmed, and (d) evaluating coping efforts and rewarding oneself. An adaptation of this coping strategy in the management of an individual who is verbally abusive and hits out at staff is illustrated in **Table 3**.

Table 3 Examples of Coping Self-Statements in the Management of a Verbally and Physically Abusive Resident

Preparing for Stressful Interaction

- I need to select an effective coping tape for my mental cassette player.
- What is it I have to do?
- We have worked out a plan to deal with this situation.
- Remember, stick to the task and don't take the verbal abuse personally.
- Watch out for his right arm.

Engaging in the Stressful Interaction

- I'm in the room, now; I need to remember, one step at a time.
- Focus on providing the care.
- There he goes, careful now, it's not personal.
- His brain isn't working right, that's why he does it.
- Take a deep breath, relax.
- This is working, it's easier than I thought.

Evaluating Interaction

- I almost lost it when he commented about my . . ..
- I could have become upset and angry.
- That deep breathing really worked.
- On the whole, I'd give myself 8 out of 10.

OR

- Didn't handle that one too well.
- Don't get discouraged. I'm new at this.
- Where did I become ineffective?
- What can I do next time?

Classification of Challenging Behaviors

Behaviors can be classified according to whether they need to be reduced or increased. Those in need of reduction are referred to as behavioral excesses, and those that need to be increased are referred to as behavioral deficits. Different behavioral techniques are applied, depending on this distinction.

Behavioral Excesses

In many instances behaviors may not be inappropriate in and of themselves, but become labeled inappropriate because of their high frequency of occurrence. Behaviors such as shouting, swearing, self-injury, constant demanding or ringing of the call-bell, verbal and physical abuse, are examples of behavioral excesses. Among techniques designed to reduce behaviors are *extinction*, *reinforcement of alternative behaviors*, and *time out*.

Extinction is the removal of reinforcement, where reinforcement is defined as any response to a given behavior. In the example in **Table 1**, the nurse's responses of inquiry, rebuke, and physical contact are all considered reinforcing of the yelling behavior. Being reinforcers, they increase the likelihood that the behavior will recur. Using extinction involves ignoring the yelling by walking away, for example. *Reinforcement of alternative behavior* involves providing reinforcement on a consistent basis for any appropriate behavior that is incompatible with the challenging behavior. Sitting quietly in the chair and saying, "Good morning," are examples of behaviors incompatible with screaming and verbal abuse respectively. In *time out*, the resident is removed from the situation in which the inappropriate behavior occurs and placed in an environment devoid of any potential reinforcers. In settings where behavioral strategies are utilized routinely, there is usually a designated time out room. In nursing homes, where space may be limited, the resident's room may double up as a time out environment. Time out falls under the classification of "punishment procedures," and normally should be used only if other interventions have failed. Occasionally, however, it may be the most prudent intervention. For example, an individual who is constantly yelling in the corridor of a nursing home may upset other residents and provoke verbally and physically aggressive reactions. These reactions to the yelling, although negative, actually reinforce the yelling. Placing individuals in time out prevents this type of reinforcement and also serves to protect personal safety. When applying time out, the individual must be informed about the length of time he is to spend in the time out environment and that time out will be terminated if he is behaving appropriately at the end of that time. A time out period of five minutes should be the rule of thumb and is usually sufficient if applied consistently.

The general strategy in managing behavioral excesses is to eliminate the positive consequences that follow inappropriate behavior, while at the same time reinforcing alternative incompatible behaviors. It is unethical to simply decrease inappropriate behaviors without attempting to replace them with appropriate behaviors. Inappropriate sexual activity and inappropriate voiding are other examples of behavioral excesses. Although they might not occur at a high frequency rate, they are labeled inappropriate because of the situation in which they occur. For example, voiding on the toilet is appropriate, but voiding in a public place is inappropriate. The general strategy aims to bring the inappropriate behavior (e.g., voiding) under the control of a particular stimulus (e.g., toilet) through repetition and training.

Behavioral Deficits

Behaviors that occur with a low frequency and are required for independent functioning are called behavioral deficits. Examples of behavioral deficits include loss of self-care skills, low activity level, and decreased social interactions. A behavioral deficit that is frequently encountered in institutional settings is decreased independence. The institutional environment can occasionally foster this decrease in independence. The fact that individuals require institutionalization often implies that their ability to function independently has been compromised in some way. They enter an institution, however, with a repertoire of preserved skills for independent functioning. Unfortunately, many of their independent behaviors are not reinforced and fall into disuse. A good example is the individual who has suffered a stroke and is left with motor deficits. He may be able to put on and button his coat, but he requires half an hour to do it. Watching an individual struggle in this way elicits caring behaviors on the part of staff who are compelled to rush in and assist the individual and may, in fact, voice mild rebuke for the length of time that the individual requires to dress independently. In this instance, what is reinforced is dependence on staff for dressing and independent behavior is discouraged by the rebuke. The individual's functional abilities decrease over time to the point of complete reliance on staff for provision of self-care activities.

The general strategy of intervention for behavioral deficits is to increase behaviors through gradual reshaping or retraining of absent or infrequent behaviors. The most frequent intervention for increasing appropriate behavior is the application of *positive reinforcement* immediately after the desired behavior has occurred. There are two main classes of *positive reinforcers*, *primary* and *secondary*. *Primary reinforcers* include such things as food and drinks which satisfy a primary physical need. *Secondary reinforcers* are social and include such consequences as praise, smiling, and verbal approval. When applied after the occurrence of a behavior, positive reinforcers increase the likelihood that the behavior will be repeated. In a typical behavior management program aimed at increasing a particular behavior, initially the behavior is reinforced each time it occurs and then later only intermittently. It is also common practice to provide primary reinforcers at the beginning of a program and substitute them with secondary reinforcers in the later stages of treatment.

The use of reinforcement depends on the individual emitting a desired behavior. Often, in the case of behavioral deficits, there is a need to intervene in order to elicit the appropriate behavior. *Shaping* and *prompting* are interventions designed to encourage the resident to emit a desired behavior. In *shaping*, a complete behavior which is not present in the behavioral repertoire of the resident, is broken down into its component parts, which are arranged in a hierarchical manner. For example, the final behavior of self-feeding can be broken down into the following steps: (a) looking down at the plate and fork, (b) touching the fork, (c) lifting the fork off the table, (d) holding the fork over the plate, (e) picking up a piece of food with the fork, (f) bringing the fork up toward the mouth, and (g) placing the fork in the mouth. Training begins with the first step, then the second, and so on, and the resident is reinforced for successfully completing each step of this behavioral sequence. Care should be taken not to progress too rapidly from one level of performance to the next, as the newly acquired behaviors may be unlearned.

Prompting is the use of physical or verbal cues to encourage a particular behavior. It is often applied during the steps of the behavior-shaping intervention, but is also applied as a discrete intervention. For example, individuals with frontal lobe dysfunction may have pathological inertia. While they have the desired or appropriate behaviors in their repertoire, they have trouble initiating them. It is not unusual for them to lie in bed for prolonged periods or simply stare into their plate without feeding themselves. Using verbal prompts (e.g., "It's time to get up") or physical prompts (e.g., guiding their hand to the utensil) helps them initiate functional behaviors.

Carrying out Behavioral Interventions

Regardless of the behavior targeted for treatment, a typical sequence of steps is followed in designing and implementing behavioral interventions. This sequence is outlined below and represents a summary of the more salient aspects of what has been discussed previously.

Defining Challenging Behavior

Challenging behaviors need to be defined in specific and objective rather than vague and subjective terms. The emphasis is on observable behaviors rather than on assumptions about what the patient is feeling or intending. For example, the vague term depression can be redefined as the "resident does not leave the room," "does not smile," "makes derogatory statements about himself," and "talks of suicide." These specific definitions are amenable to measurement in terms of frequency or duration of occurrence

Obtaining Baselines

This is a central part of any behavioral management program and serves a number of purposes. Baseline measurements yield objective evidence of the extent or severity of the problem. The frequency of occurrence of difficult behaviors is often overestimated by staff. This is not surprising, as the stress generated by these behaviors makes it seem as if they are occurring incessantly. Obtaining a baseline of a specifically defined behavior, however, gives a more accurate picture of the problem. A further function of baseline measurements is to provide a comparison for the effects of treatment. Behavioral charting continues during the intervention phase and helps determine the progress of treatment in an unbiased and objective manner, and whether progress is steady or fluctuates. Another purpose of baseline measurements is to provide important information about factors which are controlling the challenging behavior. Performing a functional analysis of antecedents and consequences of these behaviors via ABC charting provides details of events that trigger and maintain them. In many instances, it may also serve to highlight interventions that have been successful in dealing with the challenging behavior, and which can be incorporated into the management plan.

Table 4 Behavioral Management: Care Plan

NAME: Ms. C.

CHALLENGING BEHAVIORS:
1. Verbal abuse
2. Refusal of medications
3. Constant demands

ASSESSMENT: Cognitive assessment reveals problems in time orientation and estimation, attention and concentration, memory, construction, problem-solving, and mental flexibility. There is evidence of left-sided neglect.
ABC charting over a 2-week baseline period reveals seven instances of verbal abuse, two refusals to take medications, and 67 demands. The most frequent are demands for toileting, followed by demands to be helped with feeding. There are no obvious triggers for these behaviors. Responses to them are inconsistent.

NB. The challenging behaviors shown by Ms. C. are a function of the interaction between her cognitive deficits, emotional responses to her disabilities, and her premorbid personality.

MANAGEMENT PROGRAM

1. **Behavior:** Verbal abuse
   Intervention: Use extinction
   This involves withholding reinforcement by ignoring the behavior. Although it will be difficult, do not argue, reason, discuss, plead, or show that you are upset. Any reaction on your part will ensure that the verbal abuse continues.
2. **Behavior:** Refusal of medications
   When Ms. C. refuses medications, use extinction (as above). Wait one minute, then offer medication again without commenting on her refusal. If she refuses again, use extinction.
   NB. Ms. C. does not refuse her medications all the time. It is important to reinforce all instances when she complies with your request. This means, for example, spending additional time with her, performing some activity with her, or simply smiling and thanking her for cooperating.
3. **Behavior:** Constant demands
   Interventions: (for demands to be toileted)
   Place Ms. C. on a two-hourly toileting schedule. Every two hours approach Ms. C. and offer to take her to the bathroom, using a verbal prompt (i.e., "It's time to go the toilet.") Should she refuse the offer, comply with her request the next time she makes it, and then go back to the two-hourly schedule. At all other times, apply extinction.
   Interventions: (for other repetitive demands)
   Anticipate Ms. C.'s needs and meet them. Use extinction for the repetitive demands.
   Place food in her right visual space.
   Use verbal (e.g., "It's time to eat now") and physical (e.g., guide her hand to the spoon) prompts to initiate self-feeding activity. Reinforce compliance.
   Use extinction for statements of inability to perform self-feeding (e.g., "I can't," "You feed me, please").

   NB. Make sure you schedule sufficient time for Ms. C. to feed herself. If you do not, you will be pressured to rush in and help her, which will undo your attempts to increase her independence.

REMEMBER

1. Consistency of approach is the golden rule in managing challenging behaviors.
2. Reinforce all appropriate behaviors.
3. Be aware of how you label Ms. C.'s behaviors and use coping self-statements in your interactions with her.

NB. The use of self-statements follows the format outlined in **Table 3**.

Planning Treatment

There are many important considerations before starting actual treatment. Decisions have to be made about who is going to be involved in providing treatment, who will be responsible for monitoring treatment, and what reinforcers are going to be used in changing behavior. If left unattended, these issues might jeopardize the potential effectiveness of a treatment program. An example of a plan of treatment is provided in **Table 4**. The plan should form part of the resident's chart.

Beginning Treatment

Once treatment strategies have been planned, they are put into action. The golden rule of all behavior treatment programs is *consistency*. Consequences need to be provided immediately after the behavior occurs and every time the behavior occurs. In the case of behavioral deficits where the aim is to increase a given behavior, positive consequences are applied. In the case of behavioral excesses, where the aim is to reduce challenging behavior, positive consequences are withheld when inappropriate responses occur and are applied whenever incompatible appropriate responses are made. Consistency is difficult to achieve. It is made more difficult by the understaffing of nursing homes and the consequent use of on-call staff. This problem can be circumvented by instructing on-call staff about the treatment program.

Monitoring and Evaluating Treatment

As noted previously, charting of challenging behaviors needs to continue during treatment. If applied correctly, significant changes can be seen after only a few days, although in the case of behavioral excesses it is usual for the challenging behavior to escalate before they begin to decrease. If after a few weeks of treatment there has been no change in the behavior, the protocol needs to be reevaluated and adjusted. The consequences may need to be changed or may need to be applied more diligently to ensure consistency.

Case Illustration

Mr. J. was a 77-year-old widowed gentleman admitted to a nursing home following a period of hospitalization and rehabilitation for a hip fracture. Prior to admission to hospital, he had been living in his own apartment, but had required considerable assistance and supervision by one of his daughters. There was no personal or family psychiatric history. He had a diagnosis of Alzheimer's disease predating his admission to hospital. Over the course of the previous two years, he had shown progressive memory loss and inability to manage his finances. He was referred because of "increasing uncooperativeness and agitation."

Interviews with the staff revealed disagreement about the magnitude of the problem. The problem was perceived to be greatest and most urgent by the morning shift, while the evening shift did not perceive any major difficulties. The morning staff perceived the behavior as unpredictable and occurring "all the time." Whenever challenging behavior did occur, they were labeled as intentional. The staff had limited awareness of how Mr. J.'s cognitive deficits were contributing to his challenging behavior.

Cognitive Assessment

An assessment of Mr. J.'s cognitive functioning was undertaken. He was disoriented to time and place. His passive registration of information was adequate (i.e., he could repeat five digits forward), but deficits were observed when increased demands were placed on his attentional resources. He could not repeat even two digits backward or recite the days of the week backward, although he could list them correctly forward. His memory was impaired for both visual and verbal information. His immediate recall was poor (i.e., two objects out of four), and he required repeated trials to register all the information. After a delay of 5 minutes, his recall was zero, and cueing failed to enhance his performance. His language was repetitious, he had naming difficulty, and his ability to generate words was impaired. His ability to comprehend staged commands (e.g., "Do x, then y") was deficient. Drawing tasks revealed severe constructional problems. The pattern of results was consistent with his diagnosis of Alzheimer's disease.

Behavioral Assessment

"Increasing uncooperativeness and agitation" were redefined more specifically as hitting, throwing objects, scratching, and screaming. Staff on all shifts was asked to chart these challenging behaviors according to the ABC model. They were instructed to chart every occurrence of these behaviors over a one week period, with particular emphasis on their relationship to events preceding and following them. The aim was to arrive at a baseline of the frequency of these behaviors, together with the identification of factors that were triggering and maintaining them.

Results of ABC charting showed that the majority of Mr. J.'s challenging behavior occurred when he was in the process of receiving help for some activity of daily living (e.g., bathing). He was often not told what was to happen, or the instructions were too complex. While engaged in one activity, he was sometimes asked to comply with additional demands (e.g., take medications while being toileted). Charting also revealed that staff responses to Mr. J.'s challenging behavior were inconsistent and included reasoning with him, asking him to stop, or being critical.

Treatment Program

The first step was to provide the staff with feedback from the cognitive and behavioral assessments. His cognitive deficits were explained together with how they affected his ability to function and cope with the demands of everyday living. Results of ABC charting were also given to the staff. Their attention was drawn to the fact that Mr. J.'s challenging behaviors were in fact quite predictable and usually occurred when demands were placed on him to comply with some activity of daily living. The inconsistency of their response was underscored as representing the kind of intermittent reinforcement that results in strong maintenance of a behavior.

The following interventions were utilized. The staff was instructed to inform Mr. J. of their intended action using brief, uncomplicated language (e.g., "Time for a bath, Mr. J.") and to desist from making multiple simultaneous demands of Mr. J. in order to minimize the impact of his attentional, memory, and language problems. The main intervention was that of extinction. This involved ignoring (i.e., withholding positive reinforcement) the challenging behavior whenever they occurred, while at the same time reinforcing appropriate behaviors.

Figure 1 illustrates the effects of treatment over a period of three weeks. Following one week of treatment, there had been an insignificant decrease of challenging behavior. Staff was encouraged to persevere with the program, and after three weeks there was a marked reduction in the incidence of challenging behavior.

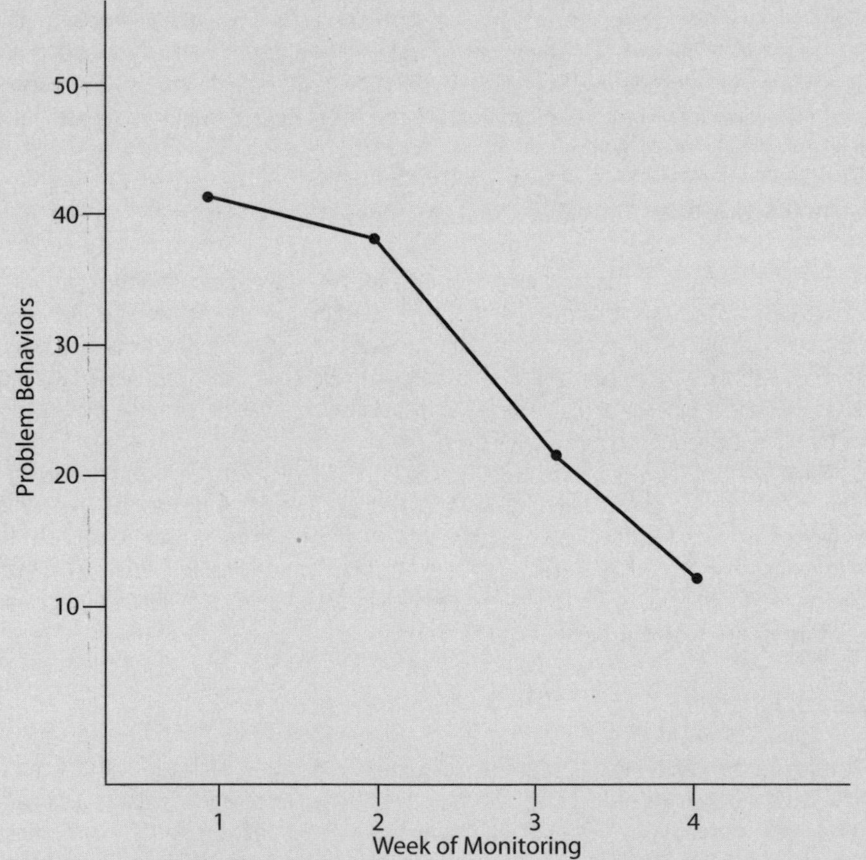

Figure 1 Results of Behavioral Management Program for Mr. J. The numbers represent the total frequency of hitting, throwing objects, scratching, and screaming.

Comment

An individualized treatment plan was developed to manage Mr. J.'s challenging behavior. It was based on a clear understanding of how his cognitive deficits were compromising his ability to cope with the demands placed upon him and awareness of how environmental factors were triggering and maintaining the challenging behaviors. Results of the cognitive and behavioral assessments led to a shift in the staff's perceptions of Mr. J.'s behaviors. Following the consistent and systematic application of reinforcement, Mr. J.'s behavior improved dramatically.

Behavior management programs require consistency and perseverance. Mr. J.'s challenging behaviors resurfaced after several months. A reassessment of his cognitive functioning did not indicate any further significant decline in his abilities. On the other hand, a review of the management protocol showed that the staff had stopped applying it consistently. Once consistency was reestablished, Mr. J.'s challenging behaviors decreased.

Case Illustration

Ms. C. was a 68-year-old single woman, a former bookkeeper and secretary, who was living with her widowed sister and awaiting placement in a nursing home. Several years previously, she had suffered a right hemisphere stroke that had resulted in a left hemiparesis. Subsequently, there was evidence of further bilateral cerebral ischemic damage. Her sister was finding it increasingly difficult to cope with Ms. C.'s challenging behaviors. These included verbal abuse, refusals to take medications, and a complete dependency on her sister for all activities of daily living. The latter was expressed in constant demands to have her sister do something for her. While Ms. C. always had been somewhat dependent, the verbal abuse was out of keeping with her premorbid personality. The sister admitted that she could probably cope with Ms. C.'s constant demands if only she were less angry, irritable, and abusive.

Cognitive Assessment

Neuropsychological testing identified a number of significant cognitive deficits. Ms. C. was disoriented to time, having particular difficulties making judgments regarding recent events. Her attention and concentration were severely impaired. Her memory for both verbal and visual information was severely impaired and she had severe constructional deficits with evidence of left-sided neglect. Her capacity for abstract reasoning and problem-solving was deficient.

Behavioral Assessment

The sister was asked to record the frequency of Ms. C.'s verbally abusive and demanding behaviors using the ABC format. She was to try and specify events that preceded the challenging behaviors, describe the challenging behaviors as objectively as possible, and record her responses to the behaviors. When she returned after one week, it was obvious that the ABC format was either not sufficiently explained or she had misunderstood the instructions. Under the C column (for Consequences), she had been recording what Ms. C. was still doing following her verbal outbursts or demands (e.g., "sister continued to ask to be toileted"), and had omitted describing her own responses to these behaviors. She was reinstructed to record what she did in response to her sister's challenging behaviors.

Results of ABC charting revealed that over the two week baseline period, there were seven occasions when Ms. C. was verbally abusive and two when she refused to take her medications. This came as a surprise to the sister. While commenting that she may have omitted some instances of verbal abuse, the sister admitted that their frequency was certainly lower than she had thought. Charting failed to reveal any obvious triggering events for the verbal abuse or refusals. Descriptions of the sister's responses to the abuse, however, showed different emotional reactions, including anger and sadness, and different behaviors, including leaving the room and crying. A total of 67 demands was recorded over the two weeks. Their frequency was underestimated, as the sister had not recorded all of Ms. C.'s demands. There was a perseverative flavor to many of the demands. Perseverative behavior is a common behavioral disturbance associated with damage to particular areas of the brain. It can be defined as repetitive responding regardless of the situation, or inability to shift one's attention from one activity or train of thought to another. In Ms. C.'s case, even though her sister had just complied with her request for toileting or a drink, this request was repeated within minutes. Toileting demands were the most frequent. While she was capable of feeding herself, Ms. C. repeatedly asked to be fed. The sister's responses to the challenging behaviors were inconsistent. They typically included pleading, bargaining, and reasoning with Ms. C., and occasionally threatening her (e.g., "I'm gonna let you starve").

Treatment Program

Ms. C.'s sister was provided with feedback of the cognitive and behavioral assessments. The effects of her attentional deficit, visual neglect, inability to keep track of information and events, and perseverative tendency on her ability to cope with the demands of her everyday environment were highlighted. She was given reading material about the impact of brain damage on the caregiver [2], and instructed in the use of self-coping statements to reduce her own level of stress.

The behavioral approach was explained. A two-hourly toileting schedule was planned in an attempt to bring Ms. C.'s demands for toileting under the control of verbal prompts on the part of her sister (i.e., "It's time for the toilet"). The sister also was instructed to anticipate Ms. C.'s needs and meet her demands prior to them being made. The main intervention was that of extinction. The sister was to ignore the challenging behaviors, while reinforcing appropriate behaviors. To compensate for Ms. C.'s left-sided neglect, the sister was told to approach her from Ms. C.'s right and also to place objects (e.g., plate of food, a cup of drink) on that side. A detailed outline of the treatment program has been presented previously in **Table 4**. The results of treatment are illustrated in **Figure 2**, clearly demonstrating the effectiveness of the program.

Comment

The sister had little appreciation of how Ms. C.'s brain dysfunction was affecting her ability to cope with demands of everyday living, and was misinterpreting many of the resulting challenging behaviors as intentional. She was also unaware of how her own inconsistent responses to Ms. C.'s behaviors were compounding the problem. Educating the sister about the nature of Ms. C.'s cognitive deficits and making her more aware of her inconsistent responses to the behaviors was essential in helping her manage them more effectively. Attention to her own levels of stress was also crucial and enhanced the effectiveness of the management program. Eventually Ms. C. was placed in a nursing home and the staff was assisted in the continued application of the management program. Ms. C.'s behavior remained manageable and did not require additional interventions.

The specificity and objectivity of behavioral management programs make them easily communicable to other staff. Valuable information about successful treatment interventions can accompany residents should a transfer to a different floor or facility be required. As in Ms. C.'s case, a clearly defined management program can also help the individual in the process of adjusting to a new environment, which is often a stressful experience.

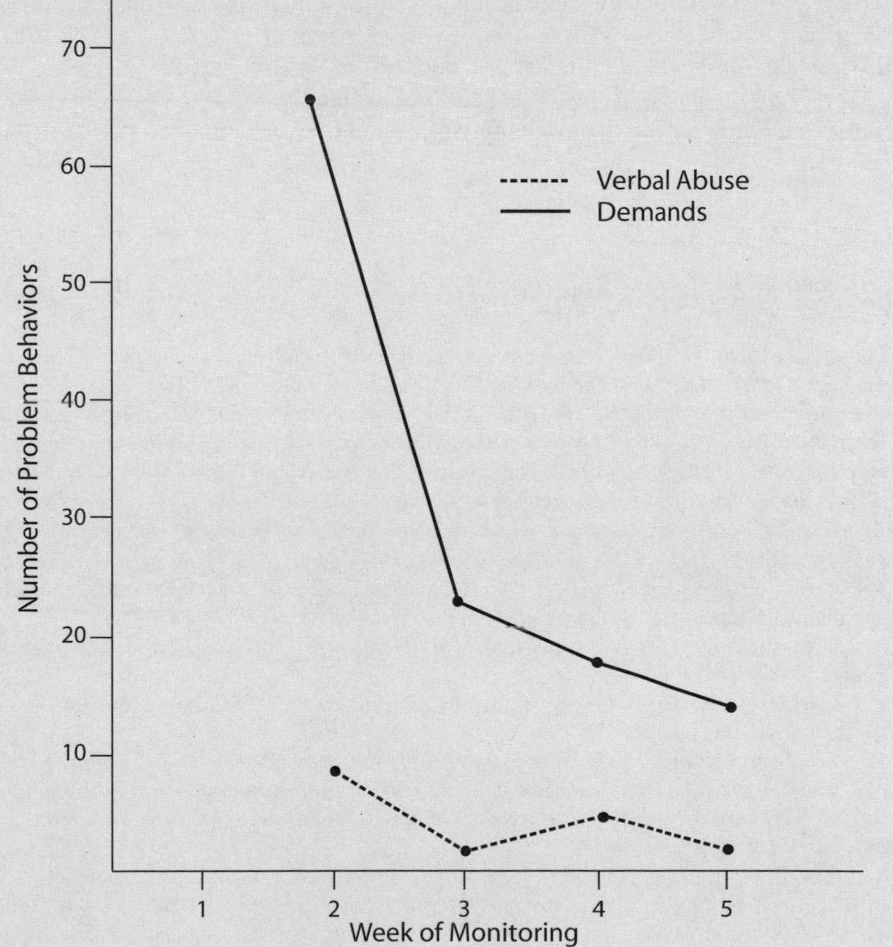

Figure 2 Results of Behavioral Management Program for Ms. C. Baseline data gathered over 2-week period. Refusals to take medications not included (only twice).

Other Nonpharmacological Approaches

The approach described in this chapter is an example of one type of nonpharmacological approach to behavior management that is best described as a *caregiver education* type of intervention. The assumption governing this approach is that increased knowledge and skills on the part of the caregiver impacts positively on challenging behaviors. Other types of nonpharmacological interventions have been utilized to manage the challenging behaviors associated with dementia, and these are the subject of two comprehensive review papers [1, 7]. These, with the assumptions regarding possible reasons for benefit in parentheses, are listed below:

- *Environmental modifications* (adapting, simplifying, or enriching some elements in the environment decreases confusion)
- *Activity programs* (provision of diversion and stimulation reduces anxiety and agitation)
- *Music, voice, and language* (music and voice are soothing)
- *Massage and aromatherapy* (touch and smell are soothing)
- *Light therapy* (exposure to light combats "sundowning")
- *Multidisciplinary teams* (the availability of a team of experts impacts positively on behavior)

Suggested Reading and References

1. Cohen-Mansfield, J. (2001). Nonpharmacologic interventions for inappropriate behaviors in dementia: A review, summary, and critique. American Journal of Geriatric Psychiatry, 9:361–381.
   This article describes different types of nonpharmacological approaches to managing challenging behaviors associated with dementia together with their efficacy and feasibility.
2. Hussian, R.A., Davis, R.L. (1985). Responsive Care: Behavioral interventions with elderly patients. Champaign, Illinois: Research Press.
   An excellent, easily readable book, which presents a practical guide for analyzing and treating challenging behaviors in elderly institutionalized individuals.
3. Josvai, E., Richards, B., Leach, L. (1996). Behavior management of a patient with Creutzfeld-Jacob disease. Clinical Gerontologist, 16:11–17.
   A case study detailing the successful treatment of inappropriate food-seeking behavior in an individual with dementia.
4. Lezak, M.D. (1988). Brain damage is a family affair. Journal of Clinical and Experimental Neuropsychology, 10:111–123.
   This article provides information about the effects of brain damage on the individual's psychosocial functioning. Although it discusses different kinds of behavioral problems that confront families, the information it contains is relevant to all who interact with cognitively impaired residents in a nursing home setting.
5. Matthies, B.K., Kreutzer, J.S., West, D.D. (1997). The behavior management handbook: A practical approach to patients with neurological disorders. San Antonio, TX: Therapy Skill Builders.
   An excellent resource book that is divided into two complementary sections. The first deals with general principles of effective management and general management techniques. The second deals with specific techniques for managing challenging behaviors related to loss of self-control (e.g., physical and verbal aggressive behaviors), physical impairment (e.g., incontinence), mood

and thought disorders (e.g., labile mood), and cognitive impairments (e.g., visual neglect, comprehension deficits).

6. Meichenbaum, D. (1985). Stress inoculation training. New York: Pergamon.
This book presents a model of treatment aimed at reducing and preventing stress. The model's principles are readily applicable to the stress produced by the challenging behaviors of nursing home residents.
7. Opie, J., Rosewarne, R., O'Connor, D.W. (1999). The efficacy of psychosocial approaches to behavior disorders in dementia: A systematic literature review. Australian and New Zealand Journal of Psychiatry, 33:789–799.
Like the Cohen-Mansfield article above, this article provides a good review of nonpharmacological approaches to management of challenging behaviors associated with dementia.
8. Palmstierna, T., Wistedt, B. (1987). Staff observation aggression scale, SOAS; Presentation and evaluation. Acta Psychiatrica Scandinavica, 76:657–663.
This article presents a rating scale for the assessment of severity and frequency of aggressive behavior, which is among the most stress-producing behaviors in nursing home settings.
9. Nilsson, K., Palmstierna, T., Wistedt, B. (1988). Aggressive behavior in hospitalized psychogeriatric patients. Acta Psychiatrica Scandinavica, 78:172–175.
Related to the reference above, this article highlights the clinical relevance and power of systematic observation and measurement of aggressive behaviors. A six-week observation period of aggressive incidents, in the absence of any planned interventions, resulted in a dramatic decrease of aggressive behaviors from week one (91) to week six (16), a decrease of 82%.
10. Spector, A., Thorgrimsen, L., Woods, B., Royan, L., Davies, S., Butterworth, M., Orrell M. (2003). Efficacy of an evidence-based cognitive stimulation therapy programme for people with dementia. British Journal of Psychiatry, 183:248–254.
This article presents the results of a single-blind, multi-centre, randomized control trial of cognitive stimulation therapy (CST) in people with dementia. Results indicate that: CST groups appear to improve both cognitive function and quality of life for people with dementia; the degree of benefit for cognitive function appears similar to that attributable to acetylcholinesterase inhibitors; and the CST groups were popular with the participants and can be conducted in a variety of settings.
11. Stokes, G. (1986 & 1987) Common problems with the elderly confused. Bicester, Oxon: Winslow Press.
An easy to read series of four practical, "how to" booklets, each one dealing with a different challenging behavior. The four topics covered by the series are "Screaming and Shouting," "Wandering," "Aggression," and "Incontinence and Inappropriate Urinating."
12. Vaccaro, F.J. (1988). Successful operant conditioning procedures with an institutionalized aggressive geriatric patient. International Journal of Aging and Human Development, 26:71–79.
This article presents the outline of a behavioral treatment program for a patient exhibiting aggressive behaviors.
13. Baycrest Centre for Geriatric Care. (1999). Dementia: Managing difficult behaviors [video tape]. (Available from Baycrest Centre for Geriatric Care, Toronto).
A 30-minute video dealing with the nature of dementia, challenging behaviors, and behavior management strategies. Throughout, the role that the caregiver plays to ensure better care is stressed.

14 Psychotherapy for the Institutionalized Elderly

Joel Sadavoy

Key Points

- The myth of aging is that the elderly, and especially the institutionalized elderly, cannot change and that psychotherapy and other forms of interpersonal intervention are of little effect. This is an erroneous concept which has been disproved over and over again.
- Psychotherapy with the elderly can be a fruitful and rewarding experience for both patient and therapist. It is to be encouraged regardless of the setting because of its role in humanizing and individualizing the lives of residents in long-term care settings.

Psychotherapy, regardless of who conducts it and for whom it is used, is characterized by a complex interplay of verbal and nonverbal interaction between usually one therapist and an individual or group of patients. Well over 200 "psychotherapies" have been described from psychoanalysis to pet therapy. While there has been considerable debate about the efficacy of specific types of psychotherapy, the evidence is gradually accumulating that interpersonal psychotherapy of various types is effective in a variety of conditions, many of which afflict the aging individual residing in an institution. Other forms of psychotherapy including cognitive, group, and behavior therapy, and treatments based on learning theory, have also been shown to be effective in certain circumstances.

Many years of research have revealed the common occurrence and severe impact of emotional disturbance in institutionalized elders [1]. Institutions for the elderly contain individuals with a substantial degree and range of psychopathology, most often dementia, closely followed by a variety of disorders including depression, anxiety disorders, psychosis, personality disorders, and others. Depression is particularly prevalent in nursing home residents. For example depressive symptoms may be found in more than half of residents [2]. These figures are not surprising when one considers the stress associated with long term care such as being forced reluctantly into a nursing home, getting used to a new environment where routines and personal freedom and choices are restricted, living with a roommate who they did not know before, loss or distancing of relationships with friends and family, and giving up most of the possessions acquired over a lifetime.

While there are many possible interventions at our disposal to deal with these problems nonpharmacological approaches like the psychotherapies are recognized as crucial and effective. Unfortunately there is good evidence that psychotherapy services are in short supply in long term care environments despite the fact that they are seen as very important and are desired by administrators of long term care facilities [3]. There are of course many practical barriers to developing and providing psychotherapeutic services in nursing homes most notably inadequate funding for training, insufficient numbers of staff to give enough time to staff to interact in these time consuming ways with residents, and few systematic guidelines on when and how to provide this type of intervention.

Despite practical problems various forms of psychotherapy have been utilized for all of the disorders mentioned earlier with enough success to warrant their more routine use in long term care. Most of the more rigorous studies have been conducted in the area of behavioral and learning therapies. While these treatments are often effective, it has been suggested that behavioral change is most long-lasting when the "pure forms" of behavioral intervention are coupled with an awareness of the overall interpersonal needs of the patient and an attempt to engage the individual as a "whole person," rather than as a symptom in need of alteration. Indeed, with regard to management of the institutionalized elderly, it is clear that treatments which preserve the humanness and individuality of the patients will be both more effective for patients and gratifying for the health care team.

Group psychotherapy for the elderly encompasses many types of intervention including psychodynamic approaches, psychodrama, exercise groups, activity groups, current event groups, etc. Many patients, even those who have a degree of cognitive impairment, can be engaged in group therapy productively. This work has been described by numerous authors [4–8]. Often, it is only when individuals come together as a group that their previous levels of isolation, and sometimes hopelessness, begin to come to light, as they express to each other their perceptions of their current state. This point was made poignantly in a paper by Leszcz et al. [7], in which they described a men's group in a home for the aged. While individuals were initially wary about exposing their feelings and expressing their emotions, they gradually began to trust each other as group cohesion developed. Only then did they begin to admit tentatively how lonely and cut off they had felt, one resident stating that he had not known that there were men in the institution like himself who were not demented.

Individual psychotherapy has been used effectively for personality disordered residents [9] and for cognitively impaired residents [10]. An important component of many psychotherapies, especially individual, is the development of a detailed intimate understanding of patients, their development, how they came to be the individuals that they are now, and the system in which they live. Personality disturbances may underlie the emergence of difficult behaviors in residents of nursing homes including behavior associated with dementia. For example, premorbid personality may affect the way in which residents behave as they become demented. Take for example individuals who, prior to their admission to a nursing home had strong needs for independence and self sufficiency. When the opportunity for personal achievement is denied in the context of the restrictive routines of the nursing home such individuals may become anxious or angry leading to difficult behaviors such as avoidance and hostility [11].

Goldfarb [12], demonstrated the effectiveness of his form of brief individual psychotherapy, characterized by short, frequent interactions with patients. His basic premise was that patients in institutions feel powerless and have suffered intense blows to their self-esteem simply by virtue of being cut off from their previous sources of gratification and interpersonal relationships. He suggested that patients will begin to feel a greater sense of value when they are able to experience the therapist as a powerful ally. In so doing, the patient is able to identify with the therapist's perceived importance and, hence, incorporate a sense of enhanced self-esteem which they have, so to speak, "borrowed" from the therapist. Goldfarb found that most patients, except for those with psychotic disorders or very severe depressions, would benefit from this type of intervention. He asserted that weekly sessions of approximately 15 minutes in duration were sufficient to induce the self-enhancing process and to modify behavior which was painful to the patient or troublesome to the staff.

To address the interplay between dementia, emotional expression, and changes in self-perception which are common in many residents of long term care facilities, interventions for the emotional and psychological aspects of dementia have included an array of psychosocial techniques. Group psychotherapy is perhaps the most common psychotherapeutic intervention used for people with dementia in residential care [13]. Key elements of group therapy that are theoretically important for effectiveness include learning new coping strategies and the therapeutic effect of group cohesion, generation of hope, and enhancement of self-esteem [14]. Group psychotherapies are reviewed in Chapter 15.

Indications for Psychotherapy

It is a safe assumption that the vast majority of individuals who live in institutions are forced to be there because of external circumstances beyond their control – cognitive and physical illness, economic disadvantage, isolation, and so on. To the extent that this is so, many individuals who are forced to reside in an institutional setting are in need of various degrees of psychotherapeutic support of one form or another. Clearly, it is patently impractical to suggest that all residents can be provided with what they need but, at the very least, an attempt must be made to establish what the needs are and respond at whatever level is possible within the limits of time, staff, and expertise.

Beginning Psychotherapy

The early contact with a patient is a delicate moment. Regardless of which form of psychotherapy is used, the therapist's goal is to establish a therapeutic relationship with the patient which is appropriate to their needs and level of impairment. The caregiver in the institution has a special and very intimate role to play with residents and patients. Many caregivers will perform very personal types of care for elders in their charge but feel uncomfortable inquiring about emotions and thoughts in the same very personal way. Sometimes elders do not want to talk about themselves but in the main they do if they are encouraged and asked. This is the first and most essential part of psychotherapy, i.e., finding out about the person who is hidden behind the mask of old age and listening carefully to them. It is important to understand that the identity of patients is contained in the relationships, accomplishments and experiences of their past and that living in a retirement or nursing home can produce a major break in the patient's sense of the continuity of her/his life. They need and want to talk about these changes and the mere act of doing so enhances their self esteem and sense of wholeness as a person. Most patients bring with them many mementos, especially pictures. The caregiver can begin the process of getting to know the patient from the inside out by asking about the relationship of the patient to these pictures.

In general, in the ordinary course of interactions such as in friendships or family contacts, feeling states are often observed but rarely elicited or inquired about. One of the unique contributions which a caregiver or therapist can begin to make in the isolated life of the cognitively intact institutionalized individual, is to recognize his/her need for emotional contact. The beginning inquiry, therefore, should not stop at eliciting practical information. Residents should be asked, for example, what it *feels* like to be in bed all the time, how they *experience* not sleeping at night, what it *means* to them when visitors come or do not come, how they *feel* about their table mates or room mate, what it *feels like* to have given up their previous homes. In undertaking this aspect of the initial inquiry, the therapist may encounter early resistance by the resident who may not be ready to expose her or himself in this way and who needs more time to trust the caregiver with knowing their uncertainties, fears and needs. This does not mean, however, that the attempt should be avoided. On the contrary, if the initial response of the resident is to pull away from the encounter, the resident should be approached again later. It is helpful to acknowledge with the resident that some feelings are difficult to talk about and that she or he may not be ready to do so, but that you, the therapist, are available to listen. This availability should be active not passive and the resident must be made aware of the therapist's willingness to talk and listen.

Areas of Inquiry

The most critical areas of inquiry, in the early stages of getting to know the resident, are issues of:

- Interpersonal satisfaction or the lack of it
- Feelings of abandonment
- Fears associated with aloneness and pain
- Alterations in the individual's self-perception

A longitudinal perspective of his or her life is of great help in understanding the individual's current behaviors and responses to the environment. While it is important to know who the person's family and friends were, what they did for a living and for enjoyment, it is of much greater value to both the resident and the therapist, to inquire about the nature of the feelings experienced in these previous relationships and activities. Eliciting memories of specific moments of intimacy, joy, or conflict will aid this process rather than relying solely on asking a general question.

Case Illustration

A 70-year-old woman was an inpatient in a psychiatric hospital. She had a lifelong history of disrupted relationships beginning with her early family life and continuing throughout her adolescence and adult life. She had never held a significant job for any length of time, nor had she ever had relationships that seemed rewarding or in any sense stable. As she grew older, even the menial and intermittent household duties which she performed in order to earn a living were no longer possible for her. She became increasingly "eccentric" in her behavior, withdrawn and uncommunicative. In addition, she developed combative paranoid behavior. A clear diagnosis was impossible because she would not communicate other than through her overt behaviors.

The staff were understandably frustrated in their efforts to deal with her. When left alone, she sat isolated, smoking one cigarette after another, rarely speaking and never confiding in anyone. With antipsychotic medication, her major symptoms seemed to settle down, but any attempts to discharge her ended in a marked return of symptoms and failure of all discharge planning. An external psychiatric consultation revealed that there were marked differences of opinion among staff on how to handle this patient. The consultant, upon reviewing the patient's history, and in discussing it with the staff of the ward, became aware that the central issue for this patient was her intense fear of living on her own. In contrast to the vast majority of individuals who end up in institutions, the institution became not only necessary but highly desirable for this patient. She saw it as her home and resisted all effort to put her back out into the cold, rejecting, and empty outside world. Once all discharge plans were abandoned, and the staff accepted the patient as an individual in chronic need of "asylum" in the best sense of the word, virtually all her symptoms remitted. The patient's need for isolation was recognized – the staff avoided intruding upon her personal space, except when absolutely essential. This treatment plan not only relieved the patient, but it also relieved the staff of their ambition to "treat" and discharge.

Comment

This example is illustrative not only for psychiatric care, but also for care of individuals in any long-term institution. There are some people who welcome the environment and thrive within it, but only on their own terms.

One should not jump to conclusions about the feelings of another. For example, a former sculptor was admitted to a home for the aged. The staff initially assumed that he was sorry to lose his creativity because he loved his work. On closer inquiry it emerged that his main gratification came not from his creations but from the admiration which he obtained from others. Such specific pieces of information about an individual will often be enough to reorient the caregiving staff to a different stance. For example, the sculptor's need for gratification produced by the approval of others was addressed by providing him the opportunity of engaging in group activity where he was able to express his opinions and be heard by others. Without knowing the particular source of gratification which he obtained in his life, it would have been easy to erroneously assume that this man's lost capacity to engage in sculpting meant that he could no longer obtain any gratification in his life.

In many instances, of course, it is not easy to replace the lost sources of gratification. In fact, it is probably safe to assume that virtually every individual in an institutional setting has had to give up most of the major and crucial sources of self-esteem enhancement and sources of intimate relationships. The task of the therapist, around this issue, is to evaluate the particular sources of grief and loss with which the individual now struggles. This is a difficult aspect of the initial inquiry. It requires the therapist to be prepared to hear the patient's pain and to be able to listen to it without judgment, and, particularly, without withdrawing from the patient. One of the things that distinguishes the therapist from the friend, family, or casual observer, is a willingness to engage with the person at the deepest level of understanding without being overwhelmed by the individual's emotional pain or driven away by it. Naturally, not all residents want or need intense personal interaction. For some patients, such a relationship has never been a part of their life and they may be either afraid of it or unable to deal with other people. Even in these cases, however, the therapist must attempt to understand what factors led the patient to push others away.

Basic Problems of the Institutionalized Elderly

The basic psychological tasks of old age include dealing with grief and loss, intense anxiety often associates with abandonment or fear of illness and pain, and various forms of depression arising from various physical or interpersonal losses and impairments in self esteem. Aging also places demands upon adaptational skills needed to deal with losses associated with physical, relational, and social decline. In the institutionalized, frail elderly particularly, these problems generally develop concurrently. It is not uncommon to find an institutionalized resident who has had major interpersonal losses and recent disabling physical illness coupled with the task of coping with the dislocation of institutional life.

Coping with New Circumstances

Residents recently admitted to institutions must learn to cope with new and often unwelcome relationships, most of which they would not have chosen. Most people find it especially difficult when they are forced into a "roommate" situation. This is akin to a shotgun marriage, forcing two people who are strangers and have virtually nothing in common to live together in very close quarters, sharing space, bathroom facilities, and the other scarce resources of the ward. The therapist can be helpful by acknowledging the situation and not trying to unduly defend it, but rather, helping the patient accept that it is a less-than-perfect solution. Caregivers in institutions, because they routinely see patients living in communal situations, often over many years, lose sight of the fact that this is an unusual and often unpleasant way to live, particularly when an individual is already struggling with physical and mental problems. Many residents react very intensely within the first month of coming into an institution – the so-called first month syndrome [15]. After that, behavior seems to settle down and the resident appears to "adapt." Most studies of institutionalized individuals are large-scale observational studies. In these reports there is rarely any data on the actual inner life of the individual, his/her conflicts, anxieties, or resentments. When one takes a closer look at newly admitted residents, the adaptation is not nearly so felicitous. "Acceptance" is often more of a giving-up, a grief process in which the individual comes to accept his or her situation and ceases rebelling against it.

Institutionalization is often provoked by crisis and once the person has been admitted to the institution, crises continue to arise. These may be personal assaults secondary to new illness, exacerbations of old problems, or external crises occurring in the family. These are particular indications for instituting psychotherapy, sometimes of a direct supportive nature, but, at other times, utilizing psychodynamic understanding in order to change the environment and the interaction with the individual. At times it may be helpful to attempt to understand the resident's inner psychological state by observing and interpreting their overt behavior [16]. The resident may be totally unable to explain verbally what she is experiencing. Especially for cognitively impaired individuals, new environments present a number of difficulties, not the least of which is that they are unfamiliar. While residents may attempt to continue to use well-learned patterns of behavior which stem from premorbid abilities, these may be no longer adaptive within the context of the institution. For example, the woman who was a tidy, meticulous housekeeper, may continue to try to maintain this type of activity in the institution. Unfortunately, this may lead her to move and tidy the belongings of other people, not realizing that she is not in her own space. The conflicts which inevitably arise will exacerbate her feelings of unreality and agitation. It is only if the staff take the time and effort to understand the meaning of the behavior and attempt to channel it in more appropriate ways (such as giving her structured repetitive cleaning or tidying tasks), that the patient will come to adapt appropriately to the environment.

While behavioral techniques may be used to extinguish such "inappropriate" activity, it is often much more humane and acceptable for staff to use the techniques of rechanneling and redirection rather than the more mechanistic approaches that *are* inherent in extinguishing behavior.

Fears About the Future

In addition to coping with loss, the elderly must often deal with a variety of fears and anxieties attendant upon facing the unknown, and an awareness of their own mortality. Interestingly, however, the elderly do not show a lot of anxiety about death. Rather, fears tend to focus on anxiety about living, uncertainties about what will happen in the future and, particularly, whether they will have pain, disability, or loss of cognitive function if that has not already occurred.

Reactions to Disability

The institutionalized elderly also must deal with adaptation to new and generally increasing, levels of dependency. Residents react with a variety of psychological responses to the various physical and other disabilities they face in old age. Some, for example, have a strong need to deny their problems. This can sometimes lead the person to resist taking necessary or appropriate measures or permitting caregiving staff to intervene. A gentle, caring, and educative stance on the part of the caregiver is necessary. The therapist should be aware of the possibility of becoming angrily confronting and feeling frustrated because advice is not heeded.

Many elderly patients become acutely anxious, fearing, for example, that they are going to be abandoned in the face of their difficulties. They assume, sometimes correctly, that others do not want to tolerate their illnesses. Frequently, they will express the fear that they are a burden, while underlying this fear is the more intense anxiety that they will be rejected. Indeed, in the face of often overwhelming illness or incurable disease, such as dementia or stroke, patients may become enraged both with themselves and their illness. They may displace this feeling onto the caregiving system. Often these angry feelings cover more basic feelings of depression and hopelessness.

Caregivers must keep in mind that many elderly patients do not understand the nature of their problems, although, when cognitively intact, they are capable of forming an understanding if educated. Ignorance about disease breeds fears and fantasies which may become overwhelming and lead to undue anxiety and depression.

Especially with chronic illnesses, withdrawal and depression are a common accompaniment. Sometimes a major affective disorder develops. More often, withdrawn behavior accompanied by sadness is a reflection of a dysthymic disorder which resembles depression but, more accurately, should be seen as a struggle to adapt to loss and grief. Similarly, patients may develop anxiety states or even panic which can be characterized by sleeplessness, frequent calls for aid and assistance or the development of a helpless importuning, sometimes demanding stance, which has been termed the "exaggerated helplessness syndrome."

Understanding and Coping with the Sequelae of Brain Impairment

In the medical institutional setting, caregivers are often faced with the long-term care of individuals who have suffered acute assaults to their cognitive functioning, for example, following a stroke. The sequelae such as dysarthria or paralysis have an obvious impact and are readily understood by staff. However, there are other disabilities which are much more difficult both to diagnose and to understand. For example, the effect of damage to the frontal lobes may spare a variety of basic motor and cognitive activities, while damaging the most sophisticated centers of intellectual functioning. Similarly, damage to the nondominant hemisphere may produce subtle deficits in visual-spatial functioning which can only be demonstrated if carefully sought out. In both circumstances individuals will feel alien to themselves, their self-image dramatically altered by their awareness that they are no longer the person they once were. This state of discomfort can only be heightened if it is accompanied by failure of the caregiver to comprehend the nature of the patient's experience. Such a failure will leave the patient not only impaired, but also isolated and often perplexed by the disability no one else seems to recognize or understand. Under these circumstances, it is imperative that the caregiver of the otherwise cognitively intact resident carefully inquire about feeling states as well as the resident's perspective on what has happened. A straightforward neurological or diagnostic stance is not sufficient at these times, because it is the personal experience, not necessarily the objective findings which are crucial to the person's day-to-day adaptation.

Interventions

Once the therapist has assessed the patient's presenting problems and determined some of the components of the psychological reaction the particular patient is struggling with, the next question is how to intervene beyond the initial assessment stage. Naturally, any effective intervention for the elderly must incorporate complete and realistic physical diagnosis with the use of pharmacology as necessary. Psychotherapeutic intervention may be very helpful, however, for many anxiety syndromes, depressive withdrawal and reactions that stem from ignorance, misinformation, avoidance, or denial.

While concurrent medication is often necessary and useful, in the context of major difficulties of adaptation and coping in old age, the relationship between the caregiver and the patient may be the most effective "medication." Psychotherapy for patients at any age, but especially for the institutionalized elderly, is based on the tenet that everyone has a basic human need to be known and understood as an individual. Illness and other alterations of life in the final stage of human development all interact to create feelings of being lost, unacknowledged, and unknown.

Techniques of Psychotherapy

It is not always possible for caregivers in a busy institutional setting to provide residents with prolonged individual time. Often contacts are brief and focused on practical issues. Where more verbal interaction with residents is specifically indicated, the caregiving staff, as already noted above, can productively attempt to work out a schedule which permits 10 to 15 minutes of time for a particular resident. Brief interventions of this sort can greatly enhance a person's self-esteem as well as providing both the individual and the caregiver with a deeper understanding of the difficulties experienced. Data on brief, intensive, individual outpatient psychotherapy suggests that three to four months of weekly contact can produce symptom amelioration in many cases [17]. The institutionalized resident may similarly respond to grief work or other forms of therapy, but the contract may have to be long-term.

If regular psychotherapy is going to be instituted, the caregiver should set aside a specific time which both he/she and the resident know will be kept free of interruptions. This is important even if the sessions are brief. Other staff should be told that they cannot interrupt the session, except for true emergencies. Therapy is most effective if conducted in a setting outside of the resident's room, where possible. If the individual is bedridden, roommates should be asked to leave if they are mobile. If not, the therapist should be sensitive to the situation; the degree of confidentiality and openness may have to be restricted.

It is the responsibility of therapist to meet the resident. The elderly in institutions are highly vulnerable to feeling that caregivers may not want to see them, and that they are a burden. The therapist should make it clear that he or she wants to see the resident. If the resident fails to come at the appointed time, the therapist should inquire what has happened and make sure that the next appointment is clearly laid out. The concept of regularity and reliability of sessions is one of the most important elements in the psychotherapeutic endeavor, but one which is often paid insufficient attention.

What Techniques Are Useful for the Institutionalized Elderly?

There are three basic approaches which are practical in psychotherapeutic management of the institutionalized elderly, even by those therapists who are not schooled in formal psychotherapy. These include supportive therapy, reminiscence or life review therapy, and cognitive therapy.

Supportive Psychotherapy

Supportive therapies are useful for all patients but are particularly important for the frail elderly. In using this mode of treatment, the therapist is most effective if he or she is active and interventionist. The therapist takes an active role in the session, engaging the patient frequently with questions which encourage the expression of feeling states, rather than eliciting practical information. For example, instead of simply asking "Did you sleep last night?" the therapist asks, "How did it feel when you were not able to sleep? What do you think about and what do you do at night during those times when you are awake?" Supportive psychotherapy also requires the therapist to be available and regular. The goals of the contact can sometimes be spelled out, for example, that the therapist will attempt to help the patient speak about his or her problems and try to work on appropriate ways of dealing with them. Often, for institutionalized residents, supportive therapy is coupled with a need for changes in the environment, changes for which the caregiver may have to advocate.

An important component of supportive therapy is simple ventilation of feeling. Patients may be encouraged to talk about their feelings, a process enhanced by very simple questions around specific issues such as, "Do you feel angry when your daughter doesn't call? Tell me about your feelings of frustration when you wake up stiff in the morning from your arthritis. Are you afraid you are going to die when you become short of breath?" and so on.

There are certain themes which will continually recur in psychotherapy, especially if there is a degree of mild or moderate cognitive impairment. Repetition is sometimes the result of a patient's need to rework the same troubling piece of material over and over, or it may be the result of the patient's inability to remember the content of sessions from one time to the next. Such repetition must be tolerated, and indeed, encouraged, since this process of repeating feelings can often be healing.

The therapist may be helpful when simply repeating back, in different words, what he or she has understood the patient has just said. This simple feedback technique is strongly enhancing of the patient's self-esteem. It is also helpful for the therapist to present alternative ways of thinking or approaching problems. While the autonomy of the patients should be respected and they should be encouraged to offer their own ideas in solving their problems, the therapist should not hesitate to discuss practical interventions with them. Unfortunately, with institutionalized elderly the degree of independent action and hence problem-solving is quite limited. However, to the extent that the person is able to think through his difficulties and come up with approaches, the accompanying sense of control over fate is most enhancing to his mental health. The elderly often feel that others, especially those who are younger, do not respect, value or seek their opinions, even on issues directly related to decisions about their own lives.

What Is the Role of Reassurance?

Reassurance must convey realistic hope. Unrealistic statements may make the therapist feel better and momentarily encourage the patient. However, patients are often exquisitely aware that reassurance can be an attempt by the therapist to "brush off" the problems. Indeed, reassurance may stem from the therapist's wish to not get closer to the patient's fears and anxieties. Reassurance is most effective when it arises from a full understanding, both of the real issues in the patient's life, and his or her emotional reactions to them. To say "I am sure everything will be all right" without being sure, creates distance and may lead the patient to avoid speaking openly with the therapist.

Reminiscence Therapy

The purpose of reminiscence therapy is to help increase the person's sense of self by encouraging what is probably a normal process of aging, i.e., life review. Most older people do have a need to reminisce and to thereby retain emotional and mental contact with a part of themselves that, in the past, was healthier and perhaps more capable of coping. The process helps to work through losses and to put the person's current situation into a lifelong perspective. This therapy is effective for virtually all, although those residents who are highly anxious and focus only on bad memories of the past, those who have suffered massive psychic trauma, and those who are deeply depressed or whose reality perceptions are otherwise distorted, should be approached with caution.

Techniques of reminiscence therapy are varied. The most straightforward and simple of these is to encourage the individual to talk about their past in vivid and emotional terms. Residents may also be asked to make audiotapes, prepare written records, or sometimes video records of their lives. This process may be even more meaningful if families are involved. Sometimes, when the resident is unable to actively participate, a family member or whole families may be interested in constructing a record of the person's life, both for their own benefit and that of the caregiving staff. The process is facilitated if residents or families contribute aids to reminiscence, such as picture albums, things they have written, or paintings, drawings, and other creative arts.

Cognitive Therapy

Cognitive therapy has been used for the elderly in a modified form and is said to be most useful for dysthymic disorders and depression [18]. The treatment is based on the idea that thoughts produce feelings rather than the other way around. Various situations provoke distorted ideas about one's self which lead to depressive conclusions, producing hopelessness and lost self-esteem. The therapeutic approach is a step-by-step method of dealing with this process. The first step is to help the individual identify the major source of depressive conflict. For example, "I am bad and useless because I cannot perform the way I used to." While there is an element of this statement which is true in that the person may not be able to do what he or she used to, there is another component which is a distortion, i.e., that they are bad and useless. The examination of the statement leads the therapist to move on to step two, that is, to evaluate, with the patient, the pros and cons of the idea and the reality component versus the fantasy. The process helps the patient correct distortions and introduces realities. For example, "this aspect of what you feel may be true, but perhaps this other element is not." In order to consolidate the learning process that goes on in cognitive therapy, the patient may be given homework comprised of testing out the truth of a new-found perspective. For example, in an institution, it may be helpful to ask a resident who is convinced of her lack of value, to risk asking for feedback about herself in various forums such as a group situation or with her family.

While the three forms of therapy, supportive, reminiscence, and cognitive, are theoretically separate, in practice the models are often productively used at the same time and sometimes in conjunction with insight-oriented approaches. The three basic therapies are not difficult to use in their simpler formats as described here and for brief interventions focused on a specific issue they do not require extensive training. As long as the caregiver and therapist attempt to understand and form a warm, caring relationship with the patient, all of the techniques are safe and useful.

Interpersonal Therapy

Interpersonal psychotherapy (IPT) is a technique originally developed for treatment of depression by Myrna Weissman and Gerald Klerman and subsequently used for the treatment of a wide variety of disorders and in a full range of ages including the elderly [19, 20]. It is based on a general theoretical principle that interpersonal issues are at the root of or exacerbate depression. The key foci of therapy include identifying and then dealing with issues arising from four areas: interpersonal conflicts, insufficient social support, role conflicts, and interpersonal losses.

Unfortunately the techniques of IPT that have been manualized and tested are largely suitable for outpatients with relatively focal problems that can be addressed in a short period of time. Essentially, IPT is one of the brief therapies, although it has also been used in longer term therapy.

Little work has been done using IPT in the elderly and virtually none has been applied to residents of long-term care institutions. The major empirical evidence for the effectiveness of IPT in the elderly has come from the work of Reynolds and his group [21, 22, 23].

They employed IPT as the psychotherapy modality in their treatment studies of depression, comparing the effectiveness of medication alone versus medication combined with psychotherapy. In these studies there was some benefit conferred by the use of combination therapy over medication alone. In the absence of further study there is no empirically proven basis for recommending the use of IPT as a discrete modality of therapy for the institutionalized elderly.

With this caveat in mind, the principles of IPT seem to be intuitively useful in conceptualizing the problems of the elderly in institutions. Interpersonal conflicts abound in this environment that forces residents into dependent interactions with staff resulting in conflicts both actual and perceived. When residents feel helpless and vulnerable, it exacerbates their reactions of depression, rage, or anxiety. Therapists can be of great assistance by helping the patient to identify the sources of conflict and tension in the environment and then working with them, as an interpersonal coach, to alter the form of interactions, confront situations in an adaptive way and to enlist necessary help. These strategies specifically target relationship problems in an organized fashion. Looking at each relationship in turn, the resident's emotional reactions are reviewed and the reality of situations is examined in order to develop a framework for understanding the issues that can be taught to the resident. Coaching then takes the form of helping the resident deconstruct incidents and feelings. The therapist then provides instruction in how to behave more adaptively. Obviously this technique is only suitable for the cognitively intact individual.

Other Therapies

Social rhythm therapy arises from a hypothesis which states that instability or disruptions in personal relationships and life's daily routine destabilize circadian rhythms, triggering episodes of affective illness like depression in vulnerable individuals [24]. When added to IPT, the social rhythms component seeks to prevent future problems in the areas of grief, interpersonal disputes, role transitions, and role deficits, by stabilizing both personal and interpersonal routines [25]. Treatment focuses on the connection between mood and the quality and regularity of social roles and relationships. The patient is asked to complete a chart designed to assess and then enhance the regularity of daily routines. For one week the patient records the time that target activities occur including meal times, bedtime, scheduled social interactions, family visits, engaging in hobbies, or leisure time pursuits. Each activity is assigned a score with higher values indicating greater regularity. The patient and therapist then work on identifying and managing potential precipitants of disruptions in the routines and rhythms. Efforts to resolve current interpersonal issues and prevent future problems in these areas are also emphasized.

Problem-solving therapy is directive and brief, usually spanning six sessions. Written lists are generated in the therapy session and homework is prescribed. The patient is asked to specify and prioritize problems whether they are thoughts, feelings of fatigue, anxiety, depression, or interpersonal difficulties. The patient and therapist assess the circumstances surrounding the problem and the patient is urged to formulate a feasible approach. A focused list of potential solutions is generated by the patient and therapist. For each solution, a set of pros and cons are drawn up, which serve to prioritize the solutions from most to least difficult to effect. Pessimism ("it has not worked before") and lack of motivation ("I forgot to practice") are addressed by taking the problem-solving approach. However, the focus is kept purposefully narrow on the initial problem that the patient identified. The aim is for the patient and therapist to focus the effort on realistic solutions. This approach has been advocated as especially useful for patients with executive dysfunction who struggle with initiating tasks or perseverating on them [26].

Reality orientation (RO) may be implemented in a variety of ways including 24 hour orientation cuing (such as visible calendars, clocks, and message boards plus staff reinforcement) or classroom interventions conducted in group formats. There may be modest improvement in behavior, social interaction, and functioning, although improvements, appear to be largely transient with the exception of some patients who may retain their improvement as long as the RO intervention is continued. Validation therapy addresses the need for individual enhancement of personal identity. The goal of validation therapies is "to stimulate energy and interaction both verbally and nonverbally, and increase each group member's sense of identity by calling up social roles from the past". Validation groups include reminiscence, active support from therapists, and activities such as discussion and singing.

Pet therapy has been used to enhance the experience of elders in long term care institutions. But caring for pets may be problematic or impossible in a facility so Libin and Cohen-Mansfield experimented with using a plush toy robotic cat and compared its effect with a live cat [27]. There was no significant difference, widening the scope for creative nonpharmacological interventions and perhaps strengthening the theoretical position that dementia-related agitation is, in part, a communication reflecting needs for comfort and contact.

Why Many Caregivers Avoid Therapy with the Institutionalized Elderly

Many individuals, including the older institutionalized resident, will at times idealize the therapist and form unrealistic expectations. Such magical ideas may cause therapists or other caregivers to feel uncomfortable because of their awareness that they are limited in what they are able to do for the person. The problems of the elderly are often chronic and not readily amenable to therapy. The caregiver and therapist must beware that they do not become unduly hopeless in the face of this chronicity.

The therapeutic contract with the institutionalized elderly individual is indefinite. Although formal sessions may become widely spaced and intermittent when a particular course of therapy has come to a natural conclusion, the nature of the problems of this population is that they will flare up and recur. The therapist must be prepared to pick up again at some time in the future, perhaps with another series of regular sessions.

All elderly residents, especially those in institutions, inevitably continue to decline. The success of psychotherapy must be viewed in the context of reestablishing the best level of emotional and psychological functioning for the person, rather than attempting to radically change the individual. Diminishing anxiety somewhat, enhancing a sleep pattern, or encouraging interpersonal relationships may be appropriate goals that the therapist can expect to achieve in certain cases.

Caregivers and therapists must be aware that guilt, anger, and frustration are normative feelings for them in treating certain of their patients, and must not let these feelings interfere with their attempts to carry on. Similarly, families are often needy, placing further demands upon the therapist. These demands may, in certain instances, lead the therapist to want to withdraw.

Whatever the therapeutic approach, and regardless of the cognitive capacity or frailty of the patient, the therapist should avoid stereotyped "rules" and always attempt to adapt technique to the patient's needs. For example, it has often been stated that the frail elderly benefit from caregivers touching and sitting close to them, and speaking in a loud voice. However, such individuals show a range of tolerance for this kind of intimate involvement. One must evaluate the resident's need for touching versus the parallel need for maintenance of a personal space. Sometimes residents miss the intimacy of touching and close involvement, while at other times they may be resentful or even panicked by such intimacy and intrusion. Similarly, the use of familiarity (first names) should be employed judiciously. Residents have spoken of feeling demeaned by the infantalizing implication of a too-casual informality imposed by caregiving staff who may view the frail elderly as "cute" or, in other ways, childlike. This stance fails to take into account the remaining "personhood" of the individual living inside the increasingly frail body and/or mind.

Special Problems of the Cognitively Impaired

Especially with the cognitively impaired elderly, the technique of reality orientation is used frequently. Such individuals are often illogical, unrealistic, and inappropriately emotional in their communications. These factors may make it difficult for therapists to interpret the meaning of the individual's behavior. When this happens, caregivers often wonder how to intervene and whether or not to correct a person's distorted reality and, if so, how to do it. Some residents are able to accept interventions and to "borrow" the staff's reality testing. In other instances, corrections of reality may lead the individual to feel rejected or humiliated. The experience of not being believed can exacerbate paranoid or other psychotic misinterpretations of reality. Correction of the person's reality, therefore, should be undertaken only after a knowledge of the individual's sensitivities has been gained.

Residents' delusional beliefs are particularly problematic for caregivers in institutions. Delusions cannot be corrected by orientation-type feedback. In this situation, a first step is to make every effort to understand the nature of the delusion. A resident, for example, may misinterpret a nurse present in the room at night as a thief coming to take the clothes which she has become convinced are being stolen from her. Such a concrete delusion is common in demented individuals, and may become entrenched and impossible to dislodge. In such circumstances, rather than trying to "reorient," it may be more appropriate to take practical steps, such as scheduling staff the resident knows well who have not been incorporated into the delusion to carry out the more intimate aspects of care. It is also important to keep the environment as predictable, structured, and simple as possible.

When residents become acutely agitated as a result of unrealistic beliefs, a simple intervention is to redirect their attention. In the case of the stealing delusion mentioned above, caregivers can reassure the resident that they will try to help locate the lost belongings shortly, while introducing another activity in the meantime to divert attention temporarily. Often, of course, no technique can prevent the overwhelming anxiety associated with reality distortions and cognitive impairment. The use of medication may be required as an adjunct. Such medications often make the resident more accessible to interpersonal techniques of intervention and should be used appropriately.

When dealing with the cognitively impaired resident individually, certain basic approaches are particularly important. As noted above, the initial stages require the establishment of an accurate and empathic rapport. In addition, the therapist must attempt to evaluate the nature of the communication difficulties to determine residents' understanding of language, memory resources, and ability to orient themselves. Often such individuals have difficulty comprehending verbal input, sometimes because of receptive problems and sometimes because of other factors such as high levels of anxiety or fear. Most importantly, the therapist and caregiver must evaluate the person's capacity to utilize interaction. Some individuals cannot be readily soothed by contact with another person, while others are easily calmed when in the presence of a familiar caregiver. Indeed, the latter is probably the more common situation. This capacity to be soothed is often the most important differentiating factor in determining whether a given demented resident will respond to psychotherapeutic interventions.

Psychotherapy of the cognitively impaired, or indeed any interaction with such residents, must take into account the often exquisite sensitivity of the person to nonverbal communication. Tone of voice or body posture may be taken as anger or rejection, even though it is not necessarily meant in that way. For example, a caregiver who addresses the resident over her shoulder while walking out of the room or unwittingly uses a patronizing tone may agitate the person, resulting in a breakdown of empathic rapport.

References

1. The American Geriatrics Society and American Association for Geriatric Psychiatry. (2003). Consensus Statement on Improving the Quality of Mental Health Care in U.S. Nursing Homes: Management of depression and behavioral symptoms associated with dementia. Journal of the American Geriatrics Society, 51:1287–1298.
2. Jongenelis, K., Pot, A.M., Eisses, A.M., Beekman, A.T., Kluiter, H., Ribbe, M.W. (2004). Prevalence and risk indicators of depression in elderly nursing home patients: The AGED study. Journal of Affective Disorders, 83:135–142.
3. Reichman, W.E., Coyne, A., Borson, S., Negrón, A.E., Rouner, B.W., Pelchat, R.J., et al. (1998). Psychiatric consultation in the nursing home: A survey of six states. American Journal of Geriatric Psychiatry, 6:320–327.
4. Akerlund, G.M., Norberg, A. (1986). Group psychotherapy with demented patients. Geriatric Nursing, 7:83–84.
5. Cox, K.G. (1985). Milieu Therapy. Geriatric Nursing, 6:152–154.
6. Lazarus, L.W. (1976). A program for the elderly at a private psychiatric hospital. Gerontologist, 16:125–131.
7. Leszcz, M., Sadavoy, J., Feigenbaum, E., Robinson, A. (1985). A mens' group psychotherapy of elderly men. International Journal of Group Psychotherapy, 33:177–196.

8. Linden, M. (1953). Group psychotherapy with institutionalized senile women. Studies in gerontologic human relations. International Journal of Group Psychotherapy, 3:150–170.
9. Sadavoy, J., Dorian, B. (1983). Management of the characterologically difficult patient in the chronic care institution. Journal of Geriatric Psychiatry, 16:223–240.
10. Sadavoy, J., Robinson, A. (1989). Psychotherapy and the cognitively impaired elderly. In D.K. Conn, A. Grek, J. Sadavoy, (Eds.), Psychiatric consequences of brain disease in the elderly: A focus on management (pp. 101–135). New York: Plenum Press.
11. Hilton, C., Moniz-Cook, E. (2004). Examining the personality dimensions of sociotropy and autonomy in older people with dementia: Their relevance to person centered care behavioral and cognitive psychotherapy. Behavioural and Cognitive Psychotherapy, 32:457–465.
12. Goldfarb, A.I. (1974). Minor maladjustments of the aged. In S. Ariet, E.B. Moody, (Eds.), American handbook of psychiatry (2nd Ed., pp. 820–860). New York: Basic Books.
13. Cheston R. (1998). Psychotherapy and dementia: A review of the literature. British Journal of Medical Psychology, 71:211–231.
14. Scott, J., Clare, L. (2003). Do people with dementia benefit from psychological interventions offered on a group basis? Clinical Psychology and Psychotherapy, 10:186–196.
15. Tobin, S.S. (1989). Issues of care in long-term settings. In D.K. Conn, A. Grek, J. Sadavoy, (Eds.), Psychiatric consequences of brain disease in the elderly: A focus on management (pp. 163–187). New York: Plenum Press.
16. Cohen, G.D. (1989). Psychodynamic perspectives in the clinical approach to brain disease in the elderly. In D.K. Conn, A. Grek, J. Sadavoy, (Eds.), Psychiatric consequences of brain disease in the elderly: A focus on management (pp. 85–99). New York: Plenum Press.
17. Lazarus, L.W., Groves, L., Gutmann, D., Ripeckyj, A., Frankel, R., Newton, N., Grunes, J., Havasy-Galloway, S. (1987). Brief psychotherapy with the elderly: A study of process and outcome. In J. Sadavoy, M. Leszcz (Eds.), Treating the elderly with psychotherapy: The scope for change in later life (pp. 265–293). Madison, WI: International Universities Press.
18. Gallagher, D.E., Thompson, L.W. (1983). Endogenous and nonendogenous depression in the older adult outpatient. Journal of Gerontology, 38(6):707–712
19. Sholomskas, A.J., Chevron, E.S., Prusoff, B.A., Berry C. (1983). Short-term interpersonal therapy (IPT) with the depressed elderly: Case reports and discussion. American Journal of Psychotherapy, 37:552–566.
20. Weissman, M.M. (1997). Interpersonal psychotherapy: Current status. Keio Journal of Medicine, 46:105–110.
21. Taylor, M.P., Reynolds, C.F. 3rd, Frank, E., Cornes, C., Miller, M.D., Stack, J.A., et al. (1999). Which elderly depressed patients remain well on maintenance interpersonal psychotherapy alone? Report from the Pittsburgh study of maintenance therapies in late-life depression. American Journal of Geriatric Psychiatry, 7:64–69.
22. Reynolds, C.F. 3rd, Frank, E., Perel, J.M., Imber, S.D, Cornes, C., Miller, M.D., et al. (1999). Nortriptyline and interpersonal psychotherapy as maintenance therapies for recurrent major depression: A randomized controlled trial in patients older than 59 years. Journal of the American Medical Association, 281:39–45.
23. Miller, M.D., Wolfson, L., Frank, E., Cornes, C., Silberman, R., Ehrenpreis, L., et al. (1997). Using interpersonal psychotherapy (IPT) in a combined psychotherapy/medication research protocol with depressed elders. A descriptive report with case vignettes. Journal of Psychotherapy Practice and Research, 7:47–55.
24. Kennedy, G.J., Tanenbaum, S. (2000). Psychotherapy with older adults. American Journal of Psychotherapy, 54:386–407.
25. Ehlers, C.L., Frank, E., Kupfer, D.J. (1988). Social zeitgebers and biological rhythms: A unified approach to understanding the etiology of depression. Archives of General Psychiatry, 45:948–952.

26. Alexopoulos, G.S., Raue, P., Arean, P. (2003). Problem-solving therapy versus supportive therapy in geriatric major depression with executive dysfunction. American Journal of Geriatric Psychiatry, 11:46–52.
27. Libin, A., Cohen-Mansfield, J. (2004). Therapeutic robocat for nursing home residents with dementia: Preliminary inquiry. American Journal Alzheimer's Disease and Other Dementias, 19:111–116.

Suggested Readings

1. Conn, D.K., Grek, A., Sadavoy, J. (Eds.). (1989). Psychiatric consequences of brain disease in the elderly: A focus on management. New York: Plenum Press.
The authors discuss the management of neuropsychiatric disorders in the elderly from a variety of different perspectives; Chapters 4, 5, 6, and 8, in particular, focus on psychotherapeutic issues.

15 Groups and Group Psychotherapy

Ken Schwartz

Key Points

- There are many types of groups in nursing homes that provide social, recreational, and cognitive stimulation.
- Psychotherapy groups that address the unique feelings and concerns of the more cognitively intact residents greatly improve the morale and quality of life of these residents.

Introduction

Nursing homes provide a maximum quality of care when they offer a range of groups that take into account the feelings, concerns, and abilities of residents. In a time of limited resources and increased needs, groups provide social and recreational stimulation to many residents at one time. Group psychotherapies also are an effective and efficient way to help residents find meaning and resolution during times of transition [1].

Empathizing and validating an individual's worth, particularly when the individual is cognitively impaired, is the foundation of any good group therapy [2]. Nonetheless, the traditional group approach needs modification because of the degree of cognitive impairment and sensory losses among nursing home residents. Group leaders must be more flexible, supportive, directive, structured, and less confrontational with group members who are frail and cognitively impaired [3]. Conversely, several factors contribute to the failure of groups in nursing homes, including the lack of pregroup planning, limited skills in leading and supporting groups, insufficient communication with the staff, and inconsistency between group goals and organizational methods [4].

Groups may led by staff of various disciplines, such as social workers, recreation therapists, nurses, physical or occupational therapists, and psychogeriatric consultants. Various types of groups [5] are mentioned in the literature on aging and institutional care (see **Table 1**).

A survey of 304 nursing homes in the United States indicates the majority offer educational, support, and therapy groups for residents [1]. Educational and support groups that address the needs of family members for information, empowerment, validation, and resources are common [1]. Family support groups deal with the feelings of family members concerning nursing home placement, especially guilt over this decision, and with emotional reactions to seeing loved ones medically and cognitively deteriorate [3]. Treatment groups for family members are less common because family members are reluctant to participate in any group that might suggest dysfunction or pathology on the part of a family member [6]. In Ontario, Canada family councils that liaise with administration and advocate on behalf of the care of vulnerable residents are now mandatory.

Table 1 Types of Groups in Nursing Homes

- Reality orientation
- Remotivation
- Poetry
- Socialization
- Educational
- Topic Specific
- Member Specific
- Reminiscence
- Support
- Growth
- Therapy

Types of Groups

Reality orientation group reinforce current details of the more cognitively impaired resident's life circumstances. In a small, structured setting to avoid overstimulation, the therapist patiently asks each group member questions about his or her surroundings, such as the date or weather conditions. Positive responses are reinforced. If more personal details are raised by the resident, such as where family members are, care is taken not to upset a resident who, for example, is not able to remember the death of a spouse.

Remotivation groups, a less common type of group, attempt to reengage a more withdrawn resident, such as an individual suffering from chronic schizophrenia.

Poetry groups provide support to residents to lessen isolation and reduce depression, or to also help adult children learn about issues related to aging parents [1].

The most common types of groups in nursing homes are social and activity groups which are led by the recreation or activity staff. They are offered to residents of all cognitive abilities who are able to sit through a group. Bingo, discussion, trivia, and music groups are examples of groups designed to improve the individual resident's quality of life by providing social, cognitive, and recreational stimulation.

Time-limited psychoeducational groups increase residents' awareness of their particular medical problem. An example is a diabetes group with goals to increase compliance with diet, increase physical activity, and help residents understand and cope with actual or potential losses associated with the illness [7]. Other examples are groups for residents with strokes or Parkinson's disease. Such programs are likely more common in the United States where presently the goal of a nursing home stay is often discharge back into the community, whereas in Canada nursing homes still provide traditional long-term care.

Reminiscence, life review, support, and psychotherapy groups are more treatment-oriented. Admission criteria to these groups is based on a clinical appraisal of the resident's cognition, mood, behavior, and ability to tolerate dysphoric affect. Residents with anxiety or depression, or with behavioral or interpersonal problems, and who possess a capacity for self-awareness and an ability to openly share with others are candidates. Residents with moderate to severe cognitive impairment are excluded because they cannot attend to what is being discussed. Residents who are paranoid, aggressive, or overly-sedated are also not included, nor is the group offered to difficult, characterologically disturbed residents who blame and devalue others.

Reminiscence groups focus on preselected topics that are relevant to the residents' pasts and allow them to get in contact with previous successes in an informal, discussion type of format [4]. Examples of topics are holidays or specific personal events, such as the first day of school, work, or marriage. Pictures may be used as an aid to stimulate discussion.

Less commonly, life review groups based on reminiscence are offered to more cognitively intact residents by therapists with more skills and familiarity with the aging process. Life review, a universal and normative process, helps people reintegrate past experiences through spontaneous or purposive memories leading to acceptance and wisdom [8]. The three most frequent themes described in group work with the elderly using a life review method were mourning, caring, and integrity [9].

Support groups are similar to psychoeducational groups in that residents are asked to participate on the basis of a shared theme, but are different in that the groups are less leader-directed so that members can interact more [7]. The purpose of support groups is to help members cope with stressful life events or transitions [5]. An example is a time-limited 16 week group for new residents to help them adjust to moving into a nursing home. Goals of support groups include encouraging emotional expression, sharing of coping skills, and promoting a sense that residents are not alone in their situations [7].

At a time of life when nursing home residents are struggling with multiple changes and losses, weekly ongoing 60 to 75 minute group meetings provide members with a sense of consistency and stability [7]. New members also benefit from being in a group with others who have already successfully adjusted to nursing home life [10].

The theoretical stance of open-ended psychotherapy groups vary according to the training of staff. Cognitive-behavioral, developmental, interpersonal, or psychodynamic approaches can be utilized, but it is the author's experience based on conducting groups in five nursing homes over the past ten years that an integrated group psychotherapy model [11] incorporating all of these approaches is best.

In an integrated psychotherapy model, appropriate historical material, or reminiscences either spontaneously produced or elicited by the therapist's familiarity with a group member are discussed when it affects the member's current life and relationships [12]. Past successes and ability to cope with previous adversity are used to confront members' dysfunctional cognitive beliefs about themselves, such as feeling worthless because they are old and institutionalized. The caring and feedback members both give and receive in the group help them again feel useful and valued.

On occasion, members are asked to try to understand that their current difficulties may be connected to their past. For example, a woman in a nursing home because of physical difficulties associated with a stroke worried excessively about getting Alzheimer's. As she became aware of how even as a child she always prided herself on her memory, she was able to appreciate why she was so anxious about what seemed to others to be just minimal cognitive difficulties. Once less anxious, she was able to accept what she could and could not do. In this way members are helped to understand how personality and emotional growth is possible at any age. As well, interpersonal conflicts that members experience with other residents in and out of the groups are examined in the sessions.

How Group Therapy in Nursing Home Works

Yalom [13] has suggested the therapeutic experience of group psychotherapy is comprised of eleven primary factors (see **Table 2**).

The factors of instillation of hope, universality, imparting of information, development of socializing techniques, interpersonal learning, group cohesiveness, and existential factors are most relevant to nursing home groups.

Table 2 Yalom's Therapeutic Factors for Group Psychotherapy

- Instillation of hope
- Universality
- Imparting of information
- Altruism
- The corrective recapitulation of the primary family group
- Development of socializing techniques
- Imitative behavior
- Interpersonal learning
- Group cohesiveness
- Catharsis
- Existential factors

Instillation of Hope

In nursing homes where hopelessness and despair are prevalent, instilling hope is a fundamental basis for creating change [14]. The combination of hopeful and optimistic therapists and residents being in a group of peers, especially with those who have successfully adjusted, builds hope for new residents that they can have a good quality of life in a nursing home.

Universality

Residents often enter a nursing home thinking they are experiencing a unique sense of despair: that they are alone in having unacceptable thoughts or feelings about themselves and others [14]. Groups provide a sense of comfort and relief as members realize "we are all in the same boat."

Imparting Information

Reality-oriented and psychoeducational groups impart information from the leader to the members. Psychotherapy groups feature more member interaction while providing one another with feedback.

Development of Socializing Techniques

Groups bring residents together in a safe, secure environment which encourages members to again use life-long social skills. A distinguishing characteristic of nursing home groups is that members are encouraged to freely interact outside the groups. This attempts to counteract the unwanted social isolation that diminishes the quality of life of many residents [10].

Interpersonal Learning

Groups provide a social environment, where through feedback and self-observation, members learn about their relational behavior with other residents and staff, which is so essential to successfully adjusting to a communal living situation [3].

Group Cohesiveness

A cohesive group has a sense of shared goals and purpose and its members feel cared for, respected, and valued. A cohesive group creates opportunities for members to assume or regain valued social roles among peers [13]. In turn, group members who value both the group and themselves begin to feel better about their living situations.

It is important for group cohesiveness that psychotherapy groups be as homogeneous as possible with respect to cognitive impairment and psychological-mindedness so that they can better address the unique feelings and concerns of the more cognitively intact residents.

In groups containing less cognitively-intact and psychologically-minded residents, therapists must be able to both verbalize what is difficult for these members to voice and to help integrate their thoughts and feelings [15]. This is usually accomplished by listening to the underlying message. For example, in one group, a seemingly irrelevant story was restated as a wish for more emotional contact and attention from others.

Existential Factors

Higher-functioning groups containing more cognitively intact members who have been together for a longer period present opportunities for members' emotional and developmental growth. Some of the members, demoralized and bitter, and unsuccessfully struggling with the late-life stage-specific issue of "integrity versus despair" [16] are given the necessary assistance to rework the unsatisfactory outcome of earlier developmental conflicts [17]. Only then are these residents better able to address the existential late-life issues pertaining to dependency, illness, and inevitability of death.

Beginning of Group Psychotherapy

Before starting any group, no matter which orientation, obtaining administrative support is a must [7]. Otherwise, when difficulties occur, the importance of the group is undermined and it becomes yet another place where members experience a lack of respect and caring at the hands of others.

It is important that a staff member who is known and respected by residents receive administrative approval to colead a psychotherapy group. It is also important that the cotherapists be familiar with the dynamics of aging and institutional living. The cotherapists need to support each other both during and after sessions because on occasion the complaints and frustration of some of the residents can be very difficult to endure for just one therapist working alone.

Although it has been suggested that smaller groups of several residents is optimal [18], large groups containing 10 or more members are advantageous in having enough members even when some are unable to attend because of illness or other commitments. Both the large group size and the outside contacts of group members help lessen their social isolation.

Examples of Common Themes in an Integrated Group Therapy

Initial sessions in nursing home groups were comprised of resident members struggling with issues of trust, autonomy, and feelings of inferiority [10]. Most members were never previously in a group or individual psychotherapy. Raised in an atmosphere where talking about feelings was construed as weakness, they were uncomfortable talking about personal issues. Often reluctant about moving into the nursing home and then experiencing frustration when staff and administration did not listen or take their concerns seriously, most members entered the group with mixed feelings. They were hopeful that the group would be a setting where they would be able to bring forth their feelings and concerns, but were also not completely trusting that the cotherapists and other group members would be able to make the group experience a good one.

A series of case illustrations are presented. They demonstrate how the group members moved from primarily expressing complaints to being able to share more personal feelings of vulnerability.

Case Illustration

Mrs. A. started an early group session complaining about the food. Mrs. B., another vocal and angry group member, joined in and said, “We deserve more for our money.” Another member stated, “I complain but no one listens.” An air of both helplessness and discouragement filled the room when Mrs. C. turned to the cotherapists and suggested, “Why don’t you two leaders go to the administration and speak on our behalf?” She then became anxious at having the staff and administration know what she was saying in the group. Members gave her their word that they would not discuss group matters with anyone outside the group.

Comment

The cotherapists understood the basis of the residents’ complaints and demands but knew that going to the administration would undermine the confidentiality and hence the integrity of the group because without assurance of “what’s said in the group stays inside the group,” personal disclosure would be jeopardized. Involving the administration would also reinforce the message that members needed outside help and could not function autonomously. Consequently, the cotherapists reminded members that although the group was not there to fix what ailed them or the institution, the group would still be helpful if members could share their complaints and feelings in an understanding and nonjudgmental setting. The cotherapists after then empathizing with the members' complaints showed their trust in the group by encouraging members to speak about their underlying feelings of demoralization, helplessness, frustration, and anger that they were experiencing when not responded to in the manner they had previously enjoyed in their lives.

Case Illustration

Tentatively at first, members started speaking of their sadness at what they had lost and their fears about losing more. The angry and vocal Mrs. B., a former salesperson in a large department store spoke proudly, but tearfully, of how she assisted customers who grew to respect and trust her. She was surprised that she could express her feelings in the group. Mrs. B. agreed with those who suggested she was able to because she had started trusting that the cotherapists and other members were interested and cared about what she had to say. She listened attentively when Mrs. D., a woman struggling with the loss of her vision, spoke about how she had to wait and wait for help. Mrs. D. stated, "I felt dehumanized. I almost wet my pants. Animals would be treated better." She received the support of the group members, one of whom asked "Did you speak up about this?" Mrs. D. said she was afraid of being mistreated and further abandoned if she spoke up and furthermore, "I was raised not to complain." The more assertive members encouraged Mrs. D. and other passive members to let others know what they were feeling because "others could not read their minds." The cotherapists agreed and suggested that they could perhaps first try speaking up in the groups. Those who did received care and attention from others.

Comment

Most group members gradually were able to share personal feelings. They became more content and also provided helpful feedback about the manner in which other members expressed themselves.

Case Illustration

As the group became more supportive and trusting of each other, the content of the group also changed. For instance, Mr. E., a 76-year-old man started complaining about the conditions in the dining room and said, "I would never have run my business this way." A couple of other members voiced their own criticisms of conditions in the dining room. Then another resident asked Mr. E. about his previous business. Surprised but visibly pleased, Mr. E. spoke with pleasure about his past. His anger dissipated as he reconnected with his previous sense of confidence and competence.

Comment

The group moved from members being united mainly through their complaints against the nursing home to being more united through their mutual interest and caring for each other. This was an important transition because it showed that residents were now recognizing each other as individuals with a past whose life did not begin or end upon entry into the facility. Members came to be regarded for who they were and still are, not just as that old grey-haired man or woman down the hall. A sense of community developed in the group and for many this carried over to outside the group.

Case Illustration

The stage was set for members in these cohesive groups to deal with the late-life challenges of coping with dependency, illness, and death, without experiencing further losses of control and dignity. For instance, Mrs. H. remarked, "I first thought using a cane was a sign of getting old and I wasn't old. Then I needed a walker. Then I imagined everyone was looking and feeling sorry for me, and now I need a wheelchair and I am trying hard not to feel sorry for myself." A member in a wheelchair spoke of similar struggles, especially because she had been previously been so active. Another member encouraged her to, "Look at what you still have and not at what you do not have. In other words, the rest of you works so help others, who cannot see or remember as well." Mrs. H. appreciated the advice because, " I did wonder if I could still be useful and independent in a wheelchair in a place like this."

Comment

Group members shared common fears of feeling worthless, of losing dignity, or of becoming difficult and demanding, which were all associated with a loss of control and autonomy over one's life [9]. The psychotherapy groups permitted sharing of members' struggles in both seeking and accepting help, because most of them were better at giving than receiving. Feelings of shame, guilt at being a burden, and lack of entitlement were expressed and needed to be either challenged or understood before members acknowledged that accepting help when needed was something they wished to become more comfortable with.

Case Illustration

The group became a place not only to deal with life, but also to deal with death as it inevitably occurred in the nursing home. Residents wanted to hear about a fellow resident's death so that they could begin to mourn the loss and were frustrated when information was kept from them by staff. For instance, Mr. O. complained, "I came into my room and my roommate was not there. It took me over a day to find out that he had died. This is supposed be a home, my community, right?"

Comment

Most members expressed relief that they could talk about death because they could not talk about this with family members. They agreed with Mrs. L. when she stated, "It is not death that I am afraid of. I led a long life, it is a long painful death and not knowing who I am that I fear." The residents who found death difficult to discuss were allowed to share their concerns about the group becoming too morbid. Usually they ended up agreeing that, "Death being part of life is okay to talk about, as long it is not the only thing discussed in the group." Sessions in which death was discussed often became "lively" discussions and the mood was one of appropriate sadness, not pessimism nor despair [10].

Difficulties in Conducting Group Psychotherapy in Nursing Homes

Despite the acceptance that groups have much to offer, this area of work remains unpopular because of challenges involved with working in a facility that lacks the will or resources to better address the mental health needs of residents [10]. For example, amplification systems to assist the hearing impaired are not purchased. Logistical problems relating to meeting times, competing activities, meeting room appropriateness and accessibility for wheelchairs, and residents who are not able to speak loudly are all difficulties [18]. Some staff attitudes may still reflect the belief that depression in nursing home is inevitable, or that the elderly are unable to change [19].

When complaints occur, the cotherapists must empathize with the resident's frustration regarding living in an institution. As well, they must point out both the advantages of living in the facility, and the difficulties residents would encounter living in their previous homes, with their current medical problems. Cotherapists occasionally must be prepared to discuss certain resident concerns with the administration to preserve the value and integrity of the group. However, administrators don't always appreciate hearing these criticisms regarding the facility. It is therefore recommended that the therapists discuss the benefits of members' new relational styles with administrators or staff, who otherwise may prefer passive, nonassertive residents [14].

A unique problem the staff cotherapist faces is balancing his or her dual roles as a social worker, and as a cotherapist. The staff role involves advocating and problem-solving, whereas in the group it primarily involves listening and understanding. Temptation must be resisted to discuss matters that arise within the group with fellow staff members.

Group work is emotionally challenging for therapists who must remember that levels of demoralization and discouragement within a group fluctuate and often relate to specific environmental and psychological stresses. Fortunately, these feelings are responsive to psychotherapeutic interventions [20]. Ultimately helping residents accept what they once thought would never be possible, that is, accepting and even liking life after entering a nursing home, results in feelings of accomplishment to be shared by both group members and therapists alike.

References

1. Mazza, N., Vinton, L. (1999). A nationwide study of group work in nursing homes. Activities, Adaptation and Aging, 24(1):61–73.
2. Feil, N. (1989). Validation: An empathetic approach to the care of dementia. Clinical Gerontologist, 8:89–94.

3. Molinari, V. (2002). Group therapy in long term care sites. Clinical Gerontologist, 25(1–2):13–24.
4. Cohen, C.S. (1995). Making it happen: From great idea to successful support group program. Social Work with Groups, 18:67–80.
5. Toseland, R.W. (1995). Group work with the elderly and family caregivers. New York: Springer-Verlag.
6. McCallion, P., Toseland, R.W. (1995). Supportive group interventions with caregivers of frail older adults. Social Work with Groups, 18:11–25.
7. Ruckdeschel, H. (2000). Group psychotherapy in the nursing home. In: V. Molinari (Ed.), Professional psychology in long term care: A comprehensive guide (pp. 113–131). New York: Hatherleigh Press.
8. Butler, R.N. (1963). The life review: An interpretation of reminiscence in the aged. Psychiatry, 26:65–76.
9. Silver, M.H. (1995). Memories and meaning: Life review in old age. Journal of Geriatric Psychiatry, 28(1):57–73.
10. Schwartz, K. (in press). Remembering the forgotten: Psychotherapy groups for the more cognitively intact nursing home resident. International Journal of Group Psychotherapy.
11. Leszcz, M. (1997). Integrated group psychotherapy for the treatment of depression in the elderly. Group, 21(2):89–113.
12. Schwartz, K.M. (2004). Concurrent group and individual psychotherapy in a psychiatric day hospital for depressed elderly. International Journal of Group Psychotherapy, 54(2):177–201.
13. Yalom, I.D., Leszcz, M. (2005). The Theory and Practice of Group Psychotherapy (5th Ed.). New York, Basic Books.
14. Ronch, J.L., Crispi, E.L. (1997). Opportunities for development via group psychotherapy in the nursing home. Group, 21(2):135–158.
15. Tross, S., Blum, N.E. (1988). A review of group therapy with the older adult: Practice and research. In: W. MacLeman, S. Saul, M. Bakur Weiner (Eds.), Group Psychotherapies for the Elderly. American Group Psychotherapy Monograph, No. 5 (pp. 3–29). Madison, CT: International Universities Press.
16. Erikson, E.H. (1950). Childhood and Society. New York: Norton.
17. Liptzin, B. (1985). Psychotherapy with the elderly: An Eriksonian Perspective. Journal of Geriatric Psychiatry, 18(2):183–202.
18. Speer, D.C., O'Sullivan, M.J. (1994). Group therapy in nursing homes and hearing deficit. Clinical Gerontologist, 14(4):68–70.
19. Zweig, R.A., Hinrichsen, G.A. (1996). Insight-oriented and supportive psychotherapy. In: W.E. Reichman, P.R. Katz (Eds.), Psychiatric Care in the Nursing Home (pp. 188–208). New York: Oxford University Press.
20. Leszcz, M. (1989). Group psychotherapy of the characterologically difficult patient. International Journal of Group Psychotherapy, 39:311–335.

Suggested Readings

1. Atchely, R.C. (1982). The Aging Self. Psychotherapy, Theory, Research and Practice, 19(4):388–396.
   This article discusses the issue of self-esteem in aging individuals.
2. Fernie, B., Fernie, G. (1990). Organizing group programs for cognitively impaired residents of nursing homes. Special Issue: Mental Health in the Nursing Home, Clinical Gerontologist, 8:123–134.
   This article discusses the benefits of homogeneous groups in nursing homes.

16 Guidelines for the Assessment and Treatment of Mental Health Issues

David K. Conn and Maggie Gibson

Key Points

- Canadian guidelines focusing on the assessment and treatment of mental health issues in long-term care homes were released in May 2006.
- The goal of these guidelines is to provide attending staff and consultants with a comprehensive approach to the care of residents with mental illness.
- General care issues are highlighted, as optimal care can reduce the incidence of behavioral symptoms. Organizational issues such as the development of the environment as a therapeutic milieu and the need for staff training are also emphasized.
- Recommendations for the screening and assessment of residents with behavioral or depressive symptoms are provided.
- Management recommendations focus on appropriate investigations, a full array of nonpharmacological interventions and the benefits versus risks of specific groups of psychotropic medications.

The Canadian Coalition for Seniors' Mental Health (CCSMH) was awarded funding in 2005 by the Public Health Agency of Canada, Population Health Fund, to lead and facilitate the development of evidence-based recommendations for best-practice national guidelines in a number of key areas for seniors' mental health. The four identified areas for guideline development were:

1. The assessment and treatment of delirium.
2. The assessment and treatment of depression.
3. The assessment and treatment of mental health issues in long-term care homes (focus on mood and behavioral symptoms).
4. The assessment of suicide risk and prevention of suicide.

Workgroups were established for the four identified areas. The workgroups evaluated existing guidelines, reviewed the primary literature, and formulated documents that included recommendations with supporting text. The four guidelines were published in May 2006 and the full documents can be found and downloaded at www.ccsmh.ca.

The Assessment and Treatment of Mental Health Issues in Long-Term Care Homes (Focus on Mood and Behavior Symptoms) Guideline is intended to promote mental health and address mental health problems (including mental disorders) in older residents of long-term care (LTC) homes. The specific focus is on depressive and behavioral symptoms.

The following individuals were members of the CCSMH LTC Homes Guideline Workgroup: Dr. David Conn (colead), Dr. Maggie Gibson (colead), Dr. Sid Feldman (group member), Dr. Sandi Hirst (group member), Ms. Sandra Leung (group member), Dr. Penny MacCourt (group member), Dr. Kathy McGilton (group member), Ms. Ljiljana Mihic (group member), Ms. Karen Cory (consultant), Dr. Ken Le Clair (consultant), Dr. Lynn McCleary (consultant), Ms. Simone Powell (consultant), Ms. Esther Roberts (consultant), Ms. Faith Malach (project director), Ms. Jennifer Mokry (project coordinator), and Ms. Kimberley Wilson (project manager).

There are several core assumptions that underpin the guideline recommendations, including the following:

1. There is a need to focus on both mental health and mental illness in LTC homes.
2. There is significant diversity in the LTC population. Each resident deserves an individualized approach to care delivery.
3. Effective mental health management requires an interdisciplinary approach.
4. Relationships among residents, family members, and staff are central in meeting mental health needs.
5. The milieu (social and physical environment) can promote or undermine mental health.

Overarching principles that promote and support the mental health of all LTC residents, whether or not they have mental health problems or mental disorders, include facility-wide commitment to: individualized, person-centered care; respect for family ties; a biopsychosocial care planning framework; a culture of caring that prioritizes quality of life; a social and physical environment that is responsive to changing needs; a focus on early intervention and prevention as well as treatment; and staff training and development as necessary to enable the provision of informed and competent care [1–3].

The LTC guideline provides recommendations to guide care for older adults living in LTC homes within two broad categories: (1) general care and (2) symptom and disorder management. The first category, general care, includes recommendations for delivering care to all LTC residents in a manner that will promote mental health. Under the second category recommendations are provided for the assessment and treatment of depressive and behavioral symptoms and disorders. Recommendations are also made that apply to the broader context of care delivery, at the facility and system level. This chapter should ideally be read in conjunction with the full-text document available at www.ccsmh.ca.

LTC Guideline Development: Method

A strategic and comprehensive review of the existing research literature on the assessment and management of mood and behavior symptoms in LTC homes was completed. A computerized search for relevant evidence-based summaries, including guidelines, meta-analyses, and literature reviews, and research literature not contained in these source documents, was conducted by librarian consultants to the guidelines project and by the Canadian Coalition for Seniors' Mental Health (CCSMH). The search strategy can be found in the original document. In addition, a list of Web sites was compiled based on known evidence-based practice Web sites, known guideline developers, and recommendations from Guideline Development Group members. This search yielded 26 potentially relevant guidelines. These were further considered by the Guideline Development Group coleads as to whether they specifically addressed the guideline topic and were accessible either online, in the literature, or through contact with the developers. Through this process 10 guidelines were selected and obtained for inclusion in the literature base for the project [1, 3, 4–11]. In addition, the search yielded several key review articles [12–15]. A supplemental literature search was also conducted. The resultant reference base includes over 200 citations. The method for developing recommendations is described in the original guideline documents. Categories of evidence were rated on a four point scale and strength of recommendations was rated from A to D based primarily on the level of evidence. Level A recommendations require randomized controlled trials or meta-analyses. The strength of each recommendation is listed in the tables below.

Recommendations: General Care

Behavioral symptoms often emerge during personal care such as bathing or dressing. Optimizing the way in which general care is provided may in itself prevent some of these behaviors. Behaviors such as agitation, restlessness, aggression, and combativeness are often an expression of unmet needs (e.g., hunger, thirst, pain, or toileting need). Care providers should try to identify when this is the case and intervene to prevent and minimize behavioral symptoms that are a reflection of unmet needs. At the same time, careful attention to assessing and understanding other factors that may be contributing to behavioral presentations (e.g., potential mental health problems and disorders, as well as other physical disorders and illnesses) is essential. The recommendations for general care can be found in **Table 1**.

Table 1 Recommendations: General Care

Strength of each recommendation is ranked from A to D. A is the highest level and D the lowest.

Family Involvement

- Encourage and support the involvement and education of the family in the institutional life of the older resident, including decision-making processes, as appropriate. [C]

Care Plan

- Individualize care plans, with due consideration to best-practice guidelines and recommendations. [D]

Communication

- Implement strategies to promote communication between care providers and residents. [B]

Dressing

- Develop an individualized approach when assisting the resident with dressing. [B]

Bathing

- Develop an individualized protocol for each resident that minimizes negative affect and promotes a sense of well-being during bathing. [A]

Activities

- Consider the need to pace activities that residents are involved in throughout the day. [B]

Mealtime

- Consider the need to develop mealtime caregiving activities to enhance nutrition and prevent behaviors that interfere with nutritional and social needs. [D]

Recommendations: Assessment

In the section on assessment, it is assumed that a facility adheres to an overarching assessment protocol that ensures compliance with both site-specific policies and statutory requirements. The recommendations speak to suggested components for the assessment protocol. There are numerous screening tools available in the literature to assist the screening process, as detailed in the full guideline. Clinical situations may require the use of customized behavioral observation techniques in addition to, or in place of, standardized scales to adequately screen for atypical or complex behaviors [16, 17]. The assessment protocol should include a triggering/decision-making algorithm to guide clinicians in determining when further detailed investigation is required [5, 18]. Although behavioral observations, self-report data, concerns expressed by others, and psychometric data should direct the assessment focus, a high index of suspicion should be maintained to ensure that less obvious factors or diagnoses that are contributing to the precipitation, maintenance, and exacerbation of depressive and behavioral symptoms are not missed. Among the medical and psychological conditions and disorders that may need to be included in the detailed investigation are, for example, pain, delirium, sleep disorders, and suicide risk [19]. The social

Table 2 Recommendations: Assessment of Mental Health Problems and Mental Disorders

Strength of each recommendation is ranked from A to D. A is the highest level and D the lowest.

Screening
- The facility's assessment protocol should specify that screening for depressive and behavioral symptoms will occur in the early postadmission phase and subsequently, at regular intervals, as well as in response to significant change. [C]
- A variety of screening tools that are appropriate to the setting and resident population should be available to facilitate the screening process. [D]
- Tool selection should be determined by the characteristics of the situation (e.g., resident capacity for self-report, nature of the presenting problem). [D]
- Screening should trigger detailed investigation of depressive and behavioral symptoms under defined circumstances. [D]

Detailed Investigation
- Core elements of a detailed investigation should include a history and physical examination, with follow-up laboratory and psychological investigations, investigations of the social and physical environment, and diagnostic tests as indicated by the results of the history and physical examination, and treatment history and response. [C]
- It is important to consider all contributing factors. Investigation of potentially contributing factors (e.g., delirium, chronic pain) should refer to clinical practice guidelines for these conditions where available. [D]
- Diagnosis and differential diagnosis should be an assessment objective where appropriate. [D]
- The end point of a detailed investigation should be the determination of the need for, type, and intensity of treatment. [D]

Ongoing Evaluation
- The treatment plan should specify the timeline and procedure for ongoing evaluation of clinical outcomes and treatment effectiveness. [D]
- Ongoing evaluation should include a history and assessment of change in the target symptoms. [D]
- Assessment of change should include quantification, preferably with the same tool that was used preintervention. [D]
- Unexpected clinical outcomes and treatment effects should trigger reassessment and potentially reconceptualization of the factors precipitating, maintaining, and exacerbating depressive and behavioral symptoms. Potential adverse reactions to treatment should be evaluated. [D]

factors and features of the physical environment that may need to be assessed include, for example, a change in the resident's social or family situation and factors in the physical environment, such as a change in room [1, 5]. Depressive and behavioral symptoms may reflect psychiatric diagnoses commonly seen in residents of LTC homes and/or medical diagnoses that are also common in this population. Assessment should be guided by awareness and understanding of relevant diagnostic criteria [20]. The need for, type, and intensity of treatment are determined on the basis of consideration of all relevant assessment information, including medical and physical findings, psychosocial findings, ratings on validated scales, behavioral analysis, risk assessment, formal diagnosis where applicable, and the perspectives and wishes of individual residents and their families. Ongoing evaluation is essential in the LTC setting, given the frailty of the population, high prevalence of comorbid conditions, and potential for rapid decline when symptoms escalate. As well, ongoing evaluation is essential to ensure that intervention objectives stay current with client-centered goals. The recommendations for assessment can be found in **Table 2**.

Recommendations: Treatment of Depressive Symptoms and Disorders

It is always important to consider the potential benefit of both nonpharmacological and pharmacological interventions in the treatment of depressive symptoms and disorders. The psychological and social intervention recommendations provided in these guidelines are grouped together based on the effects or goals they hope to achieve. This approach reflects recent understanding that "common factors" underlie various interventions, and a focus on these might be the best strategy for further development in this field [21]. Given the complexity and uniqueness of LTC settings, we have included interventions that would be delivered by mental health clinicians, as well as other care providers, family, and volunteers. LTC homes differ in their resources, and residents differ in the extent to which family and friends are available and willing to be involved in care. This section takes an aspirational approach to the task of identifying psychological and social interventions that can contribute to the treatment of depressive symptoms of residents in LTC homes, recognizing that the reality of what is available may differ. The appropriateness and effectiveness of different interventions will vary for different stages in the progression of dementia, and individualized assessment and care planning informed by the dementia care literature are essential [22]. The resident's capacity to understand and willingly engage in the intervention should be carefully considered to avoid unintended outcomes, such as increased agitation or distress. Selection of an appropriate antidepressant medication for nursing home residents should be based on (a) the history and experience of the resident; (b) other medical comorbidities; (c) side-effect profiles of the antidepressants; and (d) potential drug-drug interactions. It is important to obtain a history of bipolar illness as the treatment of bipolar depression will likely require the use of a mood stabilizer. Psychotic symptoms associated with depression rarely respond to antidepressant medication alone and usually require the addition of an antipsychotic medication. A full discussion of the pharmacologic management of depression can be found in the companion document, *National Guidelines for Seniors' Mental Health: Assessment and Treatment of Depression* [23]. The recommendations for treatment of depressive symptoms and disorders can be found in **Table 3**.

Recommendations: Treatment of Behavioral Symptoms

Psychological and social interventions should generally be used before initiating pharmacologic treatment; however, in urgent situations, or when symptoms are severe, it is appropriate to initiate pharmacologic and nonpharmacologic interventions together. Resi-

Table 3 Recommendations: Treatment of Depressive Symptoms and Disorders

Strength of each recommendation is ranked from A to D. A is the highest level and D the lowest.

General Treatment Planning
- Consider the type and severity of depression in developing a treatment plan. [B]

Psychological and Social Interventions
- Social contact interventions, including interventions that promote one's sense of meaning, should be considered where the goal is to reduce depressive symptoms. [C]
- Structured recreational activities should be considered where the goal is to engage the resident. [C]
- Psychotherapies should be considered where the goal is to reduce depressive symptoms. [B]
- Self-affirming interventions (e.g., validation and reminiscence therapies) should be considered where the goal is to increase a sense of self-worth and overall well-being. [C]
- Consider the impact of comorbid dementia in developing a treatment plan. [C]

Pharmacologic Interventions
- First-line treatment for residents who meet criteria for major depression should include an antidepressant. [A]
- Appropriate first-line antidepressants for long-term care home residents include selective serotonin reuptake inhibitors (e.g., citalopram and sertraline), venlafaxine, mirtazapine, and buproprion. [B]
- For residents with major depression with psychotic features, a combination of antidepressant and antipsychotic medications is appropriate. [B]
- Residents with a first episode of major depression responding well to antidepressant treatment should continue on full-dose treatment for at least 12 months. Residents who have had at least one previous episode of depression should continue with treatment for at least two years. [A]
- The treatment of depressed residents with a history of bipolar mood disorder should include a mood stabilizer such as lithium carbonate, divalproex sodium, or carbamazepine. [B]
- Residents with severe depression not responding to medications should be considered for a trial of electroconvulsive therapy. (These residents will likely require transfer to a psychiatric facility.) [B]
- Psychostimulants (e.g., methylphenidate) may have a role in treating certain symptoms that are commonly associated with depression (e.g., apathy, decreased energy). [C]

dents with moderately severe symptoms may also benefit from medication. The selection of specific behavioral interventions should be based on a solid behavior analysis (e.g., the ABC approach which tracks antecedents, behaviors, and consequences). Moreover, it is important to note that the process of behavior analysis can in itself have beneficial effects, often through the changes in staff behavior that follow from increased understanding [17].

Regarding medications, the best evidence from placebo-controlled trials in LTC homes would support the use of atypical antipsychotics for severe behavioral symptoms, with or without psychosis [1, 24]. Clinicians should carefully evaluate the risks versus the benefits of psychotropic medication in each resident and obtain informed consent. In consideration of the potential risks, many experts in the field believe that the use of antipsychotics in individuals with dementia should be reserved for residents with severe agitation or psychosis, where severity is evaluated on the basis of the degree of danger, suffering, or excess disability [25]. Clinicians should aim for the lowest possible effective dosage. Despite the limited evidence for the effectiveness of antidepressants in the treatment of behavioral symptoms they are widely used and some patients seem to respond to them. Combination pharmacologic therapy for residents with severe behavioral symptoms may be necessary

Table 4 Recommendations: Treatment of Behavioral Symptoms

Strength of each recommendation is ranked from A to D. A is the highest level and D the lowest.

Psychological and Social Interventions
- Social contact interventions should always be considered, especially where the goal is to minimize sensory deprivation and social isolation, provide distraction and physical contact, and induce relaxation. [C]
- Sensory/relaxation interventions (e.g., music, snoezelen, aromatherapy, bright light) should be considered where the goal is to reduce behavioral symptoms, stimulate the senses, and enhance relaxation. [B/D]
- Structured recreational activities should be considered where the goal is to engage the resident. [C]
- Individualized behavior therapy should be considered where the goal is to manage behavior symptoms (e.g., contextually inappropriate, disturbing, disruptive, or potentially harmful behaviors). [C]

Pharmacologic Interventions
- Carefully weigh the potential benefits of pharmacologic intervention versus the potential for harm. [A]
- Appropriate first-line pharmacologic treatment of residents with severe behavioral symptoms with psychotic features includes atypical antipsychotics. [B] Antipsychotics should be used only if there is marked risk, disability, or suffering associated with the symptoms. [C]
- Appropriate first-line pharmacologic treatment of residents with severe behavioral symptoms without psychotic features can include (a) atypical antipsychotics [B] and (b) antidepressants such as trazodone or selective serotonin reuptake inhibitors (e.g., citalopram or sertraline) [C].
- Pharmacologic treatment of residents with severe behavioral symptoms can also include (a) anticonvulsants such as carbamazepine [B] and (b) short- or intermediate-acting benzodiazepines [C].
- Appropriate pharmacologic treatment of residents with severe sexual disinhibition can include (a) hormone therapy (e.g., medroxyprogesterone, cyproterone, leuprolide), (b) selective serotonin reuptake inhibitors, or (c) atypical antipsychotics. [D]
- Appropriate pharmacologic treatment of behavioral symptoms associated with frontotemporal dementia can include trazodone or selective serotonin reuptake inhibitors. [B]
- Appropriate pharmacologic treatment of residents with behavioral symptoms or psychosis associated with Parkinson's disease or dementia with Lewy bodies includes (a) cholinesterase inhibitors [B] or, as a last resort, (b) an atypical antipsychotic with less risk of exacerbating extrapyramidal symptoms (e.g., quetiapine) [C].
- Pharmacologic treatments for behavioral symptoms or psychosis associated with dementia should be evaluated for tapering or discontinuation on a regular basis (e.g., every 3–6 months). Ongoing monitoring for adverse effects should be undertaken. [A]

if monotherapy of a sufficient dose and duration is unsuccessful. It is important to be aware that certain behaviors are unlikely to respond to medications (e.g., wandering, exit-seeking behavior, and excessive noisiness). The recommendations for treatment of behavioral symptoms can be found in **Table 4**.

Recommendations: Organizational and Systems Issues

Organizational issues focus on internal policy and procedures, such as human resource practices, whereas system issues focus on community context and partnerships. Best-practice guidelines can be successfully implemented only with adequate planning, the allocation of required resources, and organizational and administrative support. Organizations implementing recommendations for best practice are advised to consider the means by which the implementation and its impact will be monitored and evaluated. The recommendations regarding organizational and systems issues can be found in **Table 5**.

Table 5 Recommendations: Organizational and Systems Issues

Strength of each recommendation is ranked from A to D. A is the highest level and D the lowest.

Organizational Issues

- LTC homes should develop the physical and social environment as a therapeutic milieu through the intentional use of design principles. [D]
- LTC homes should have a written protocol in place related to staffing needs specific to the care of older residents with mood and/or behavioral symptoms. [C]
- LTC homes should have an education and training program for staff related to the needs of residents with depression and/or behavioral concerns. Ideally, dedicated internal staff would be available to provide leadership in this area, including the development and delivery of best practices. [C]
- LTC homes should have a written protocol in place related to the administration of medication by paraprofessional staff. [D]
- LTC homes should have a written policy in place regarding the use of restraints. [D]

System Issues

- LTC homes should obtain mental health services from local practitioners or multidisciplinary teams, with interest and expertise in geriatric mental health issues. [D]
- Administrators and managers within LTC homes should be prepared to advocate with local, provincial, and national policy makers and funding agencies to promote the health and well-being of older residents. [D]
- LTC homes should have a process in place that ensures adherence to the ethical and legislative rights of the older resident. [D]
- LTC homes should ensure adequate planning, allocation of required resources, and organizational and administrative support for the implementation of best-practice guidelines. [D]
- LTC homes should monitor and evaluate the implementation of best-practice recommendations. [D]

Conclusion

Caring for residents in LTC with mental health problems is often challenging. Concern about the quality of care around the globe led to the recent formation of an International Psychogeriatric Association (IPA) Task Force on Mental Health Services in Residential Care Homes (www.ipa-online.org). Early discussions suggest that similar issues are relevant in almost all countries. These issues include inadequate staffing levels, lack of staff training regarding mental health issues, aging and poorly designed LTC homes, failure to identify and assess residents in a timely fashion, inappropriate use of psychotropic medications, and limited availability of mental health consultants. The guidelines note that although it may be difficult to implement all of the recommendations, given the challenges outlined above, each facility should strive to adopt as many as possible.

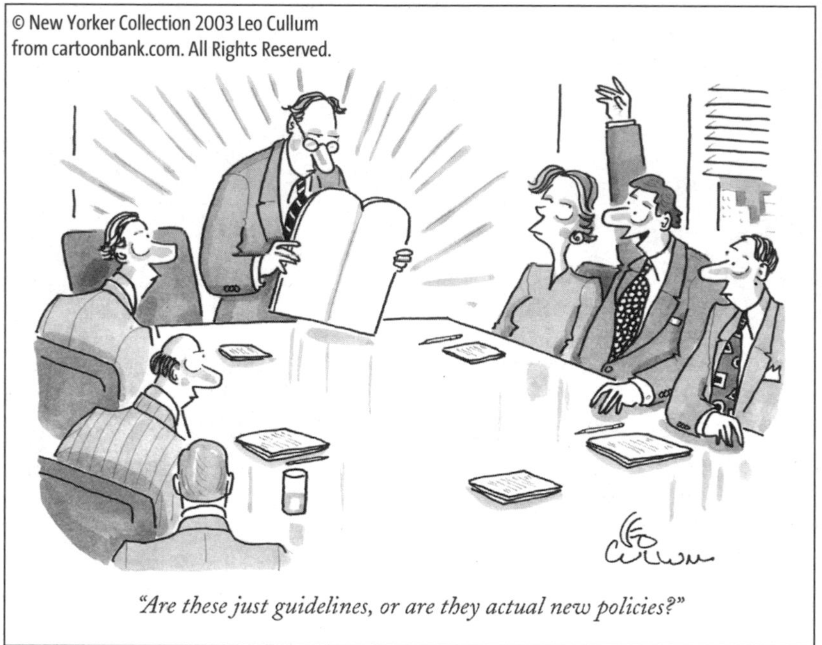

"Are these just guidelines, or are they actual new policies?"

References

A full list of references used in the guideline may be found with the full-text document: Canadian Coalition for Seniors' Mental Health (CCSMH). National Guidelines for Seniors' Mental Health: The Assessment and Treatment of Mental Health Issues in Long Term Care Homes. Toronto: CCSMH; 2006. Available at www.ccsmh.ca.

1. American Geriatrics Society and American Association for Geriatric Psychiatry (AGS/AAGP). (2003). Consensus statement on improving the quality of mental health care in U.S. nursing homes; management of depression and behavioral symptoms associated with dementia. Journal of the American Geriatrics Society, 51(9):1287–98.

2. British Columbia Ministry of Health. (2002). Guidelines for best practices in elderly mental health care in British Columbia. Victoria, BC: British Columbia Ministry of Health.
3. Registered Nurses Association of Ontario (RNAO). (2004). Caregiving strategies for older adults with delirium, dementia, and depression. Toronto: Registered Nurses Association of Ontario. Available at www.rnao.org/Storage/11/573_BPG_caregiving_strategies_ddd.pdf.
4. Alexopoulos, G.S., Jeste, D.V., Chung, H., Carpenter, D., Ross, R., Docherty, J.P. (2005). The expert consensus guideline series: Treatment of dementia and its behavioral disturbances. Postgraduate Medicine: A Special Report. Minneapolis, MN: McGraw-Hill.
5. American Medical Directors Association (AMDA). (2002). Depression: Clinical Practice Guidelines. Columbia (MD): AMDA. Available at www.amda.com.
6. Doody, R.S., Stevens, J.C., Beck, C., Dubinsky, R.M., Kaye, J.A., Gwyther. L. (2001). Practice parameter: Management of dementia (an evidence-based review). Report of the Quality Standards Subcommittee of the American Academy of Neurology. Neurology, 56(9):1154–1166.
7. Futrell, M., Melillo, K.D. (2002). Evidence-based protocol: Wandering. The University of Iowa Gerontological Nursing Interventions Research Centre: Research Dissemination Core; Available at www.guideline.gov/summary/summary.aspx?doc_id=3250&nbr=002476&string=iowa.
8. Gerdner, L. (2001). Evidence-based protocol: Individualized music. The University of Iowa Gerontological Nursing Interventions Research Center: Research Dissemination Core. Available at www.nursing.uiowa.edu/centers/gnirc/protocols.htm.
9. McGonigal-Kenney, M.L., Schutte, D.L. (2004). Nonpharmacological management of agitated behaviors in persons with Alzheimer's disease and other chronic dementia conditions. Iowa City (IA): University of Iowa Gerontological Nursing Interventions Research Center, Research Dissemination Core. Available at www.guideline.gov/summary/summary.aspx?doc_id=6221&nbr=003992&string=iowa.
10. Registered Nurses Association of Ontario (RNAO). (2003). Screening for delirium, dementia and depression in older adults. Toronto: Registered Nurses Association of Ontario. Available at www.rnao.org/Storage/12/645_BPG_DDD.pdf.
11. Thiru-Chelvam, B. (2004). Bathing persons with dementia. Iowa City (IA): University of Iowa Gerontological Nursing Interventions Research Center, Research Dissemination Core. Available at www.guideline.gov/summary/summary.aspx?doc_id=6220&nbr=003991&string=iowa.
12. Cohen-Mansfield, J. (2005). Nonpharmacological interventions for persons with dementia. Alzheimer's Care Quarterly, 6(2):129–45.
13. Forbes, D.A., Morgan, D.G., Bangma, J., Peacock, S., Pelletier, N, & Adamson, J. (2004) Light therapy for managing sleep, behavior, and mood disturbances in dementia. Cochrane Database of Systematic Reviews, 2:CD003946.
14. Hemels, M.E., Lanctot, K.L., Iskedjian, M., Einarson, T.R. (2001). Clinical and economic factors in the treatment of behavioral and psychological symptoms of dementia. Drugs and Aging, 18(7): 527–550.
15. Tilly, J., Reed, P. (2004). Evidence on interventions to improve quality of care for residents with dementia in nursing and assisted living facilities. Chicago (IL): The Alzheimer's Association.
16. Lundervold, D.A., Lewin, L.M. (1992). Behavior analysis and therapy in nursing homes. Springfield (IL): Charles C Thomas Publishers.
17. Rewilak, D. (2001). Behavior management strategies: An update. In D.K. Conn, N. Herrmann, A. Kaye, D. Rewilak, B. Schogt (Eds.), Practical psychiatry in the long term care facility: A handbook for staff, 2nd edition (pp. 199–221). Toronto: Hogrefe & Huber Publishers.
18. Morris, J.N., Hawes, C., Murphy, K., Nonemaker, S. (1995). Long term care resident assessment instrument user's manual, Version 2.0. Baltimore (MD): Health Care Financing Administration.
19. Canadian Coalition for Seniors' Mental Health (CCSMH). (2006). National guidelines for seniors' mental health: The assessment of suicide risk and prevention of suicide. Toronto: CCSMH. Available at www.ccsmh.ca.

20. American Psychiatric Association (APA). (2000). Diagnostic and statistical manual of mental disorders, 4th edition, text revision. Washington: American Psychiatric Association.
21. Niederehe, G. (2005). Developing psychosocial interventions for depression in dementia: Beginnings and future directions. Clinical Psychology: Science and Practice, 12:317–320.
22. Teri, L., McKenzie, G., La Fazia, D. (2005). Psychosocial treatment of depression in older adults with dementia. Clinical Psychology: Science and Practice, 12:303–316.
23. Canadian Coalition for Seniors' Mental Health (CCSMH). (2006). National Guidelines for Seniors Mental Health: Assessment and Treatment of Depression. Toronto: CCSMH. Available at http://www.ccsmh. ca.
24. Ballard, C., Waite, J. (2006). The effectiveness of atypical antipsychotics for the treatment of aggression and psychosis in Alzheimer's disease. Cochrane Database of Systematic Reviews, 1:CD003476.
25. Weintraub, D., Katz, I.R. (2005). Pharmacologic interventions for psychosis and agitation in neurodegenerative diseases: Evidence about efficacy and safety. Psychiatric Clinics of North America, 28:941–83.

17 Planning Mental Health Educational Programs

Susan Lieff and Ivan Silver

Key Points

- Educational programs for caregivers in nursing homes need to be individualized to the setting in which they are taught.
- Administrative support for continuing education is critical to the compliance with and success of the programs.
- The outcomes of nursing home educational programs outcomes are enhanced if clinical educational support is available on site.
- Any educational intervention must begin with an assessment of the intended audience's perceived needs, which should be complemented by other measures aimed at identifying nonperceived and misperceived needs.
- Educational programs should maximize opportunities for learners to actively engage in learning and interact with teachers; their content should be based on material which is meaningful to the learners' context.
- Evaluation of an educational program is essential. Information gathered in the process of evaluation provides both evidence of the program's effectiveness and guidelines for ways in which future programs could be modified to better meet the learning needs of the target audience.
- Learning can and should be fun.

Increasingly, as home care services for the elderly expand, those who ultimately require residential care in a nursing home have much more severe and complex mental health and physical problems. As a result, caregivers are being challenged to understand these conditions and their relationship to each other and to develop appropriate treatment plans for their patients. The need for continuing education in the assessment and treatment of mental disorders of nursing home residents and their families has become a priority for all disciplines. A recent study of the learning needs of social workers in nursing homes identified that the most relevant function they performed was assessing residents' social and emotional needs and that the primary obstacle to carrying out this function was lack of training and education [1, 2]. Similarly, the biopsychosocial process of aging has been identified as the number one educational priority of nursing personnel working in nursing homes [3]. A recent survey of its membership conducted by the Canadian Academy of Geriatric Psychiatry identified primary care physicians working in long-term care as the priority target audience for a psychiatric educational program [4]. This chapter discusses some of the key factors that need to be addressed in the planning of mental health educational programs in nursing homes.

The Nursing Home as a Teaching and Learning Environment

The need for educational programs to be individualized to the setting in which they are to be implemented is critical to the development of educational programs in nursing homes. All care facilities have a structure and an administration that must be understood and accommodated in order for an educational program to be successful. Any new educational endeavor must take into consideration issues such as shifts that occur over a 24 hour period, administrative support, efficient use of time available, accessibility to staff within the nursing home, funding, motivation of, and incentives for, attendees.

The first step toward educating care providers in a nursing home is the establishment of a relationship between the educator and the staff in order to facilitate communication and the development of trust, factors which are critical to any program of teaching and learning. In an ideal circumstance the educator is a mental health clinician who provides a consultation service to the home. This maximizes the one-on-one or group "teachable moment" opportunities around cases that the consultant is seeing. Making the material meaningful for learners by utilizing their own cases enhances their ability to learn. In addition, having the opportunity to apply principles learned "at the bedside" with the benefit of feedback from a consultant is invaluable. A number of studies have discussed the value of the onsite psychiatrist [5, 6, 7] or specialist nurse clinician [8, 9] in communication with allied health professionals in the nursing home, teaching general principles learned from individual cases, understanding difficult behaviors, and improving patient care because of increased knowledge and skill and changes in attitudes.

The important role of the nursing home's administrator in the support and facilitation of training cannot be overstated. Differences in the success rates of mental health training programs have been demonstrated based on the degree of support offered by administration in different facilities [10]. The administrator can facilitate an educational program by encouraging nursing supervisors to support a program, publicizing the program, communicating the program's value, encouraging staff to attend, encouraging release time from duties, providing compensation, and creating incentives and rewards for successful completion of the program such as certificates, personnel file letters, and write ups in newsletters. In one study a weekly lottery for all staff who met performance objectives was utilized; the prizes included a free lunch in the cafeteria, permission to arrive at work 30 minutes late, permission to leave work 30 minutes earlier, or one additional break during the shift [11].

Outside funding for nursing home education programs from government and private foundations may be available. The privately funded Teaching Nursing Home Program in the United States linked nursing homes with schools of nursing in the 1980s. The program succeeded in improving the quality of nursing care in these homes and in enhancing research into the needs of nursing home residents. Although this program was primarily directed at undergraduate students, changing a nursing home into a more academic environment had the effect of enhancing the quality of care [12].

Because care providers and support staff in long-term care facilities are adult learners with varied backgrounds, education, and learning styles, a variety of formats needs to be utilized in order to motivate them, maintain their attention, and encourage interaction and reflection [13]. Creating a safe, nurturing, and fun learning environment can be facilitated by enthusiastic educators, games, simulations, positive attitudes, constructive feedback to students, and the use of humor [14].

Key Elements in Planning a Teaching Program

All education activities, large or small, in a nursing home can be structured according to the following key elements (see **Table 1**): (a) needs assessment, (b) program development, and (c) evaluation.

Table 1 Key Elements in Planning a Teaching Program

(a) Needs Assessment	– Who wants it? – What do they want/need to learn? – Where/when should it take place? – Why is this important for them? – What format do they prefer?
(b) Program Development	– Who are the targeted participants? – What is the curriculum? – Where/when will it take place? – How will it be delivered? – Who will teach it?
(c) Evaluation	– Did they come and were they satisfied? – Did they learn something (knowledge, skill, attitude)? – Did they modify or change their behavior? – Did the residents of the nursing home do better? – What is the cost/benefit?

Needs Assessment

In determining the curriculum for a teaching program in a nursing facility a distinction must be made between what are perceived, unperceived, and misperceived needs. Perceived needs are those that care providers are consciously aware of. For example, they may appreciate the need to learn about how to bathe the resistive patient. A focus group or survey with open ended questions is often used to identify perceived needs. Asking staff to describe a current clinical issue that they would like help with generates a lot of useful information. This type of qualitative evaluation of needs also provides information about what sort of issues (i.e., who wants the program and why) motivate prospective participants. Alternatively, an itemized survey would provide information about perceived needs but would be limited by the surveyor's ability to anticipate what these needs are.

Unperceived and misperceived needs are those that the psychiatric consultant believes are learning issues that the care provider is unaware of (e.g., use of prn medication for agitation or misdiagnosis of psychiatric problems). These may be identified through chart audits, a review of psychotropic utilization in the nursing home [15], the literature on psychiatric illness in the nursing home, or the clinical experience of the consultant. Information about all three types of need is essential for the development of a comprehensive and useful educational program. Other information, which also is necessary and lends itself to a survey, concerns suitable times, locations, and preferred learning methods.

Program Development

The needs assessment helps to identify, not only the learning issues, but also the target audience. These factors guide decisions about the type of educational program that needs to be developed. If the priority learning issues and learning objectives (e.g., the behavioral management of screaming patients) are of interest and relevance to all disciplines, a multidisciplinary participation may make sense. If the identified learning need is discipline specific (e.g., psychotropic management of agitation in dementia), then a more selected and discipline specific attendance would be more appropriate. A variety of mental health training programs in nursing homes, targeting either specific care providers or having a multidisciplinary participation including not only health professionals, but even housekeeping, maintenance, and clerical staff have been described [10, 12, 13]. They all reported positive outcomes in knowledge and/or performance of participants. The multidisciplinary program reported positive outcomes regardless of discipline. It seems that the success of any program is in part determined by the ability of the program to meet the needs of the identified participants. As much as possible, the program must be individualized to the needs of the target group.

Prior to developing the program the learning objectives should be clearly defined. Objectives can be conceptually organized into knowledge, skill, or attitudes. They need to be stated in behavioral terms that indicate the expected outcome of the program and can be readily measured at the end of the educational intervention. For example, a learning objective can be stated as follows: "At the end of the program, participants will be able to develop a strategy for the evaluation and management of an agitated nursing home resident."

The actual operational format of the program must take into consideration the number of participants, the accessibility of the program to participants, the scheduling of the program, and the amount of time allocated to individual educational or training sessions. For example, if the program is targeted to nursing staff on site, then a convenient time may be for a one hour group program on the unit beginning one half hour before change of shift and ending one half hour after change of shift. Alternatively, the learning needs may be more efficiently met with individual structured learning assignments with feedback. Programs which are onsite, easily accessible (e.g., staff coverage available, scheduled around change of shift), and mandated as a requirement are more likely to be attended. *Train the trainer* methods have been employed when on site training is not an option for the majority of staff [16]. Using this methodology one staff member, chosen as an "opinion leader," may be trained to be an expert consultant who, in turn, will educate colleagues. Open-ended longitudinal educational programs are more likely to have a lasting effect on staff behavior and patient outcomes [17]. A single educational intervention, while perhaps increasing short-term knowledge, is unlikely to result in any detectable change in behavior of staff [18].

The program should integrate adult learning principles into its format. Essential to this conceptualization of learning is the recognition that participants come to a program with a foundation of knowledge, skill, and attitudes. The format or process of the program should endeavor to modify or expand what is already known by the learner to accommodate the new material [19]. This can be achieved by applying the following principles of effective teaching and learning [20]. Teachers need to:

- Be knowledgeable in the subject matter
- Actively involve the learner
- Maximize interactions between teachers and students
- Have students take responsibility for learning
- Utilize a variety of teaching methods (e.g., workshops, seminars, role playing, individual assignments)
- Make the material meaningful to their context (e.g., by using clinical vignettes)
- Utilize constructive, positive, and descriptive feedback
- Create an atmosphere of collaboration and cooperation

A variety of workshop and seminar formats have been described that employ these principles [21]. The method should be selected to suit the objectives. For example, if development of a skill is the goal, then participants must have the opportunity for practice of the skill with feedback. If the goal is to develop an understanding of a problem, then a problem based or case based seminar may be more appropriate. Didactic presentations can be useful to provide needed information, generate reactions and stimulate debate, but need to be kept brief to allow for audience reactions, questions, and interaction. Reading relevant material prior to the actual teaching or training session facilitates learning, but only if the participants actually do it. It can be useful to provide the readers with focused questions that highlight the learning issues in the material or for them to present a synopsis of the material to a colleague, learning group, or class. Nothing makes material clearer than having to teach it to someone else.

Demonstrations can be useful in modeling skills but only if there is an opportunity for the participants to practice and receive constructive feedback. This can be achieved by direct observation of the participant through role playing, use of a video tape, or use of simulated patients. If a group skill is the focus, then having a small group observed by a larger group surrounding them can be informative. In this "fish bowl" technique, the inner circle practices certain strategies while the outer circle provides them with constructive feedback.

Small group methods which generate reactions and responses from participants in an open way have the benefit of actively engaging the participants, allowing them to learn from each other, and informing the teacher of their connection with the topic. Examples of these methods include:

- *Brainstorming* – Members of a group generate as many ideas as they can on a given topic (e.g., all possible causes of agitation in a demented individual); an important rule is that all ideas are accepted without judgment about their worth, usefulness, etc.
- *Buzz groups* – Participants are divided into small groups of two to six members and then assigned a time limited task (e.g., "In the next ten minutes, discuss how you would educate a family member about her/his parent's depression")
- *Think/Pair/Share* – Participants are initially asked to think about a problem for a couple of minutes and then are invited to form pairs and share the problem with their partners. Subsequent to this, they are invited to share their discussion with the other pairs in a larger group in order to generate further discussion.
- *"Stand up and be counted"* – Participants are initially asked to reflect on a clinical problem or discuss it in pairs. They are asked to commit themselves to an opinion on a problem and stand up in front of the area on a Likert scale (a scale that has several anchor points ranging from "strongly agree" to "strongly disagree" with intermediate ratings in between) that most closely reflects their opinion. The facilitator then interviews different individuals who are positioned at different points of the scale, encouraging debate and discussion from the entire group and then summarizing at the end.
- *Games* – Participants are divided into teams and instructed to compete in games that have learning objectives. Learning games increase motivation and can be entertaining.

Case-based and problem-based learning has become an increasingly popular method for engaging the learner in medical education. This model can be applied in a variety of ways. The structured case is one in which a group(s) is presented a case and then is left the task of discussing it for 5 or 10 minutes. Next, the teacher either visits each group to listen and give feedback on its solutions and approaches or may solicit feedback from the groups so that they can hear from each other and expand the discussion beyond their individual group. Another case based method is to give the group a case with specific questions for discussion and apply the same method. Alternatively, role playing of a problem can be useful in simulating the context and "testing" the solutions. Case based methods can also be utilized for individual learning programs that have similar requirements.

For those learners who require more flexibility or may not be able to secure time away from their clinical responsibilities, internet or CD-ROM based programs may be more appropriate. Electronic mail may also serve as a vehicle for ongoing communication between students and teachers as part of an educational program or part of the follow-up to it.

Finally, and most importantly, learning can and should be FUN. A learning environment, which is stimulating, active, nurturing, and enjoyable enhances learning and increases motivation to learn, both with respect to both the current and any future educational program.

Programs that employ a variety of teaching methods over an extended period of time with opportunities for knowledge to be applied and skills to be observed and reinforced have been shown to be the most successful at demonstrating observable changes in behavior and patient outcomes. In the nursing home studies mentioned earlier, there typically was an on-site clinical nurse specialist available to the nursing home for follow up to the educational program. One study, which assessed the effects of one week of classroom teaching based on a variety of teaching methods, followed by clinical nurse specialist visits on site over six weeks, demonstrated increased knowledge, communication skills, and teamwork of participants [22]. In another study a combination of onsite teaching and ongoing consultation by a nurse specialist was associated with lower depression scores in residents of a nursing home over a six month period [23].

Evaluation

The evaluation of an educational program serves not only to measure the effectiveness of the program but also to modify the program so that it is consistent with the learners' needs and expectations. Several outcomes are typically selected when evaluating the impact of an educational program. These may include measures to assess (1) the participants' satisfaction with or perception of the program, (2) changes in the participants' degree of knowledge, skill, or attitude, (3) changes in the participants' actual performance or behavior in the clinical setting, (4) changes in the mental health status of individuals receiving care from the participants, and (5) the cost-benefit ratio associated with the program [24, 25].

The easiest outcome to measure is the participants' satisfaction with or opinion of the educational program. Measures of satisfaction or opinion include questions about the speakers, workshops, facilities, as well as attendance figures. It may be more useful measuring satisfaction weeks or months after a program in order to accurately reflect its impact. Competency or learning measures are those that measure any changes in knowledge, skills or attitudes in the test setting or learning environment. This may be evaluated by such methods as pre/post tests, touch pad technology, questionnaires, or verbal feedback. It bears stressing that an increase in knowledge or level of skill demonstrated in the test setting or learning environment does not necessarily translate into behavior change in practice [26]. For this reason, it is important to use measures which assess the real life performance or behavior of participants in the actual clinical setting. Such measures provide a more accurate and reliable estimation of change as a result of the training program. One study, for example, evaluated the impact of an educational program on the communication skills and handling of mentally impaired residents once the participants had returned to front line duties [10]. Patient or health care outcome measures are those that evaluate changes in patients or residents receiving care from staff members who have completed the educational program. Any changes that do occur in the recipients of care are deemed to represent the impact of the educational program on the participants' job performance.

One study examined the impact of an educational intervention on the level of depression in residents of nursing homes; only residents in nursing homes whose staff had participated in the intervention showed a reduction in their depression scores [23]. Cost benefit analyses are those that evaluate the economic impact of an educational intervention in terms of the health care costs in a system. Psychotropic drug utilization, absenteeism because of injuries, and the ordering of tests are examples of costs that could serve as indicators for the effectiveness of an educational intervention.

References

1. Brown, M. (1999). Psychosocial functions and training needs of social workers in nursing homes: A survey. Continuum Jan-Feb, 19:7–13.
2. Green, R.R., Vourlekis, B.S., Gelfand, D.E., Lewis, J.S. (1992). Current realities: Practice and education needs of social workers in nursing homes. Journal of Gerontological Social Work, 18:39–54.
3. Hirst, S.P., Metcalf, B.J. (1986). Learning needs of caregivers. Journal of Gerontological Nursing, 12:24–28.
4. Conn, D.K., Silver, I.L. (1998). The psychiatrist's role in long-term care. Canadian Nursing Home, 9:22–24.
5. Bienenfeld, D., Wheeler, B.G. (1989). Psychiatric services to nursing homes: A liaison model. Hospital and Community Psychiatry, 40:793–794.
6. Sakauye, K.M., Camp, C.J. (1992). Introducing psychiatric care into nursing homes. The Gerontologist, 32:849–852.
7. Streim, J.E., Oslin, D., Katz, I.R., Parmelee, P.A. (1997). Lessons from geriatric psychiatry in the long-term care setting. Psychiatric Quarterly, 68:281–307.
8. Smith, M., Mitchell, S., Buckwalter, K.C. (1995). Nurses helping nurses: Development of internal specialists in long-term care. Journal of Psychological Nursing, 33:38–42.
9. Smith, M., Mitchell, S., Buckwalter, K.C., Garand, L. (1995). Geropsychiatric nursing consultation as an adjunct to training in long-term care facilities: The indirect approach. Issues in Mental Health Nursing, 16:361–376.
10. Chartok, P., Nevins, A., Rzetelny, H., Gilberto, P. (1988). A mental health training program in nursing homes. The Gerontologist, 28:503–507.
11. Stevens, A.B., Burgio, L.D., Bailey, E., Burgio, K.L., Paul, P., Capilouto, E., Nicovich, P., Hale, G. (1998). Teaching and maintaining behavior management skills with nursing assistants in a nursing home. The Gerontologist, 38:379–384.
12. Mezey, M.D., Mitty, E.L., Bottrell, M. (1997). The teaching nursing home programme: Enhancing educational outcomes. Nursing Outlook, 45:133–140.
13. Phillips, R.M., Baldwin, B.A. (1997). Teaching psychosocial care to long-term care nursing assistants. The Journal of Continuing Education in Nursing, 28:130–134.
14. Inglis, A.D., (1992). Ten common sense teaching strategies for effective inservice presentations by staff nurses. The Journal of Continuing Education in Nursing, 23:263–266.
15. Conn, D.K., Ferguson, I., Mandelman, K., Ward, C. (1999). Psychotropic drug utilization in long-term care facilities for the elderly in Ontario, Canada. International Psychogeriatrics, 11:222–233.
16. Smith, M., Mitchell, S., Buckwalter, K.C., Garand, L., Albanese, M., Kreiter, C. (1994). Evaluation of a geriatric mental health training program for nursing personnel in rural long-term care facilities. Issues in Mental Health Nursing, 15:149–168.
17. Davis, D., Thomson O'Brien, M.A., Freemantle, N., Wolf, F.M., Mazmanian, P., Taylor-Vaisey,

A. (1999). Impact of formal continuing medical education. Journal of the American Medical Association, 282:867–874.
18. Cohen-Mansfield, J., Werner, P., Culpepper, W.J., Barkley, D. (1997). Evaluation of an inservice training program on dementia and wandering. Journal of Gerontological Nursing, 23:40–47.
19. DeLay, R. (1996). Forming knowledge: Constructivist learning and experiential education. Journal of Experiential Education, 19:76–81.
20. Tiberius, R., Tipping, J. (1990). Twelve principles of effective teaching and learning for which there is substantial empirical support. Unpublished paper.
21. Tiberius R., Silver I.L. (1998). Guidelines for conducting workshops and seminars that actively engage participants. Unpublished paper.
22. Feldt, K.S., Ryden, M.B. (1992). Aggressive behavior: Educating nursing assistants. Journal of Gerontological Nursing, 18:3–12.
23. Proctor, R., Burns, A., Stratton Powell, H., Tarrier, N., Faragher, B., Richardson, G., Davies, L., South, B. (1999). Behavioural management in nursing and residential homes: A randomized controlled trial. The Lancet, 354:26–29.
24. Dixon, J. (1978). Evaluation criteria in studies of continuing education in the health professions: A critical review and a suggested strategy. Evaluation and the Health Professions, 1:47–65.
25. Casebeer, L., Raichle, L., Kristofc, R.E., Carillo, A. (1997). Cost benefit analysis: Review of an evaluation methodology for measuring return on investment in continuing education. Journal of Continuing Education of the Health Professional, 17:224–227.
26. Parker, K., Parikh, S.V. (1999). Application of Prochaska's transtheoretical model to continuing medical education from needs assessment to evaluation. Annals of the Royal College of Physicians and Surgeons of Canada, 32:97–99.

Suggested Readings

1. Chartok, P., Nevins, A., Rzetelny, H., Gilberto, P. (1988). A mental health training program in nursing homes. The Gerontologist, 28:503–507.
   This paper is a useful outcome study of a multidisciplinary mental health education intervention in a number of nursing homes.
2. Tiberius, R., Silver, I.L. (1998). Guidelines for conducting workshops and seminars that actively engage participants.
   An excellent resource for ideas about what format a workshop should have. This is now available at the website of the Association for Academic Psychiatry: www.aapsych.org. Click on Resources for Teaching, and then click on Teaching Skills.
3. Dixon, J. (1978). Evaluation criteria in studies of continuing education in the health professions: A critical review and a suggested strategy. Evaluation and the Health Professions, 1:47–65.
   A classic and often quoted reference on the conceptualization of evaluation in health care education.
4. Hamilton, P., Harris, D., Le Clair, K. (2005). Putting the P.I.E.C.E.S. together: Learning program for professionals providing long-term care to older adults with cognitive/mental health needs.
   Contact office@piecescanada.com or go to www.piecescanada.com. Excellent resource from a Canadian train the trainer program.

18 Helping the Nursing Staff: The Role of the Psychogeriatric Nurse Consultant

Alanna Kaye and Anne Robinson

Key Points

- Working alone or in conjunction with other mental health professionals the psychogeriatric nurse consultant assists staff in the process of understanding and caring for residents, especially those with psychiatric/behavioral problems. Extensive psychiatric clinical experience, education, and collaborative style contribute to the efficacy of the role. It is important that front-line staff feel understood, supported, and valued by the consultant.
- Types of help include:
  - Assisting with crisis management
  - Developing consistent models of care
  - The provision of ongoing support
  - The acknowledgment and management of staff grief
  - Identification of educational needs and systems issues
- Assisting direct caregivers requires a long-term commitment from the nurse consultant to remain engaged and supportive as long as the problem lasts.

The provision of high quality patient care and job satisfaction for personnel are two goals common to all institutions. Statistics Canada reveals that the rapidly aging population is projected to last until the year 2031, when 23–25% of the total population will reach the age of 65 years. This is double the current population of thirteen percent [1]. The trend for increased diagnosable psychiatric disorders in long-term care facilities continues, and the rate of behavioral disorders may be as high as 76% [2]. The nursing staff make up the vast majority of professional caregivers and their work is often physically and mentally arduous. Unlike other health care professionals, nurses remain with their residents throughout their shift and are unable to escape the unrelenting nature of behaviorally disordered residents. This leads to increased stress levels and a need for support. Although other mental health professionals can be of assistance to nursing staff, this chapter will address the unique role of the psychogeriatric nurse consultant with a particular emphasis on increasing the quality of patient care by the provision of clinical teaching and staff support.

The evolution of the nurse's role currently encompasses a variety of leadership positions, including consultant, educator, clinical leader, coach, mentor, clinician, clinical nurse specialist (CNS), advanced practice nurse, nurse practitioner, and registered nurses (RNs) assuming a leadership role. The College of Nurses of Ontario [3] describes leadership as part of the standard of practice for RNs, and indeed facilities are looking to expand the leadership responsibilities of RNs to encompass part of the role of the psychogeriatric nurse consultant in an effort to utilize resources more effectively, increase the autonomy of the nurse's role, and meet current nursing standards with respect to leadership. There are, however, many considerations to expanding the scope of this leadership role. Formal/informal education and promotion of critical thinking has often been encompassed by the roles mentioned above, integrating four domains of practice. Woodward et al. [4] describe these domains as expert practice; professional leadership and consultancy; education, training, and development; and practice and service development. They further suggest that educational preparation as well as professional experience in change management is important to the success of the individual to integrate the various components of the role. Moreover, Woodward et al. further contend that these nursing roles are not readily accepted within multidisciplinary settings, which speaks of the need for individuals in these capacities to have the ability to negotiate organizational issues [5]. It is our position that success in a role of this nature requires a complex blend of personal characteristics inherent in the role of mentor/coach, combined with specific clinical expertise and education in the area, and a clear mandate of support from organizational administration to field systems issues that may impact on the delivery of nursing care.

Pajarillo et al. define the consultation-liaison nurse consultant as a "certified psychiatric and mental health nurse at the advanced level, focusing on the emotional, spiritual, developmental, cognitive, and behavioral responses of clients who enter the health care system" [6]. Within this definition, the psychogeriatric nurse consultant's role encompasses a consultative, collaborative, and educative relationship with nurses as well as other health care providers. If employed by a facility, the psychogeriatric nurse consultant would perform functions within the administrative realm as well, such as consultation, performance improvements, and research.

Stolz Howard links the roles of nurse clinician and mental health consultant in an attempt to define the function of the psychogeriatric nurse consultant [7]. These functions include:

- Responding to staff requests for assistance with specific nursing interventions in the provision of care.
- Assisting staff to extract and co-ordinate information from their nursing assessments to further understand a problem.
- Assisting them to integrate their knowledge of the resident's behavior with the theory that behavior has meaning.
- Providing support for the staff around difficult clinical issues through care-planning conferences, educational programming, and remaining involved with the staff/client for the duration of the problem.
- Identifying aspects of a problem which may be systems-related and may be impacting

on the clinical situation. Facilitating problem-solving sessions to reduce the effect of these issues on the staff/residents is an important component of this role.
- Providing weekly supportive counseling to residents which then assists staff to care for the residents in their own milieu.
- Providing didactic teaching sessions to aides, registered nursing assistants, registered nurses, and other multidisciplinary team members in accordance with the biopsychosocial model.
- Helping staff to consider and identify possible underlying psychiatric syndromes.
- Facilitating staff and families to work as collaborative partners in difficult situations.
- Helping staff to determine which residents may need referral to a psychiatrist or a psychologist. (We are aware that in many institutions such consultations may be difficult to obtain).

Unique to psychiatry, liaison has been defined as "the process of facilitation of the relationship that exists among the patient, the adjustment to the illness, the consultee(s) and the hospital/ward milieu" [8]. Liaison is a central function of the psychogeriatric nurse consultant's role. Intimate knowledge of the conflicts and stresses that staff encounter working in institutions promotes a sense of collegiality and identification by staff with the consultant in the formation of a trusting relationship, which is essential to effective liaison work. The credibility of the psychogeriatric nurse consultant is enhanced when clinical experience and theoretical knowledge are conveyed in a supportive manner. This can have a calming influence during a crisis and should communicate to staff that their work is valued.

Case Illustration: "How could she say that to me?"

Mrs. B. was a 79-year-old widow who had been admitted to the institution with moderate cognitive impairment. She had no family or friends. While staff had noted her to be "moody" at times, they had nevertheless taken an interest in her. As time progressed, Mrs. B. became more verbally abusive. Staff requested assistance from the nurse consultant as they were having increasing difficulty providing care and dealing with the insults. Investigation revealed a woman whose cognition was severely impaired. Although she was able to engage in brief conversations, she was disoriented to the time, place, and person, and had little short-term memory. She was noted to be highly impulse-laden. Staff agreed to meet over a 6-week period to review her status and discuss strategies in the provision of her care.
The first three sessions were emotionally intense. Staff were offended by the resident's obscene and insulting remarks. They were angry and bewildered, wondering why she would attack those who had cared for and befriended her. They had difficulty accepting her increased cognitive impairment as the cause of her disinhibition, commenting, "But many times we can talk and I know that she knows me. She's not that impaired." These reactions were not unlike those experienced by family members who are unable to believe the person they love is irrevocably changed. When reviewing the case with the nurse consultant, the anger and helplessness felt by staff was evident during various role-playing situations. The anger, once released, appeared to dissipate and subsequently staff began to report a change in Mrs. B.'s behavior. They noted a decrease in the number of insults and developed a higher tolerance of her salty language during the delivery of care.

Comment

The clinical support groups facilitated expression and exploration of feelings, and helped the staff to provide a high level of care. Change is a slow process and often there is a disparity between intellectual understanding and integrated "knowing." The facilitation by the nurse consultant of the sharing of knowledge and mutual support fosters the integrating process, which results in changes in staff attitudes and responses.

Why Do Staff Need Help?

Nurses in long-term care are in a unique position. Their tasks are clearly defined, but the satisfactions are often nebulous. The nurse's inner sense of satisfaction is often derived from the knowledge and experience of giving within a highly sensitive, intimate, and therapeutic context. However, these positive energizing feelings can be severely diminished when the nurse is confronted with unrelenting racial slurs, aggression, accusations, sexual disinhibition, and preseverative noises. These have been described in the chapters on depression, dementia, suspiciousness, and characterologically difficult individuals. It must be noted that nurses are not dealing with these situations in isolation. Given the frequency with which these behaviors are encountered, it is not unusual for a nurse to have sole care for eight or more residents exhibiting these behaviors on a single shift.

In addition, nursing staff assist and interact with the many family members on the unit. Since family dynamics, coping styles, and abilities will affect communication, staff must be prepared to deal effectively with a barrage of complaints, anger, and accusations that they "aren't doing enough." (see Chapter 19, Understanding and Helping the Family). Situations are often seen by both families and staff in black or white terms. In reality uncertainty abounds during the process of clinical care and decision-making. Ethical, moral, legal, professional, and personal issues often blend to produce a total picture of great complexity. Nurses, therefore, need a highly developed sense of tolerance to be able to deal simultaneously with the varied physical and emotional demands, expectations, and ambiguities. These strengths and abilities to nurture are rarely valued by society or the institution in which nurses work. The nursing profession has traditionally emphasized technological skills and higher education rather than the less tangible personal qualities necessary to provide comprehensive, humane care to the elderly. Attitudes must change if gerontological nursing is to flourish and we are to retain and attract caring staff. To accomplish this shift in attitude, specific types of support are required.

Case Illustration

Mrs. Q. was a 92-year-old widowed woman admitted to the institution as a result of diminished physical activity following a myocardial infarction. A friendly, outgoing, and "feisty" woman, she soon made friends with members of the treatment team, sharing with them fascinating stories of her life and travels. Difficulties began for Mrs. Q. when a resident who was somewhat noisy was admitted. She took an immediate, intense dislike to him and demanded that he be moved to another part of the institution. When this could not be arranged, she was offered the opportunity to move to a different section of the unit when room became available. She was incensed with the thought of being inconvenienced by this man and became more intensely agitated. She threatened to kill him if he was not relocated. The nurse consultant, who had been seeing her regularly for some time, attempted to work with her and the staff with regard to the management of her anger. The necessity to control physical outbursts was explained and appropriate alternatives were reinforced. Despite these efforts, Mrs. Q. remained enraged with her coresident and attempted to throw objects at him from afar. The need to set firm, clearly defined limits of acceptable behavior became critical. She was then given the opportunity to work with staff towards the goal of maintaining her self-control. She was informed that the alternative would be possible certification and transfer to a psychiatric unit where she could be assisted in regaining her self-control. Two days later, Mrs. Q. threw a can of tuna at the resident screaming, "I'm going to kill you! I don't care what anyone says." Arrangements were then made for a brief admission to the psychiatric unit and she was placed on constant care until the transfer. Despite the need to follow through on limit-setting, staff became very uneasy, perceiving her admission to psychiatry as a punishment and questioning the validity of the decision. Several sessions with the staff were arranged to help them understand the management approach and Mrs. Q. was transferred. Upon her return, staff felt more comfortable with the idea of setting limits in order to preserve an individual's dignity and comfort. Mrs. Q. was subsequently able to remain on the unit maintaining her relationships without further loss of control. As no medications had been used, it appeared that the management plan, with its clear delineated expectations and consequences, had assisted her in achieving self-control.

Comment

In situations such as these, quick action is required to follow through on a particular care plan. As illustrated, Mrs. Q had a good understanding of her situation, the consequences, and some degree of control over her actions. The dual interventions of applying external controls when necessary as well as supporting and educating staff were important factors in the successful outcome. These actions enabled the care plan to be carried out in a manner which left the dignity of all parties intact and promoted the continuity of the warm relationship between the resident and the staff upon her return.

Types of Help

Assisting with Crisis Management

One of the problems that arises in institutions is how to handle situations where a resident or family member is out of control. Understanding is not enough. The clarity, consistency, and follow-through necessary to contain certain unacceptable behaviors may be perceived by staff at all levels as punitive. It is important to assist staff to be consistent, while maintaining an empathic approach. The subjective sense of being out of control creates great discomfort, loss of dignity, and may damage helpful relationships.

Developing Consistent Models of Care

Provision of care in a long-term care setting differs from that in acute care settings. Although this may seem obvious, these differences are often a source of misunderstanding between residents, staff, families, and administrators. All four groups require help in identifying possible differences in goals if difficulties are to be minimized. The consultant can assist in clarifying some of the issues that arise. The difference between the "care versus cure" models of care combined with increasing desires of the resident (or substitute decision-maker) to participate in decisions creates the basis for a variety of potential problems.

Case Illustration

Mrs. H., a severely demented woman, wailed loudly and incessantly if left alone, even for brief periods. Despite all attempts to meet her needs, her wailing could not be easily diminished. The use of small doses of a phenothiazine was attempted and was successful in reducing the extreme agitation. Mrs. H.'s daughter, however, began to berate the team physician for this use of medications, telling him that he and the nursing staff were "incompetent and unable to handle the simplest task of keeping mother company." Unable to tolerate her mother's cognitive impairment, the daughter continually harangued the staff until finally medications were reduced. The team began to withdraw from the situation and referred to Mrs. H.'s daughter as manipulative and "wanting her own way." The wailing escalated once again, sending the relatives of coresidents to the administrator to "do something" about the noise. Miscommunications and unrealistic expectations from all parties added to the confusion about Mrs. H.'s management. The nurse consultant, liaising with all members of the treatment team and administration, facilitated a clarification of issues and the setting of realistic goals. Once these things had been accomplished, the team felt supported and empowered to help the daughter understand and accept the need for a transfer to a floor with other residents like her mother and the need for some pharmacological interventions to reduce Mrs. H.'s agitation.

Comment

This vignette also raises the issue of whether it is acceptable for staff to have emotional reactions to intense situations, within the parameters of professional behavior. The fact that the problems encountered in chronic care facilities are long-term in nature cannot be overlooked. Unlike in acute care settings residents cannot be "cured" and sent home, for the institution has become their home. As a result, awareness and empathy among all parties concerned becomes a more critical aspect to the philosophy and expectations of those involved in long-term care.

Acknowledging and Managing Staff's Grief

There are frequent discussions about the resident's and family's losses and grief, yet little attention is paid to the grief experienced by the staff. The long-term relationships formed with residents and visitors are highly valued and their loss can be understandably distressing. The perpetual decline and relentless losses can become overwhelming and affect the ability to work effectively with this population. There is a great emotional demand upon staff and unless the cumulative losses are acknowledge and managed, "burnout" can occur. Staff meetings to discuss recent losses can be an effective method of working through such losses.

Case Illustration: The Provision and Maintenance of Ongoing Frontline Support

The case of Mrs. Y. illustrates the need, not only for support of staff, but also the day-to-day intervention in the care of certain residents with multiple needs.

Mrs. Y., an 80 year-old widow was admitted to a home for the aged when she became increasingly frail and incapacitated as a result of multiple physical problems. Although she had been a strong, successful woman, she had suffered many losses and traumas during World War II. She responded to her increasing infirmity by becoming needy, helpless, clingy, and demanded to be "taken care of." She perceived the staff's attempts to encourage independence as rejection and lack of caring. This produced catastrophic-like reactions in her and increased the intensity of her demands.

She was often agitated, highly anxious and complained constantly of physical problems. Staff could no longer tolerate her incessant demands or determine which symptoms required intervention.

The nurse consultant was asked to assist with the management of Mrs. Y.'s anxiety. Intervention and care planning required both individual counseling and increased staff support. Mrs. Y. was seen one to three times weekly for supportive counseling. Over the months and years, she found great comfort in having the consultant's complete attention. As the trusting relationship grew, she would save many of her complaints for the consultant, and reduced her demands on the staff. In addition, she was able to acknowledge her grief over the many losses she had suffered, both past and present. She was able to regain some sense of her strengths as she spoke of her past achievements and derived satisfaction from this.

Supportive sessions with the staff helped to increase their understanding of Mrs. Y.'s behaviors, balance the need for independence and dependence, and allowed staff to share their frustration and feelings of "never being able to do enough to please her." A consistent routine of care was implemented. Over the years, Mrs. Y. was able to attend programs and outings (albeit with much persuasion). Staff became attuned to the subtle changes in her behavior, which signaled a physiological change requiring medical intervention. Over the 4 years until she died, the long-term, mutual support between the staff and consultant enabled them to provide the necessary care for Mrs. Y. and to maximize her quality of life.

Comment

This case illustrates that the problems encountered in long-term care institutions are rarely short-lived. In order to maintain high quality care in the face of unremitting demands and demeaning personal slurs, support to staff must be available for as long as the problem exists.

Case Illustration

Mr. M. was an 81-year-old man living in a home for the aged. He had lived there for many years and was loved for his warmth and gentle wit. As the years passed, staff noted that he was becoming more demanding, forgetful, and needy. He required constant reassurance that staff would continue to provide care. As it became increasingly difficult to look after him, staff discussed the possibility to moving him to another floor with a higher staff-to-resident ratio. In discussions with the nurse consultant, staff shared their feelings as they watched Mr. M.'s slow decline and their guilt around proposing his transfer. Several weeks after these discussions, staff decided they would not transfer him but would continue their attempts to care for him. They acknowledged that the open exchange and realization of their feelings had been a factor in their decision. Having developed a close relationship with Mr. M., they would continue to provide their care and support until he died.

Comment

One of the risks involved in developing relationships with the elderly is the reality of eventual loss. In an attempt to "maintain professional distance," actual personal distancing in the form of avoidance of the resident, or precipitous transfers, may occur. By openly acknowledging sadness and grief within the safety of a peer group, this team was able to subsequently make decisions based on the resident's actual needs.

Identification of Educational Needs

Current trends indicate that the residents admitted to long-term care facilities are older, more frail, and more cognitively impaired than in the past. Consequently, increased knowledge of dementia is required to provide comprehensive care. As needs are identified by the nursing managers, the nurse consultant can develop and implement a unit-based educational package to meet these requirements. For example, didactic educational sessions are created to teach an understanding of how cognitive impairment translates into the behaviors seen on the unit. Management strategies are outlined, case examples are used, and role-playing may be utilized as a mechanism to reinforce communication techniques.

Summary

In the authors' experience, the psychogeriatric nurse consultant can be effective only when the delicate balance between assistance and preservation of the dignity of the staff is maintained. Staff must be able to experience the consultant as being committed to, and valuing, front-line work. One of the dilemmas faced by professionals other than nurses providing consultation to direct caregivers is that they may be perceived as being critical, with no knowledge of what it is like to provide intrusive, intimate care which often provokes intense reactions from the residents. The relationship between staff and the nurse consultant evolves over time and becomes a mutual learning experience. Thus, the role of the psychogeriatric nurse consultant encompasses support to staff via direct patient care in the form of supportive counseling of residents, assistance in identifying, and resolving systems issues that impinge upon resident care and nursing staff, informal/formal education, and mentoring/coaching of nursing staff in critical thinking as it applies to the psychogeriatric symptomatology exhibited by the residents. As Tobin accurately points out, "Maintaining staff tolerance is not an easy task . . . it can only be accomplished if staff are supported and nourished by administration so that they can withstand personal abuse" [9].

References

1. Statistics Canada. (December 15, 2005). The Daily. Retrieved on October 22, 2006 from www.statcan.ca.
2. Santmyer, K.S. (1991). Geropsychiatry in long-term care: A nurse centered approach. Journal of the American Geriatric Society, 39:156–159.
3. College of Nurses of Ontario. (2002). Compendium of standards of practice for nurses in Ontario. Professional standards for registered nurses and registered practical nurses in Ontario (pp. 14–16). Toronto: College of Nurses of Ontario.
4. Woodward, V.A., Webb, C., Prowse, M. (2005). Nurse consultants: Their characteristics and achievements [Electronic Version]. Journal of Clinical Nursing, 14(7):845–54.
5. Woodward, V.A., Webb, C., Prowse, M. (2006). Nurse consultants: Organizational influences on role achievement [Electronic Version]. Journal of Clinical Nursing, 15(3):272–280.
6. Pajarillo, E.J., Sers, A.J., Ryan, R.M., Headley, B., Nalven, C. (1997). Consultation-liaison psychiatric nursing in long-term care. Journal of Psychosocial Nursing and Mental Health Services, 35:24–30.
7. Stoltz Howard, J. (1978). Liaison nursing. Journal of Psychosocial Nursing and Mental Health Services, 4:35–37.
8. Lewis, A., Levy, J. (1982). Psychiatric liaison nursing: The theory and clinical practice (pp. 4–15). Reston, VA: Reston Publishing Co.
9. Tobin, S. (1989). Issues of care in long-term settings. In D.K. Conn, A. Grek, J. Sadavoy (Eds.), Psychiatric consequences of brain disease in the elderly: A focus on management (pp. 181–182). New York: Plenum Press.

Suggested Readings

1. Pajarillo, E.J., Sers, A.J., Ryan, R.M., Headley, B., Nalven, C. (1997). Consultation-liaison psychiatric nursing in long-term care. Journal of Psychosocial Nursing and Mental Health Services, 35:24–30.
   Good, easy to read description of the role, with effective case studies to illustrate the main points.
2. Stoltz Howard, H. (1978). Liaison nursing. Journal of Psychosocial Nursing and Mental Health Services, 4:35–37.
   Although an older reference, it remains a classic in describing the process of establishing and defining the role of the psychiatric liaison nurse. Clear and easy to read.
3. Santmyer, K.S. (1991). Geropsychiatry in long-term care: A nurse centered approach. Journal of the American Geriatrics Society, 39:156–159.
   Focuses on the kinds of problems referred to a psychiatric consultation-liaison team and common interventions emphasizing interpersonal and environmental adaptations.

19 Understanding and Helping the Family

Etta Ginsberg-McEwan & Anne Robinson

Key Points

To understand and help the "institutionalized family" staff need to:

- Consider the family system as the client.
- Recognize how disruptive chronic illness and institutionalization will be to the family system.
- Teach families about disease, its course, and the possible effects on their relative and themselves.
- Support and assist families by teaching them in areas that are new for them, such as how to visit and respond to a demented or unresponsive relative.
- Encourage their participation in planning and providing care and the setting of goals for care and living.

Changing the model of care in a long-term care facility from one that focuses on the resident alone to one that considers the resident and the family means that members of the family are also considered to need care. Unlike an acute care hospital, a long-term care facility is a place where the individual goes to live. Here intimacies of family life unknown to strangers become institutional knowledge. Family styles of interaction are divulged and discussed as families struggle to cope with the intrusion of the institution into family life and the demands of chronic illness. Staff become involved as observers and participants in the family's struggle to adapt. When care includes family members and it becomes clear that their contribution to care is valued by the staff, there is frequently a decrease in the worry, guilt, and anxiety of the family.

Gates suggests that shifting perceptions of care to all members of the family, leads to an increase in the overall quality of care [1]. This shift in focus assists staff in their struggle to understand, first, the family's ambivalence and pain in giving over care to strangers, and second, their struggle to encompass the idea of their relative as old and sick.

Burnside states that the mutual participation required by staff and families is often unfamiliar territory for both groups [2]. Misunderstandings and competitions occur as everyone struggles to work together and plan care. Social workers and nursing staff working collaboratively can do much to enhance the care of families and decrease the difficulties of institutionalization. The communicating of family history and observations of day to day interactions by the family allows staff to feel involved with their resident and the family.

Institutionalization: A New Phase In Living

We are born, we go to school, we go to work, we marry, we have children, we have grandchildren, we retire: and we hope for a peaceful death. We move through these chapters of life prepared by preceding generations and by a whole host of rituals that mark the critical moments of passages in the life cycle. Institutionalization is the most recent phase of living; it is becoming a way of life as people live longer, develop chronic diseases, and as families are frequently unable to provide care at home. The entire family structure undergoes a reorganization. The forced removal of an individual from his lifelong context places him in an alien situation. Few enter an institutional setting willingly. Most enter because of complicated illness and the depletion of resources. There is no ritual to prepare us for this passage and what a passage!

Developing a New Institutional Identity

Upon entering the institution, the family enters a totally new developmental phase and moves slowly, cautiously, fearfully – and with trepidation. It is a time of crisis. It is the final chapter for the ill relative. **Table 1** lists some of the issues facing the family when a relative is admitted. The family unit appears to be in an identity crisis. Their familiar roles, for example, husband, wife, son, daughter, do not seem to be easily understood by the institutional staff. The family member who is placed in the institution has never had a lesson in "how to behave as a patient." Preston discusses identity as being essential to orientation. "It tells a man, in terms of society, what he is and might be, how worthy he is and what he should do" [3]. Upon entering the institution, the individual and his family take on a "new" identity. There is a feeling of inner chaos, bewilderment, and apprehension. Whereas there may be relief in finally sharing the caregiving burden, family members are uncertain of what to expect.

On occasion, families may encounter rigid institutional responses. Verbal and nonverbal messages to the family tell them to step aside, leave the room, go home, come back tomorrow at 11:00 a. m., and not before 11:00 a. m., or remain until 8:00 p. m., and no later. Family members must leave the room when staff are giving direct care to their relative. Family members who have been the primary caregivers for years feel shut out. Hopefully there is some degree of flexibility and institutional rules can be discussed and negotiated.

The ill family member may be placed in the position of almost total dependency. He resigns himself to acquiescing to every recommendation of the health care team; he sleeps,

Table 1 Issues Facing Families when a Relative Is Admitted to an Institution

1. Feelings of guilt and anger for "abandoning" relative to strangers
2. Partial loss of role, as wife or husband, son or daughter, mother or father
3. Loss of supportive family member, e.g., parent's emotional support and wisdom; spouse's emotional, social and financial support, and physical tenderness
4. Fear of relative's impending death
5. Fear of relative's rejection and anger
6. Lack of knowledge about institutional, medical, and nursing care and fear of asking questions
7. Financial burdens

awakens, attends to personal needs, eats; and struggles to live within the rules and regulations of the "world of the sick." In the "world of the sick," you are addressed by your first name, you are called "honey," "dear," – you are patted on the head, you are told to smile, brighten up. Staff and families wanting to comfort and reassure, instead, may become unintentionally patronizing. Sometimes you are dressed in a white gown which is in reality, symbolic of the shroud – that which is worn by the dead. In a way, part of you feels dead. If your body is twisted with disease, if your eyes have a vacant stare, if you utter something that is totally incomprehensible, if you cry out, all eyes avoid you or you are quickly reassured that all will be okay. But the individual and family know all is not okay. A strange environment; strangers speaking a new language – the institution language of "do's" and "don'ts." Privacy disappears and the family have become part of the public domain.

The Patient Remains Part of the Family Unit

The ill member enters the institution with his family. At first this may sound overwhelming and unreasonable. Of course the entire family does not "live" in the institution. The family's lifelong relationships, values, conflicts, legacies, and loyalties enter the institution. This rich history impacts on the patient. Personal history should not be ignored by staff as it is critical to care and treatment. Successful institutional adjustment is dependent upon maintaining the family's integrity. Staff reactions may reflect their own family backgrounds. Every staff member has a separate identity/uniqueness within his/her family history tree.

"Ties of kinship, marriage, and sustained intimacy create special psychological and moral bonds in our lives. Families, a term virtually impossible to define precisely in American society at present, are composed of these ties and bonds, and constitute a distinctive social space, a space where rules and expectations apply that are somewhat different from those in impersonal, public places and in transactions among strangers" [4]. The institution is an impersonal public place and staff members are initially strangers.

"Family life, and especially the moral obligations that family members have toward one another, are challenged by severe chronic illness in two ways; first by the burdens imposed on families by chronic care; and second by virtue of the fact that severe chronic illness in a family can pose a crisis for our traditional moral expectations concerning family life" [4].

"Honor thy Mother and Father" is clearly and strongly stated in the Ten Commandments. The noted poet, Emily Dickinson, said: "Hold your parents tenderly, for the world will seem a strange and lonely place when they are gone" [5].

And the playwright, Marsha Norman stated: "One of the problems for daughters and sons is that you come into life with an unpayable debt, the mortgage of all time" [6]. The giving of life establishes an everlasting link with the past and the future. And whether it is said aloud or not, there is a traditional wedding vow: "In sickness and in health, till death do us part."

Case Illustration

Mr. and Mrs. Y. were married 50 years when Mr. Y.'s 10-year history of Parkinson's disease necessitated nursing home placement. Mrs. Y. had provided her husband with personal care over the past five years when he could no longer attend to his needs. Mrs. Y. visited her husband every day and remained through lunch and supper to feed him. Staff were pleased with Mrs. Y.'s feeding help. However, when Mrs. Y. freshened up her husband every night with a sponge bath and a change of pajamas and stayed until her husband fell asleep, the staff became upset. They said that Mrs. Y. was disobeying the rules and staying beyond normal visiting hours. The staff felt that Mrs. Y.'s behavior implied that their care was somehow inadequate.

Comment

These kinds of issues must be discussed and negotiated so that the family and staff can participate together in the best possible care, with staff understanding the threat that their "laying on of hands" poses to Mrs. Y.

Family System and the "Institutional Family System"

The family system has to interact with the "institutional family system." The latter is a highly bureaucratic and political system which takes staff months and years to comprehend. Yet, we expect families to negotiate the new system within a matter of a few days. Think of all the members of the "institutional family:" administrators, nurses, doctors, social workers, recreationists, occupational therapists, physiotherapists, language pathologists, lab technicians, X-ray technicians, dieticians, housekeeping staff, and maintenance staff. The patient and his/her family have suddenly taken on a whole new assortment of relatives.

There are now two family systems; the family of origin is at a vulnerable intersection of life. The ill member feels he or she has failed the family by becoming a burden, and failed society at large by being unproductive, while families feel they have failed the ill member by placing him/her in an institution. Family ties have been ruptured by illness.

Case Illustration

Myra, aged 43, single, had to seek nursing home placement for her 75-year-old widowed mother, Mrs. X., who suffered a serious stroke that left her paralyzed with impaired speech. She remained cognitively alert. Mother and daughter lived together all their lives and were devoted with strong bonds.
Mrs. X. was widowed at an early age and had raised Myra. They shared the same interests. Myra was determined to fix up her mother's room so that it resembled, in part, the home they once shared. Myra brought in pictures, a bed pillow, a favorite bed-side lamp, a blanket, a small chair, and numerous stuffed animals which belonged to Myra herself. Myra moved in a few items of her own clothing to place beside her mother's clothing in the closet. The staff were annoyed and politely asked Myra to remove most of the personal items. She could leave a picture or two and one or two stuffed animals. Staff said that this was an institution and all must be orderly and easy to clean. Myra refused and Mrs. X. was upset with the staff's anger and their threats to pack everything up in boxes.

Comment

The empathy that Myra required was an understanding that this was the last chapter in her life with her mother and that the separation, emotionally and concretely, was too painful for her at the time of admission. After several family meetings in which the focus was mutual understanding, it was possible to reach an acceptable compromise. Staff sometimes take on a powerful and controlling role rather than a partnership of care with the family. Questions posed by families as a result of their anxiety may result in defensive and self-protective responses. It is helpful for staff to listen carefully and address with sensitivity the concerns of the family. Questions tend to be seen as challenging rather than indicative of family's fears and concerns.

The "institutional family" is equally vulnerable. They are mourning the loss of the resident who vacated the bed, almost always someone who had died. Staff are expected to start all over again, sometimes in less than 24 hours. Staff then must direct their energies toward a new family without having grieved for the family that is gone.

The family of origin and the institutional family meet at a time of crisis for both. Staff are expected to be supportive and families are expected to be grateful that they are relieved of caring for their relative. Both groups report stressful encounters. **Table 2** lists some of the major issues which potentially cause conflict between staff and families.

Staff may pass negative judgments about the family's behavior, becoming defensive, self-protective, and at times fearful of losing their jobs. Staff believe the family to be powerful because of their potential access to the administration. It is difficult in the face of threats of a lawsuit, but important to understand that a family's outburst may be due to feelings of helplessness. Staff's behavior of defensiveness and uncertainty adds to the family's fears of whether their relative is being provided with the best care. Their relative is now living in a community of "the many sick" and each must wait his/her turn to be washed, repositioned, toiletted, fed, etc. And the major change – "who will love my relative with the tenderness and who will plant the good-night and good-morning kiss?"

Table 2 Major Issues Causing Potential Conflict Between Staff and Families

1. Institutional policies and procedures taking precedence over maintaining the family relationship
2. Tight scheduling for washing, dressing, feeding, bathing, and toiletting resulting in lack of flexibility
3. Lack of understanding the uniqueness of the family's relative
4. Staff feeling families ought to be grateful for their care
5. Poor communication around day-to-day events
6. Personal care given by families often discouraged
7. Strict adherence to visiting hours
8. Staff competing with staff for "the love" of the family

Understanding behavior does not relate just to the behaviors of the families. It is equally important and at times more helpful for staff to understand their own behaviors and reactions. For example, it is possible to over-identify with a family or to be at loggerheads because of negative feelings about one's own family.

Dynamics of Family–Staff Relationships

The caring by the wife in the family is primarily taken over by the nursing staff who tend to every conceivable need of the husband. This includes physical needs and a special form of intimacy that may result from bodily care. We must be exquisitely sensitive to the threat that "hands on caring" poses to the woman. The reality is that the husband's care is managed, directed, and controlled by a host of staff, who are predominantly women: nurses, social workers, recreationists, dieticians, lab technicians, physiotherapists, occupational therapists, etc. The wife of 40 or 50 years feels as if she is an unwelcome guest. If she visits too often, the relationship is perceived as "enmeshed" or she is "controlling." If her visits are not frequent, she may be perceived as "rejecting." The adult children are caught in the middle having a mother who is "at sea without an anchor" and who is struggling to learn to negotiate with all these newly acquired concerns. The wife is potentially in conflict with the female staff for "the love" of her husband. The nursing and social worker staff, not understanding what is happening, may view the husband as a victim of an aggressive wife.

Staff Perceptions

In resident care conferences, the staff rarely discuss their own reactions in terms of identifications, cultural/ethnic differences, and expectations. Families are simplistically described in negative or positive terms. Team conferences need to reflect an understanding of the person and their family life, rather than being a discussion of medications and problems alone. We pathologize far too quickly and too much. Families enter a fish-bowl where every piece of behavior is scrutinized, discussed, and documented.

It is time for us to recognize that it is all right for both the institutional staff and the family to be unsure. Until this era of institutionalization families were generally in control and the primary caregivers. At the heart of every struggle with a family is the issue of who is in control. We need to move toward a partnership. We have to learn from families who are the socially evolved caregivers of the aged and from the ill themselves. Aging begins at conception and is a continual process from birth to death. This generation of older people and their families are the pioneers in institutionalization. We must learn to avoid singling out this end of the continuum as abnormal.

"It is difficult sometimes not to see the older person as victim, the family as enemy, and staff as saviours. Such a rescue fantasy serves only as an impediment to service. Instead, with the entire family as a unit of attention, focus must be placed on understanding the family's feelings about placement, on easing guilt if it is there, on lending a vision of help, that as partners, families and institution will do what must be done to ease the pain" [7].

Helping Families

Funding to ensure more than basic physical care for residents is often not a serious priority for long-term care institutions. Mental health consultation and care and social workers are frequently unavailable. Nevertheless, direct care staff frequently possess a considerable degree of knowledge about the people for whom they provide care. Observations of family and interactions, requests for care from different members of the family and social occasions within the facility all provide an opportunity for observing family dynamics and styles. Family differences of opinion abound! It is not uncommon for staff to overhear or be told:

DAUGHTER #1:
Mother would like to be independent: She has always made her own decision.
DAUGHTER #2:
No, she's sick, she should have everything done for her.

OR

DAUGHTER:
You don't visit often enough to know what is going on.
SON:
Well, it's better than wearing myself out like you and then not being of any use.

OR

GRANDDAUGHTER:
I told the staff to get her up whenever she asks.
DAUGHTER:
Oh no! She needs her rest, besides they won't put her back to bed.

Families struggle with their new roles and are often unaware of the subtle pressure they exert on staff to favor their relative at the expense of other residents, for example:

> *You don't understand, my mother needs more help than the others. She never asked for help before, if she is asking now, you need to help her.*
> OR
> *My father says his food is always cold, feed him first.*
> OR
> *He's always the last to get up.*

When the ramifications of what they are asking for are pointed out, families are surprised. They certainly do not mean for others to be neglected, they just want their relative cared for as they would care for him.

Distressed that their once independent relative is now dependent, families sometimes criticize or make demands for care that are not fully considered. To deal with the chronic illness of a family member requires restructuring of the image of the person that one has held for years. This is a painful process, since no one willingly gives up the image of their parent as they once knew them. It is important to families that they share with staff who mother or father used to be – or "the person behind the illness." They want and need staff to know and understand that the person being cared for was once very different. Unless this is understood by direct caregivers, conflict and misunderstandings arise between staff and families.

How can this process be made easier? Families need assistance and education to understand the ravages of chronic illness.

Management

The family, once involved, need help in understanding the underlying disease, its progression, and what they can expect over the next months/years.

For example, in dementia:
- What is it?
- How does it manifest itself?
- Will the person get better?
- What are the stages?
- Does everyone go through every stage?

This knowledge helps families in understanding and surviving the changes in their relative. The information then needs to be translated into the very situations that they are likely to experience. They need to know that:
- Their relative will remember sometimes and sometimes not (and that this is not purposeful forgetting, it is a part of the disease process).
- As a result of forgetfulness, the resident will perhaps begin to accuse staff of taking money, clothing, or not providing food.
- Family members themselves may be accused of neglect and not caring and of stealing or attempting to steal funds.

By arming families with knowledge of the nature of the illness and how it manifests itself, visiting itself may then become less anxiety-provoking. Concrete assistance in how to visit alleviates family distress, particularly when the resident is suspicious and accusatory.

Suggestions for Families when Visiting

- Use statements – don't ask questions of someone whose memory is impaired.
- Have a visitors' book or calendar that all visitors sign and comment that the particular person was visiting.
- Have a family album of pictures with names if possible (don't ask the resident continually – Who is this? or Do you remember . . .?).
- Just walk or sit together, it is all right not to talk.
- Listen to familiar music together, play cards.
- If suspicions are present, listen for a short time – do not argue or try to logically prove a point. Distract by suggesting a trip to the snack bar or a walk.
- Ask staff what they have found helpful.

During visits, family members often give idiosyncratic information to direct caregivers. This information needs to be valued, passed from shift to shift and written in the plan of care. For example:

> *But nurse, I told the staff yesterday morning that my mother never wore nail polish. She doesn't like it, she always said it made her feel claustrophobic. How could they let anyone put it on her – I told them!*

Case Illustration

Mr. A. cannot tolerate his wife's deteriorating condition and he continually berates staff, barring some from entering the room and insisting on choosing the caregivers who will be allowed to provide care. He demands copious supplies and repeatedly insists that the doctor be called immediately. He accuses staff of not doing enough, but won't allow them to provide the necessary care. No matter what they do, it is never good enough. The entire team is tired and discouraged as this vicious cycle of behavior is repeated. Threats of lawsuits, rudeness, and racial insults become common place. Often heard threats include: "What's your name? – See I'm writing it down. I'm reporting you to the administration. You're negligent in your duty!"

Comment

It is important to understand that Mr. A.'s behavior reflects his own feelings of helplessness with regard to being unable to help his wife. When these feelings escalate, he becomes abusive and out of control. The staff can help him to regain control by maintaining control themselves and by defining for him the boundaries of acceptable behavior.

Such an oversight confirms the family's worst fear. The person behind the illness is not really known. The family feels that they must be vigilant and staff wonder what all the fuss is about. Understanding that family vigilance is designed to preserve the dignity of the relative, rather than reacting with anger or indignation, helps staff to work collaboratively with the family in planning care and to work in partnership to provide this care. To facilitate collaboration it is useful to have one identified staff member on the day and one on the evening shift with whom the family can spend a few minutes. This contact reassures the family that they have someone to talk to about their relative who will know the details of their care. This is particularly helpful when there is an absence of resources and for those families who experience a great deal of difficulty with the institutionalization of their relative.

There are those family members whose difficulties in dealing with placement of their relative in a long-term care facility cause tremendous concern, anger, and dismay. Staff and the family, unable to work together, struggle daily. These are the exceptions, but at times it can feel as if they are the rule.

Management Suggestions

- A clearly written plan of care by the treatment team must be developed and adhered to by all – including the administrators. The plan must then be discussed with the family.
- A weekly update of the resident's condition by the physician may help lower Mr. A's anxiety.
- the social worker (if there is one) can provide active support to the husband.
- A contact staff member on each shift can be appointed to meet briefly with Mr. A daily (5–10 minutes).
- Allowing rudeness to continue does not help Mr. A. He will be hated by staff and will be seen not as a participant, but rather as an adversary in his wife's care. Tell him quietly that when he is calmer you will talk (but not now) and walk away. Do go back later in the shift when he is calmer. The same approach applies to rudeness over the telephone.

Misunderstandings arise if families, residents, and staff are not aware of and/or do not agree with the goals and plan of the treatment team. Understanding these goals, how they are arrived at, and, participation in the formulation of future goals (1) allows the family to be active participants, (2) helps to ensure a smoother working relationship, and (3) results in better care for all members of the family.

References

1. Gates, K. (1986). Dementia: A family problem. Gerontion, 1/2:12–17.
2. Burnside, M. (1980). Psychosocial nursing care of the aged (p. 235). New York: McGraw Hill Book Company.
3. Preston, R.P. (1979). The dilemmas of care: Social and nursing adaptations to the deformed, the disabled and the aged (p. 38). New York: Elsevier North Holland.

4. Jennings, B., Callahan, D., Caplan, A.L. (1988). Ethical challenges of chronic illness (pp. 1–11). Hastings Center Report, February/March.
5. Luce, W. (1978). Belle of Amherst (A play based on the life of Emily Dickinson). Boston: Houghton Mifflin.
6. Gussow, M. (1983). Women playwrights – New voices in the theater. New York Times Magazine, 5(1):40.
7. Solomon, R. (1983). Serving families of the institutionalized aged: The four crises. In G.S. Getzel, M.J. Mellor (Eds.), Gerontological social work practice in long-term care (pp. 83–96). New York: The Haworth Press.

Suggested Readings

1. Preston, R.P. (1979). The dilemmas of care: Social and nursing adaptations to the deformed, the disabled and the aged. New York: Elsevier North Holland.
   This book addresses the health professional's adaptations to caring for the sick. It is a vision of the "world of the ill" viewed from that of the well.
2. Fischer, L.R. (1986). Linked lives. Toronto: Fitzhenry and Whiteside.
   Focuses on the enduring bond between mothers and daughters throughout the life-cycle.
3. Edelson, J.S., Lyons, W.H. (1985). Institutional care of the mentally impaired elderly. New York: Van Nostrand Reinhold.
   A book full of humanity and compassion, it demonstrates the art of making institutional life bearable for patients, families, and staff.
4. Goodman, R., Jackson, L. (2006). Visiting with elders, 2nd edition. Toronto: Baycrest Center for Geriatric Care. Available at www.baycrest.org/documents/baycrest_visiting_online.pdf.
   A useful guide for families on how to make visits as mutually satisfying as possible.
5. Duncan, M.T., Morgan, D.L. (1994). Sharing the caring: Family caregivers' views of their relationships with nursing home staff. Gerontologist, 34:235–244.
   Study suggesting that families desire emotionally sensitive care in addition to technically competent performance of tasks.

20 Legal and Ethical Dimensions

Michel Silberfeld

Key Points

- Respect for the integrity of the dependent adult means being concerned to preserve the person's autonomy, tempered with a protective attitude in the areas of functioning where the person is impaired.
- Obtaining consent and assessing competency ensure that residents are given respect protecting them from unwanted intrusion.
- Standards exist for appointing substitute decision-makers and for guiding their choices for individuals who are not competent to choose for themselves.
- Involuntary admissions to long-term care settings are acceptable only if the decision to admit is thoroughly justified. Competent residents who express the desire to leave the nursing home are free to discharge themselves in most circumstances.
- Involuntary intervention is required only to preserve life and to restrain in situations of danger. The use of physical restraint has declined dramatically. Medications are often used to control dangerous behavior and avoid the use of restraints. Institutions should have policies governing the use of restraints.
- The resident's personal finances are best handled outside the institution to avoid potential conflicts of interest.
- Many controversial issues arising in nursing homes are addressed at the individual level. They can also be a subject of public debate. These include lifestyle and sexual issues as well as the use of forced feeding and resuscitation.
- An open dialog between those involved can resolve most disagreement. Consultants can play a useful mediating role. Conflicts that cannot be otherwise resolved can and at times must be taken to a legal authority.

Preserving the dignity of dependent adults is an issue which is increasingly being raised by professionals and caregivers alike. This is a welcome development from which nursing home residents are likely to benefit. Clearly, respect for the integrity of the person is an important part of chronic care that contributes directly to well-being. Some institutions have taken the step to set up ethics committees or some equivalent review body to make hard ethical decisions more consensual.

Respect for the integrity of the person means preserving to the utmost a person's autonomy, facilitating the exercise of self-directed choices to the limits of the person's ability. Respect also requires a protective attitude toward those areas of functioning where the person is impaired. A judicious evaluation of the person's best interests may not always be in line with the interests of the staff. It is difficult for caregivers to recognize themselves as having interests that are not shared equally by those for whom they care. Staff is highly motivated to help. Some of the reward from helping, however, comes from the sense of mutuality that develops in the relationship. At times it can appear that this mutuality is disrupted if there is a disagreement on an area of common interest. This is regrettable and mistaken. Mutuality can be enhanced by "agreeing to disagree." This result is consistent with a high level of respect.

Obtaining consent is the procedure designed to promote respect for autonomous choices. Some people are not capable of making such self-directed choices. Assessment of competency is the evaluation required to determine who requires a substitute decision maker and in what circumstances. Substitute decision-makers for incompetent residents are not unconstrained in their responsibilities. It is a common fear that if one becomes incompetent, substitute decision-makers will be free to do anything they please. This is not so. Standards for surrogate decision making are imposed to protect the incompetent.

There are circumstances where the wishes of residents can be overridden. This is necessary to protect them and to uphold certain values which have greater precedence. Some of these circumstances that occur commonly in nursing homes will be examined. The object of this examination is to clarify the current solutions to these thorny problems. Many issues remain controversial and incompletely resolved.

Sometimes residents' wishes are overridden not be design, but inadvertently. The regulations and requirements of a nursing home can impose lifestyle restrictions which can be as intrusive as enforced treatment. Not enough attention has been paid to the lifestyle implications of institutionalization. Nursing homes can help residents deal with their fears concerning the restrictions they may have to accept in order to have their dependency needs met.

These general comments can be amplified for a number of specific issues.

Consent

The self-governing choices of all persons merit respect and freedom from intrusion. In obtaining consent, caregivers ensure that respect is given. This requirement is imposed by law as a further safeguard and warning against unwanted intrusion.

The laws of consent derive from the common law on assault. None may touch another person without his/her explicit agreement. In the health care field this translates into: No treatment or procedures may be applied without explicit agreement. To make the nature of this agreement more explicit the law defines a valid consent as the understanding of the matter for which consent is being sought and a clear appreciation of the consequences of both giving and withholding consent.

The general thrust is clear. A person must have the opportunity to make an informed choice, and to formulate their own intentions. In other words, valid consent occurs when a person makes a voluntary and considered choice. A voluntary choice is free of coercion. Persuasion on the part of others is part of normal caring, providing it is not intended to overcome a person's natural inclinations.

There are frequent circumstances in the nursing home where it is difficult to ascertain whether residents have formulated their own considered choice. A sensitive caregiver will be alert to and respectful of a competent refusal, as well as open to the possibility of an incompetent assent, which may simply be the absence of direct refusal. Agreement itself is not a sign of consent or competency. It is a mere jest to say that the competent are those who agree with us, while all others are incompetent.

Clearly there is a need for staff to exercise professional judgment and execute professional responsibility. Caregivers are always informal assessors of competency. They must determine whether there is any reason for doubt. If there is such a reason, it is their responsibility to solicit an expert opinion toward a formal determination of competency. Formal assessments of competency are medical-legal acts that have considerable legal and other implications. Decision guidelines regarding assessment of competency are outlined in **Figure 1**.

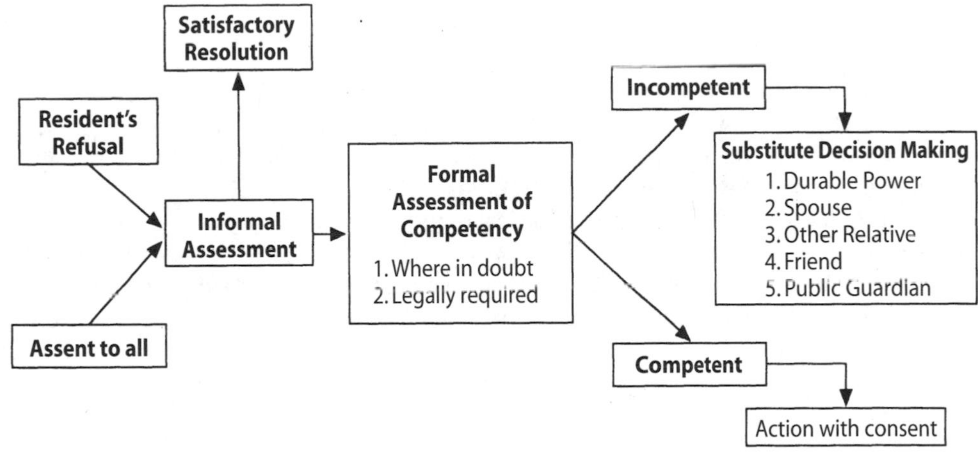

Figure 1 General Decision Guidelines.

When people agree to enter into a long-term facility, it is sometimes considered that they have thereby given tacit consent for routine care. Explicit consent would then only need to be obtained for intrusive major interventions such as surgery. If routine care is opposed, consent and competency to give consent must be considered. Making the assumption that tacit agreement for routine care is part of the decision to enter a nursing home may be erroneous, however, and could lead to problems in care provision. Explaining the routines and general care provided upon admission may assist in uncovering latent competency issues which need to be addressed early.

Substitute Decision-Making

Someone is assigned to make choices for a person deemed to be incompetent. Who should that be? There is a growing consensus that those who are most familiar to the incompetent person should make the choice: spouse, family, friends, caregivers, and lastly, if none other is available, the public guardian. Familiarity with the incompetent person is thought to ensure both care (if not love) and the potential for a choice in line with the incompetent person's wishes or enduring values. In some circumstances family may have interests which come into conflict with this responsibility. Where this can be demonstrated, another substitute decision-maker is appointed. More and more people will leave advance directives specifying who shall serve for them as substitute decision-makers in the event that they should become incompetent. Where such directives exist, they should be honored for the most part. Sometimes conflict will arise between substitute decision-makers and caregivers. Such conflict, if it cannot be resolved by dialog, should be taken to a higher authority. In some places a court hearing is required.

On what basis does one choose for another? Substitute decision-makers are enjoined (in Ontario for example) to choose, "as the person would have chosen for themselves." This may be difficult to do with confidence in the absence of an advance directive. Caring and familiarity do help, yet a great deal of uncertainty can remain. Making decisions can be felt as a burden by substitute decision-makers. Assistance can be received from caregivers. However, caregivers can feel at times that their authority is undermined by the presence of a substitute decision-maker. Sometimes the caregivers themselves have the responsibility of substitute decision making. The best health care interest of the resident is the required standard for their choices. Of course, the perception of best interest can vary. When resolving discrepant perceptions, courts have considered whether due care is evident in the choice (in accordance with professional standards) made, and whether the choice was reasonable.

Involuntary Institutionalization

A person who is found incompetent to choose her place of residence can be admitted involuntarily to a nursing home. In many localities, involuntary institutionalization requires sanction from a court even if there is an appointed substitute decision-maker. There is a formal process to reflect the policy that coercion be the last option exercised. Often other less coercive solutions can work if the effort is applied. Those admitted involuntarily often settle into their new environments to their own satisfaction in due course. Nevertheless, involuntary institutionalization is often painful to those involved. The pain created is acceptable only if the decision to admit is thoroughly justified.

It is important to distinguish those who are admitted involuntarily to a psychiatric facility. Psychiatric patients committed involuntarily lose their freedom of movement. They retain all other rights including the right to refuse treatment (unless they are incompetent in that respect as well). By contrast, people who are incompetent to choose their place of residence lose their right of choice with regard to shelter only. For that purpose they are treated like minors (children) whose choice is governed by their parents (surrogate decision makers).

Discharging Self

It is common for nursing home residents to express a desire to return to a previous familiar environment. This occurs most frequently soon after admission during the adjustment period. If there is conflict about the leaving, and a friendly dialog cannot resolve it, then the person who wants to leave is free to do so. However, there are two exceptions.

First, persons putting themselves in serious danger by leaving have to be protected. This obligation is reinforced by statutes (such as the Mental Health Act in Ontario). Acts such as this provide the authority to detain persons at serious risk of harm. Acting on this authority would usually result in the person being transferred to a psychiatric facility for further evaluation.

Second, there are persons who are incompetent to make discharge decisions, i.e., to choose their place of shelter. Persons thought to be incompetent to make the discharge decision should be informed of this. An expert should be called in to evaluate the person's competency in this respect. If the person is competent and involuntary hospitalization is not warranted, discharge is the answer. If the person is found to be incompetent a substitute decision-maker will be assigned to make the choice. In some localities this will require a court application or the court itself may make the decision. Where a court appointed guardian exists, the guardian can decide the place of shelter. In some localities, however, even court appointed guardians cannot override the wishes of their incompetent charges without a further court appearance. Knowledge of the law, expertise in assessing competency and involuntary hospitalization are required. In many circumstances, however, with a willingness on the part of caregivers to avoid confrontation an informal solution can be found.

Involuntary Intervention

Involuntary intervention is required in only two general circumstances: to preserve life and to restrain in situations of danger. Involuntary treatment can occur even if consent is withheld only in the situation described. However, other involuntary interventions can occur for public health reasons. Mass vaccination and other attempts to stem the spread of communicable disorders do lead to involuntary intervention. Tacit consent is usually presumed.

In an emergency where treatment is required to preserve life, involuntary treatment is given according to the same guidelines as would be followed in an emergency room. Can a competent person refuse life-saving treatment? Decisions made in an emergency situation have the potential for regret due to heightened emotions. Medical staff are duty bound by their professional oath to preserve life. Yet some people do refuse urgent life-saving treatment. Court decisions do not give clear guidance, though, in the case of a Jehovah's Witness, an Ontario court upheld the right to refuse blood even if life-sustaining. On balance, giving treatment is preferred. Physicians are likely to be concerned about being negligent of their professional duty if they do not act. If they proceed, they may still be liable to charges of assault. Financial penalties for assault have been granted against physicians who have given life-saving treatment. The patient is compensated for the assault even when the court declares the physician to have acted properly.

Occasionally physical restraint may become necessary when working with nursing home residents. Today many nursing homes have moved toward a restraint-free policy. Prescribed medications can sometimes reduce dangerous behaviors and avoid the need for restraints. Clearly, a shortage of staff is not a sufficient cause for the application of restraints. Facilities should have a policy in this regard that has been approved by an ethics committee. The lawyers for the institution should sanction the policy. A small institution can borrow policies from another in the same jurisdiction. Sometimes there are guidelines imposed by health authorities.

Restraint is the same as involuntary confinement, and the same criteria apply: presence of a serious risk of bodily harm (to self, to others, or both) and absence of voluntary solution. Restraint is a temporary measure until a better solution can be found. Restraint may be required to properly evaluate an agitated patient so that a definitive treatment can be applied. When restraints are applied, it should be only for a specified period of time with a built-in mechanism for review after a set time.

Forced Feeding

Many residents in a nursing home are too debilitated to feed themselves and need assistance. Some of them may not even have a recognizable desire to eat. Helping with feeding is routine care so long as it involves feeding by mouth.

Some residents are not cooperative and may even reject feeding. For the caregiver responsible for feeding, this is a test of the ability to care, perhaps in the face of "meaningless" opposition. Not only is feeding difficult but there are risks of aspiration pneumonia and its sequelae. These risks are an additional burden to those responsible for feeding the patient.

A reason must be sought when a resident is refusing food by mouth. If late stage dementia is the sole cause, forced feeding with a nasogastric tube is sometimes considered. This is an intrusive, though life sustaining treatment. It is likely that such a resident would be deemed incompetent.

Substitute decision-makers sometimes ask to discontinue nasogastric food and fluids based on arguments about poor quality of life. The latest U. S. Supreme Court pronouncement on the Cruzan case have set a very strict standard. There must be clear and convincing evidence that the person (at some point when competent) requested discontinuation of feeding should they end up in such a situation. Inference from relatives and friends is insufficient. This very high standard is not applied everywhere. In the Conroy case, it was stated that the burdens of living with forced feeding must be shown to outweigh the benefits beyond a reasonable doubt. It is possible that continuing treatment (feeding) might be considered inhumane in the presence of severe and uncontrollable pain. Some have suggested a less restrictive criterion such as medical futility for withdrawing food and fluids from persons who remain in a chronic "vegetative" state. These decisions remain controversial.

Resuscitation

Efforts to resuscitate a resident in a nursing home usually lead to the resident being transferred to an acute care facility. Most nursing homes have the expertise to provide basic life support, but it is rare for them to have the equipment to sustain cardiopulmonary functioning.

The model for medical care in nursing homes is frequently similar to acute care. The staff are geared to treat the onset of new illness in the same way as it might be done in an acute care hospital. There is some discontent with this approach. Nursing home treatment, it is said, should be modeled on palliative care. Care, comfort, and quality of life should override simple prolongation of life. Resuscitation should not invariably be performed. It should be a judgment call. Residents and their relatives should be able to instruct the facility that resuscitation is not wanted after a certain point. Several studies show that resuscitation efforts in nursing home populations almost always fail to prolong life to a meaningful degree [1, 2]. Some argue that resuscitation is a medical treatment that should not be offered if it is not medically indicated.

Some facilities would like to have blanket policies advocating no resuscitation for anybody under any circumstance. People would be forewarned about the institutional policy upon entry to the facility. Unfortunately, residents may not have an alternative choice of placement even if they object to the resuscitation policy. Medical discretion perhaps should prevail over a blanket policy.

Matters are complicated by a common reluctance to discuss resuscitation with residents and relatives. This reluctance is both regrettable and understandable. These are painful choices to contemplate, especially on admission. Nevertheless, it is best if residents can participate and concur with the choice offered. Significant others can be involved in the discussion if the resident is agreeable. The discussion and those present at the time can be documented in the chart. Clear documentation results in an effective directive that is known to all involved.

Disputes may occur. A competent resident who gives a clear and informed advance directive should expect that directive to be honored when it comes to resuscitation. Relatives who object to the directive given should be directed to the resident. A caregiver can object but the resident's competent wishes ultimately prevail. The substitute decision-maker should be consulted for an incompetent resident. Where the medical staff and the substitute disagree without resolution, an appeal to legal authority is the next step. Staff may have to put forward the best informed and most reasonable views about the value of resuscitation. A competent resident or caring other usually retains the balance of discretion. How and under what circumstances people choose to die is not a decision which belongs to caregivers in the nursing home. However, the courts can supervene if a poor decision is contemplated and this can be demonstrated.

The most secure decisions with respect to resuscitation are arrived at through dialog, openness to persuasion leading to mutual agreement. Where there is mutual respect, an adversarial resolution can be avoided. Despite widespread publicity, the number of cases that have come to court is minuscule; the ones that do usually involve the withdrawal of life support after resuscitation has been instituted.

End of Life Care

Chronic irremediable illnesses, such as those found in nursing homes, have led to the view that a palliative care model should be adopted. The adoption of the palliative care model would promote end-of-life care emphasizing comfort measures. This viewpoint has led to questioning the active treatment of terminal episodes, such as pneumonia.

Finances

Persons entering a nursing home may request their personal finances to be handled by the facility. Sometimes a nursing home will require a person to turn over the management of their personal finances as a condition of admission. The potential for a conflict of interest in these circumstances is great. For example, the home may wish to spend on supplementary care. When staff is short, money for a private duty nurse or attendant makes this choice attractive. The resident may wish to preserve much of his estate for his family or other beneficiaries. This illustrates only one of many potential conflicts of interest when the institution takes control of personal finances.

Personal finances are best managed outside the nursing home by the assignment of a durable power of attorney to a trusted person, some paid assistant such as a lawyer, or through voluntary assignment to the public trustee (responsible government authority).

Trying to meet the costs of nursing home care can give rise to conflicts for residents. Long-term care is often very long indeed; the accumulated costs can be prohibitive. Some residents feel that they should not be forced to divest themselves completely to meet the costs. There are also objections to relatives being coerced to underwrite the costs with threats of withdrawal of service. For example, a resident may feel very guilty that the cost of care results in poverty for their family.

Lifestyle Restrictions

Nursing homes require structure in order to function. Programming of residents' activities is one of the components of such structure. However, scheduling people can remove their sense of discretion and effectiveness. Loss of control over one's daily activities has been documented as the most frequent cause of demoralization in nursing homes. Good programming, however, can help residents continue to feel effective. Respect for residents can be demonstrated by flexibility and by active efforts to allow residents to exercise discretion whenever possible. This should be a valued goal of programming. Input from residents should be the rule rather than the exception when it comes to their daily activities.

Couples are often forced into separation when one member is admitted to a nursing home. This separation is as difficult and painful as any forced loss of a loved one. The loss of intimacy cannot be recovered by visits alone. Nursing homes seldom permit enough privacy for true intimacy. Toward the end of life this is a sorry loss indeed. It is a shame that couples cannot be admitted as such more often. Many would be willing. Where they are not willing to live together this direction should not be taken. It is sometimes better for couples to live apart despite their stated wishes if one partner's dementia puts the other at risk of abuse.

The desire for sexual relations among the elderly residents of a nursing home cannot be denied. For consenting adults, privacy should be available. Concerns can arise about new liaisons occurring in the nursing home. Children or a spouse may raise objections. Is the resident being sexually exploited, or exploiting others unwittingly as a result of his/her dementia? These are difficult questions. How elderly and demented individuals construct their social world is very poorly understood. It may be a separate question regardless of handicap whether the search for sexual intimacy should be interfered with.

Case Illustration

An elderly woman with Alzheimer's disease had lost control of her ability to swallow effectively. The health care team was considering tube feeding because of the resident's otherwise good state of health. The resident's daughter was a single mother of three children who was very burdened emotionally and financially by her mother's care. She objected to starting tube feeding and sought legal assistance to impose her point of view. In order to push her viewpoint she claimed her mother was not capable of making this decision for herself. Prior to reaching a court battle, the daughter was offered financial relief, and was reassured that the health care team would feed her mother in a manner not requiring her additional help. The conflict was satisfactorily resolved.

Comment

This case illustrates the complex interplay between competency issues and the availability of resources. Once the resource problem had been addressed, the conflict leading to a competency assessment was resolved. The mother's choice was not the issue, but only mistakenly became a point requiring resolution.

Avoidance of the deeper questions has been the approach so far. This cannot remain the case. As more people anticipate their old age and the possibility of confinement to a nursing facility, the lifestyles they can expect will increasingly become a subject of public debate.

Fear of Liability

Clinical opinions about competency seldom lead to litigation. The little litigation that occurs has mostly to do with the consequences for estates. However, the fear of litigation remains among health care providers. This is remarkable since the most contentious difficulties usually arise in acute care settings and not in nursing homes. Residents themselves are unlikely to be able to launch a claim that their capacity has been misjudged.

The fear of liability is a problem of perception. The persons feared are family members. When family has been consulted about the assessment of capacity they usually do not complain. Yet, the problem of perception can result in health care providers becoming reluctant to rely on the residents themselves, and thereby being driven to request capacity assessments further eroding the resident's autonomy.

Whereas legal suits in the provision of nursing home care are unlikely, regulatory sanctions are more frequently applied. Regional and local government authorities do regulate numerous aspects of care within nursing homes. Violations of basic standards of care can lead to penalties or closure of the facility. Perhaps regulatory sanctions have not been used sufficiently to advocate for better standards of care. For both the individual caregiver and the nursing home, the best way to manage a risk is with the explicit use of protocols. Clear criteria for contentious situations can be articulated and taught to staff. Documentation is a further way to reduce the risk. The act of accounting in writing for the outcome of

Case Illustration

An elderly man was transferred to a long-term care facility from an acute care bed after his family (two daughters) had signed the papers of admission. On admission, it became apparent that he did not want to be in long-term care. In addition he did not appear to be incompetent to make his own decision. The administrator of the long-term facility requested a competency assessment. In the course of the assessment, the daughters admitted they had been precipitous. They withdrew their father's home from the sales market, and used his ample resources to provide the in-home assistance he required. Just invoking due process was sufficient to dissolve the conflict between this man and his daughters.

Comment

Estate issues are the visible expressions of family dynamics. The sale of the home was the daughter's way of settling emotional accounts with her father. The challenge posed to all of them by the competency assessment forced the children to reconsider their indebtedness to their father.

situations serves as a double safeguard. It gives a record that can be examined in the future, and it fosters thoughtfulness in the interpretation of events. Unfortunately, documentation can sometimes become a way to vindicate one's actions.

Another effective way to reduce risk is the use of consultants. For example, a geriatric psychiatrist or other mental health professional who is not part of the health care team can play a useful role as a mediator between caregivers, a resident, and family. Even if the outcome of mediation remains the same, the opinion of an uninterested party is reassuring. It indicates that the problem was recognized and due care was taken to come to a suitable resolution. The law does not require more, particularly in situations recognized not to have clear-cut solutions.

References

1. Bedell, S.E., Delbanco, T.L., Cook, E.F. (1983). Survival after cardiopulmonary resuscitation in the hospital. New England Journal of Medicine, 309:570.
2. Gordon, M., Hurowitz, E. (1984). Cardiopulmonary resuscitation of the elderly. Journal of the American Geriatric Society, 32:930–934.

Suggested Readings

1. Silberfeld M, Fish A. (1994). When the mind fails: A guide to dealing with incompetency. Toronto: University of Toronto Press.
   This book is a layman's guide to all the issues surrounding incompetence.
2. Silberfeld M. (1994). Assessing competence in the geriatric patient. The Canadian Journal of Geriatrics, 10(7):19–23.
   This article reviews the general protocol for assessing competence, and some tips and traps of doing so.
3. Lazar, N.M., Greiner, G.G., Robertson, G., Singer, P.A. (1996). Bioethics for clinicians: 5. Substitute decision-making. Canadian Medical Association Journal, 155(10):1435–1437.
   This article reviews in brief the appointment of substitute decision makers and the process of surrogate decision-making.
4. Caplan, A.L. (1985). Let wisdom find a way. Generations, Winter 1985:10–14.
   This paper reviews the ethical complexities of competency assessments. It is a concise clearly written statement of the major ethical conflicts with a proposal to consider the values of elderly residents as authentic.
5. Fader, A.M., Gambert, S., Nash, M., Gupta, K.L., Escher, J. (1989). Implementing a "do-not-resuscitate" (DNR) policy in a nursing home. Journal of the American Geriatrics Society, 37:544–548.
   This paper describes the introduction of DNR orders in a Nursing Home. It also discusses the major considerations leading residents and their surrogates to their choices.
6. Arras, J.D. (1988). The severely demented, minimally functional patient: An ethical analysis. Journal of the American Geriatrics Society, 36:938–944.
   This paper explores a description of quality of life considerations that may enter into a decision to withdraw food and fluids.

7. Kapp, B.M. (1988). Forcing services on at-risk older adults: When doing good is not so good. Social Work in Health Care, 13(4):1–12.
The inter play between ethical principles is reviewed when social intervention is refused by residents. The rights of older residents are distinguished from the interests of professional caregivers.
8. Evans, L. (1989). Tying down the elderly. Journal of the American Geriatrics Society, 36:65–74.
This paper reviews the controversial complexities of the application of restraints.
9. Ersek, M., Wilson, S.A (2003). The challenges and opportunities in providing end-of-life care in nursing homes. Journal of Palliative Medicine, 6(1):45–57.
10. Hogstel, M.O., Curry L.C., Walker, C.A., Burns, P.G. (2004). Ethics committees in long-term care facilities. Geriatric Nursing, 25(6):364–369.
11. Van der Steen, J.T., Ooms, M., van der Wal, G., Ribbe, M.W. (2002). Pneumonia: The demented patient's best friend? Journal of the American Geriatrics Society, 50(10):1681–1688.
12. Verweij, M. (2001). Individual and collective considerations in public health: Influenza vaccination in the nursing home. Bioethics, 15(5–6):536–346.
13. Verweij, M.F., van den Hoven, M.A. (2005). Influenza vaccination in Dutch nursing homes: Is tacit consent morally justified? Medicine, Health Care and Philosophy, 8(1):89–95.

Index